Incest-Related Syndromes of Adult Psychopathology

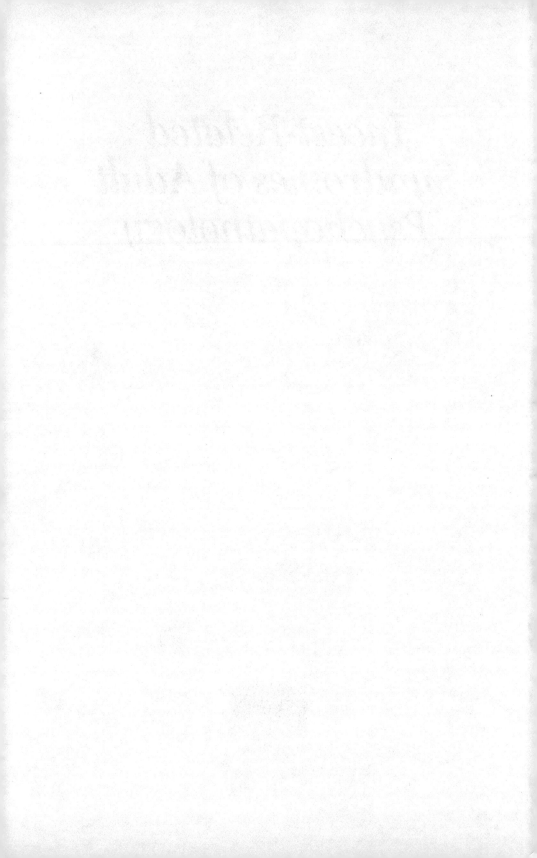

Incest-Related Syndromes of Adult Psychopathology

EDITED BY
RICHARD P. KLUFT, M.D.

Washington, DC
London, England

Copyright © 1990 American Psychiatric Press, Inc.

ALL RIGHTS RESERVED
Manufactured in the United States of America
First Edition

93   92   91   4   3   2

American Psychiatric Press, Inc., 1400 K Street, N.W., Washington, DC 20005

The paper used in this publication meets the minimum requirements of the American National Standard for Information Sciences—Permanence of Paper for Printed Library Materials, ANSI Z39.48-1984.   ∞

Library of Congress Cataloging-in-Publication Data
Incest-related syndromes of adult psychopathology / edited by Richard P. Kluft.—1st ed.
    p.   cm.
    Based on a symposium held at the 140th Annual Meeting of the American Psychiatric Association, in Chicago, Ill., in May of 1987.
    Includes bibliographical references.
    ISBN 0-88048-160-9 (alk. paper)
    1. Adult child sexual abuse victims—Psychology—Congresses. 2. Incest victims—Psychology—Congresses. I. Kluft, Richard P., 1943–   . II. American Psychiatric Association. Meeting (140th : 1987 : Chicago, Ill.)
    [DNLM: 1. Child Abuse, Sexual—psychology—congresses. 2. Incest—psychology—congresses. 3. Mental Disorders—etiology—congresses.
WM 610 I36 1987]
RC569.5.A28I53   1990
616.85'83—dc20
DNLM/DLC
for Library of Congress   90-85
                                                                                   CIP
British Cataloguing in Publication Data
A CIP record is available from the British Library

Contents

To Estelle, David,
and Jacqueline

Contributors

Bennett G. Braun, M.D.
Medical Director, Dissociative Disorders Program and Inpatient Unit, Rush North Shore Medical Center, Skokie, Illinois

Coral Cole, M.A.
Psychotherapist, Julian Center, Indianapolis, Indiana

Philip M. Coons, M.D.
Associate Professor of Psychiatry, Indiana University School of Medicine; Staff Psychiatrist, Larue D. Carter Memorial Hospital, Indianapolis, Indiana

Catherine G. Fine, Ph.D.
Program Coordinator, Dissociative Disorders Program, The Institute of Pennsylvania Hospital, Philadelphia, Pennsylvania

Jean M. Goodwin, M.D., M.P.H.
Professor of Psychiatry, Medical College of Wisconsin, Milwaukee, Wisconsin

Judith Lewis Herman, M.D.
Associate Clinical Professor of Psychiatry, Harvard Medical School, Boston, Massachusetts

Richard P. Kluft, M.D.
Clinical Professor of Psychiatry, Temple University School of Medicine; Senior Attending Psychiatrist and Director, Dissociative Disorders Program, The Institute of Pennsylvania Hospital, Philadelphia, Pennsylvania

Richard J. Loewenstein, M.D.
Senior Psychiatrist, The Sheppard and Enoch Pratt Hospital, Baltimore, Maryland

Victor Milstein, Ph.D.
Professor of Psychology/Psychiatry, Indiana University School of
Medicine; Psychophysiologist, Larue D. Carter Memorial Hospital,
Indianapolis, Indiana

Terri A. Pellow, M.D.
Assistant Professor of Psychiatry, Indiana University School of
Medicine; Staff Psychiatrist, Larue D. Carter Memorial Hospital,
Indianapolis, Indiana

Frank W. Putnam, M.D.
Chief, Unit on Dissociative Disorders, Laboratory of Developmental
Psychology, National Institute of Mental Health, Bethesda, Maryland

Diane H. Schetky, M.D.
Private Practice, Rockport, Maine

Rosalyn Schultz, Ph.D.
Assistant Clinical Professor, Department of Psychiatry, St. Louis
University Medical School, St. Louis, Missouri

David Spiegel, M.D.
Associate Professor of Psychiatry and Behavioral Sciences, Stanford
University School of Medicine, Stanford, California

Michael H. Stone, M.D.
Professor of Clinical Psychiatry, Columbia College of Physicians and
Surgeons; Research Coordinator, Middletown Psychiatric Center, New
York, New York

Acknowledgments

This book began as a symposium at the 140th annual meeting of the American Psychiatric Association, in Chicago, Illinois, in May 1987. Sensing the importance of this topic to contemporary American psychiatry, the American Psychiatric Press, Inc., encouraged its conceptualization as a book and has demonstrated a sustained interest in seeing *Incest-Related Syndromes of Adult Psychopathology* through to completion. For this, I am deeply grateful on a personal basis, both as the editor of the book and as a clinician who recognizes the critical importance of its subject to the understanding, diagnosis, and treatment of psychiatric patients. I will express as well to the American Psychiatric Press, Inc., the gratitude of those many patients who have been victims of incest, who often have felt that mental health professionals have been poorly equipped to appreciate and respond to the importance of the relationship of their incestuous exploitation to their subsequent difficulties.

Those who endeavor to explore, investigate, and treat the impact of incest rapidly recognize the arduous demands of working in this field. Spending a good percentage of one's time in the intensive treatment of the victims of abominable acts is a grueling and demanding task with an inherently high risk of secondary posttraumatic distress. The study of incest is a reluctant little field, one we can all agree heartily that we wish had no need to exist. As Judith Herman has said: "Incest is not a topic that one embraces; one backs into it, fighting it every step of the way" (1981, p. vii). Therefore, I acknowledge with pleasure the tremendous friendship, comradeship, nurture, and mutual support that I have found among both the scientific investigators and the clinicians I have met who share an interest in this area. Many of them and their contributions are represented in this book. My debt to them, both those who have written chapters here and those who have not, is immense and unrepayable.

A special note of acknowledgment is due both to two colleagues and friends whose support and help I have drawn on excessively and unconscionably, Bennett G. Braun, M.D., and Catherine G. Fine, Ph.D., and to Ms. Elizabeth A. Klein, whose help as typist, commentator, and cheerleader has been invaluable.

The writing of a book can consume a great deal of time and energy. I am grateful to my wife, Estelle, for her understanding and tolerance in the course of this project, and to my son David and daughter Jacqueline, who respected and supported my efforts.

Finally, I acknowledge not only the many patients who had the courage to tell the story of what they had endured and to wrestle the demons of their past into submission in the course of psychotherapy, but also the totally unanticipated candor and generosity of many colleagues and friends who, when they learned I was working on this book or when they read parts of the manuscript in preparation, shared their own experiences with incest. It is because of them, and in respect for their disclosures, that I decided to publish "On the Apparent Invisibility of Incest: A Personal Reflection on Things Known and Forgotten" (Chapter 2), which was originally written as a personal document to "clear my head" preparatory to the completion of this project.

Richard P. Kluft, M.D.

REFERENCE

Herman JL: Father-Daughter Incest. Cambridge, MA, Harvard University Press, 1981

CHAPTER 1

Introduction

Richard P. Kluft, M.D.

A CONTEMPORARY OVERVIEW

The importance of real trauma to the development of psychopathology is increasingly recognized. Among the most deleterious of real traumata is incest, the sexual exploitation of a child by another person in the family, who stands toward them in a parental role, or in another relationship invested with significant intimacy and authority. Incest is a social problem of major proportions. Extrapolating from Russell's (1986) landmark study, which admittedly may be somewhat skewed toward underreporting, as many as 160,000 women per million in the United States may have been incestuously abused before they reach the age of 18, and as many as 45,000 per million may have been incestuously exploited by their own fathers.

Incest-Related Syndromes of Adult Psychopathology attempts to consolidate findings that bear on the clinical presentations of adult patients who have suffered childhood incestuous exploitation. Although there are many accounts of incest now available from the lay literature (Armstrong 1983; Bass and Davis 1988; Bass and Thornton 1983), there is much less about how incest presents in such a manner that it and its impact can be minimized, discounted, or denied or appear to play such a peripheral role in a clinical situation that its importance remains unrecognized. Because the study of the incestuous experiences of boys and their long-term consequences is a rather new and undeveloped field of inquiry in comparison to the exploration of the incestuous experiences of girls and their sequelae, *Incest-Related Syndromes of Adult Psychopathology* focuses almost exclusively on the plight of the female victim of incest. This in no way is meant to deny or minimize the plight of the male incest survivor.

Recognition of the presentations of incest survivors becomes a matter of great importance to the mental health professional. Not only is incest a prevalent concern that inevitably will be encountered among those persons seeking help (although many will not and/or cannot acknowledge this), and as such requires extensive study, but increasing evidence is accumulating to the effect that incest victims are overly represented among those seeking psychiatric care. One study (Beck and van der Kolk 1987) demonstrated that incest victims constitute a substantial proportion of those psychiatric patients who become chronically institutionalized in state hospitals. Another showed that incest had occurred in the majority of those who suffer multiple personality disorder (Putnam et al. 1986). Increasingly, incest is associated with a considerable subgroup of those who are diagnosed as having borderline personality disorder (Stone, Chapter 9, this volume) and with posttraumatic sequelae (Coons et al., Chapter 10, this volume; Donaldson and Gardner 1985). These are only a few examples from a rapidly expanding literature.

Despite a growing awareness both of the scope of incest as a problem and its increasingly appreciated (but not inevitable) connection to subsequent psychopathology, its importance is all too often overlooked in the consideration of the unique individual who comes, seeking help, to the office of the mental health professional. Not only are incest victims often reluctant to share their experiences until they become comfortable with their therapists (DeYoung 1981), but their presentation is not necessarily straightforward (Gelinas 1983). Instead, they may manifest a wide range of symptoms and syndromes that may be understood as "disguised presentations" of incest (Gelinas 1983). Since these symptoms and syndromes are not recognized as suggesting an incest history, and themselves may become the focus of their subsequent treatment

> If this [disguised presentation] becomes the focus of treatment, the history of incest remains hidden and the negative effects are not available for treatment. Treatment continues to focus on the disguised presentation but becomes increasingly frustrating and relatively unsuccessful. . . . The patient is then at risk for becoming a repetitive treatment seeker while the intrapsychic, interpersonal and intergenerational negative effects become more and more elaborated. (Gelinas 1983, p. 326)

It is difficult to overstate the importance of these observations. The discovery of the connection between what had been previously refractory symptoms and an incest experience may turn a frustrating or stalemated treatment into a process that can bring about impressive growth and change. It may succeed in preventing a patient from becoming a treatment failure with regard to what was erroneously assumed to be her condition. It may place her in the situation of having a rather complex but prognostically more optimistic variety of posttraumatic stress disorder (conceptualized in the wider rather than in the more narrow phenomenological sense of this term). It is hardly surprising to discover that the patient who is understood correctly has a much better chance to receive appropriate treatment.

It has been my clinical experience that a large majority of the patients referred to me for the evaluation of a treatment failure, a prolonged stalemate, a therapist-patient misadventure, or sustained diagnostic uncertainty have been incest victims. This is all the more striking because until 1987 I had never written, lectured, or made a scientific presentation about incest, reducing the likelihood that these patients somehow were referred to me because of my interest in incest. I think particularly of the many mental health professionals whom I have treated who had not disclosed their incestuous experiences to their previous therapists, or had in some way excluded these experiences from their conscious awareness until the recollections became available once again in the course of treatment.

Tragically, the unrecognized or hidden victim of incest has long been the clinical norm. Recognition has been the rare or aberrant event. Writing in the authoritative *Comprehensive Textbook of Psychiatry*, 2nd Edition, Henderson (1975) estimated that the true prevalence of incest was 1 per 1 million population. Recalling Russell's (1986) data above, this means that the mental health professions were proceeding with prevalence figures that represented 1/160,000 of the overall population of incest victims (.00000625%) and 1/45,000 of those who suffered father-daughter incest (.0000222%).

In contrast, Herman's (1981) review suggested that between one-fifth and one-third of all women have experienced some form of childhood sexual encounter with an adult male, that between 4% and 12% have had some sort of sexual experience with a male relative, and that 1 in 100 may have had some sort of sexual experience with her father or stepfather. The Kinsey et al. (1953) data, for example, documented a 5% incidence of incest in a study population of "normals." Finkelhor (1979) found a 1% prevalence of paternal incest in his study of 800 women at New England colleges.

The long-standing belief that incest is rare has exerted a pernicious effect on the mental health of generations of women. As noted earlier, the true incidence of incestuous experiences in men is a far more obscure subject, but it stands to reason that it, too, has been grossly underreported and seriously underestimated. Herman (1981) offered a trenchant historical social exploration of the forces that contribute to the underrecognition of this problem from a feminist perspective. Goodwin (1985) addressed the forces within clinicians and society that predispose them toward the denial of such unpalatable realities as incest, child sexual abuse, and the syndromes that follow in its wake.

Now that it is seen that incest is a commonplace event instead of an unusual and remarkable occurrence and that it takes place despite the ostensible repugnance that is assumed to exist toward it, both within individuals and society, a painful realization must be faced. There must exist powerful forces that compel individuals toward it and divert still others from confronting it, forces more powerful, to many, than the entire weight of the venerable traditions and the onus of the publicly stated and openly reinforced moral fabric of our society. The study of these forces has been impeded by the failure of the mental health field and the social sciences to identify and address this problem until quite recently.

Incest means "the sexual exploitation of a child by an older person in a parental role" (Goodwin 1982, p. ix). Herman (1981) defined incest "to mean any sexual relationship between a child and an adult in a position of paternal authority" (p. 70) and sexual relationship "to mean any physical contact that had to be kept a secret" (p. 70). Russell (1986) defined incestuous abuse as

> any kind of sexual contact or attempted contact that occurred between relatives, no matter how distant the relationship, before the victim turned 18 years old. Experiences involving sexual contact with a relative that were wanted and with a peer were regarded as nonexploitive and hence nonabusive. (p. 41)

These definitions share in common several factors. The first is the disparity of age or power (and hence the relative status and degrees of freedom) of the participants. The second is the notion of consequent de facto exploitation of the weaker by the stronger party (often stated in the discussion of these definitions rather than in the words quoted above). The third is that the normative obligations inherent in a prescribed social role have been abrogated by the parental/authority/stronger individual, who has a differential power advantage. Finally, in connection with these factors, a sexual event occurs or is attempted.

The modern study of incest is young but well underway. Unfortunately, it is primarily the study of female victims that has been accelerated. This is probably due to several factors. First, evidence indicates that more females than males are incestuously exploited. Second, males seem less comfortable in reporting and dealing with their experiences of sexual exploitation. Third, the feminist inspiration and orientation of many recent contributions has led to an understandable emphasis on the difficulties of women, and to a differential research interest in that direction. Hopefully, the study of exploited males will advance with similar vigor in the near future. Reinhart (1987) noted much of the literature in this area; recently Hunter (1990) and Law (1990) have made useful contributions. However, throughout this volume, the emphasis on the female incest victim will, by necessity, be far more pronounced and explicit.

MAJOR THEMES IN THE STUDY OF INCEST

To place *Incest-Related Syndromes of Adult Psychopathology* in context, it is useful to review and offer selective illustrations of several of the major themes in the contemporary study of incest. My reading suggests that six areas of concern can be identified: 1) demonstrating the reality of incest reports, 2) establishing the prevalence and epidemiology of incest, 3) studying the social forces that bear on incest, 4) exploring the noxious impact of incest, 5) outlining the clinical phenomenology that follows incest, and 6) offering a framework for the study of incest. An additional topic that follows naturally from the study of incest per se is treating the sequelae of incest.

The Reality of Incest Reports

Herman and Schatzow's (1987) landmark study is a more powerful argument than the entirety of the heated literature that surrounded the publication of Masson's (1984) study of Freud's repudiation of the "seduction theory." Herman and Schatzow elegantly demonstrated that patients' accounts of childhood sexual abuse, whether they were always accessible or recovered in the course of therapy, could be supported by corroborating evidence in the majority of cases. Of their patients, 74% obtained confirmation of their sexual abuse from another source, and another 9% obtained statements that indicated a strong likelihood that their suspicions were on target. Most strikingly, "the majority of patients who did not obtain corroborating evidence of abuse were those who made no attempt to do so" (p. 11). On the basis of these findings, "the presumption that most patients' reports of childhood sexual abuse can be ascribed to fantasy no longer appears tenable" (p. 11). Simply stated, most incest allegations can be documented. Herman and Schatzow's study appears destined to become a classic reference in psychiatry.

The Prevalence and Epidemiology of Incest

The prevalence and epidemiology of incest has been the subject of two ground-breaking studies, those of Russell (1986) and Wyatt (1985). Russell, who explored the experience of a carefully selected community sample of San Francisco women, found that 16% of her sample had experienced at least one incestuous event and at least 5% had experienced an incest event with the biological father. She described types of incest events that had been little studied in the literature. By classifying the types of experiences, the perpetrators, the impact of the events on the interviewees, and numerous other measures, Russell was able to lay a more objective foundation for the future study of incest, conclusively dispel innumerable myths that had surrounded the condition, and provide scholars with a rich data base and valuable food for thought. Wyatt, whose impressive materials have not been reported as extensively, had findings strongly consistent with those of Russell.

The Social Forces That Bear on Incest

The study of the social forces that bear on incest is a crucial dimension that undoubtedly will be explored in depth and breadth in view of the newer findings in the field. One of the most powerful contributions to this area of endeavor is Herman's (1981) *Father-Daughter Incest*, which offers a strong feminist perspective and outlines the potential for the abuse of power inherent in a patriarchal society. Like any strong statement of a theory, time and the findings of others will place it in a new perspective; indeed, Russell's (1986) data hint at other dimensions than power as major determinants. Nonetheless, the feminist viewpoint has demonstrated a lasting vigor and proven to be a valuable orientation in the appreciation of the incest problem.

The Noxious Impact of Incest

Demonstrating the noxious impact of incest is of crucial importance because there has been a tradition, reviewed by both Herman (1981) and Russell (1986), of minimizing incest's effects, of declaring concern for its sequelae as "a tempest in a teapot." A growing literature, pioneered by Landis (1940), Lukianowicz (1972), Spencer (1978), and Rosenfeld (1979), summarized by Herman, and augmented by numerous studies reviewed and cited in this volume, is implicating incest in the etiology of a number of mental disorders and demonstrating its connection to a wide variety of difficulties in living. Russell's survey documents that although some survive incestuous abuse relatively intact, even those forms of incest usually assumed to be fairly benign have had a deleterious impact. At this time, even by using relatively gross measures, the preponderance of evidence is that incest is a harmful and detrimental experience.

Furthermore, it is my impression that as the study of posttraumatic stress disorder accelerates, the less dramatic restrictive symptoms of this condition (Horowitz 1976) will be explored in increasing depth. When restrictive symptoms are better operationalized and more energetically inquired after, it will be seen that many of the supposedly asymptomatic survivors will prove to have symptoms and residual difficulties that earlier studies did not consider. I continue to be impressed in my observations of allegedly "asymptomatic" incest survivors that the trajectory of their lives has been altered unfavorably by the incest experience, and that when the "negative symptoms" of ego constriction and the like are considered as well as more dramatic and intrusive symptoms, they show the scars of what has befallen them. The shattering by trauma of the basic assumptions described by Janoff-Bulman (1985)—that one is invulnerable, that the world is meaningful, and that one can perceive one's self positively—exact a heavy toll in areas of function that may not be inquired after in a standard interview or mental status examination.

The Clinical Phenomenology That Follows Incest

Outlining the clinical phenomenology that follows incest is crucial if clinicians are to increase their index of suspicion for the possibility that incest may play a role in a given patient's difficulties. This is the major focus of *Incest-Related Syndromes of Adult Psychopathology*, which attempts to consolidate the findings of the recent literature and build on them. However, one of the foundation contributions to this area of study is Goodwin's (1982) book, *Sexual Abuse: Incest Victims and Their Families*. In the clinical studies that constitute the majority of her book, Goodwin offered many observations of extreme value that drew connections between both syndromes and problematic behaviors and the incest histories of her patients. This is the area of study that brings the comprehension of the incest problem home to the diagnostician who attempts to find the central theme underlying the diversity of the psychopathology with which he or she is presented.

A Framework for the Study of Incest

A further major area is the attempt to systematize the study of incestuous abuse. In this area, the extensive work of Finkelhor is widely cited and respected. Finkelhor (1984) offered the observation that all factors relating to sexual abuse could be grouped into one of four preconditions necessary to be met before sexual abuse could occur:

1. A potential offender needed to have some motivation to abuse a child sexually.
2. The potential offender had to overcome internal inhibitions against acting on that motivation.
3. The potential offender had to overcome external impediments to committing sexual abuse.
4. The potential offender or some other factor had to undermine or overcome a child's possible resistance to the sexual abuse (p. 54).

This rather terse and affectively neutral framework encourages objectivity and discourages the elaboration and representation of single-factor theories as more comprehensive than they are in fact.

Treatment of the Sequelae of Incest

From the study of incest follows naturally the study of the treatment of the sequelae of incest. It is heartening that a number of excellent works have been published in recent years that offer useful advice to the clinician who is confronted with the incest victim. Among these are Courtois' (1988) *Healing the Incest Wound* and my own (1989) *Treatment of Victims of Sexual Abuse*. There is reason for optimism with regard to the treatment of the incest victim.

THIS VOLUME

After this general introduction to the field of incest, *Incest-Related Syndromes of Adult Psychopathology* will address a series of more focused topics. In Chapter 2, I attempt to speak to these concerns by demonstrating how, to the nonparticipant, incest can appear so decentered with respect to one's point of view that it becomes virtually unrecognized or derealized. Next, in Chapter 3, Diane H. Schetky, M.D., reviews the accumulated literature on the long-term effects of childhood sexual abuse, observing that one major problem in that literature is the frequent failure to distinguish between the incestuous and the extrafamilial sexual abuse of children.

In Chapter 4, Jean M. Goodwin, M.D., M.P.H., traces a continuity between the circumstances of the child and the adult incest survivor and moves toward describing a syndrome characterizing the incest victim. In Chapter 5, Richard J. Loewenstein, M.D., explores the complex relationship between sexual abuse and the somatoform disorders. In Chapter 6, Frank W. Putnam, M.D., explores the impact of childhood sexual abuse on the formation and function of the "self."

Rosalyn Schultz, Ph.D., describes the impact of incest on aspects of the adolescent passage in Chapter 7. Catherine G. Fine, Ph.D., explores the impact of incest on cognition from both a theoretical and clinical point of view in Chapter 8.

The contribution of posttraumatic origins, especially the impact of incest trauma on the development of borderline personality disorder, is the subject of Chapter 9, by Michael H. Stone, M.D. In Chapter 10, Philip M. Coons, M.D., Coral Cole, M.A., Terri A. Pellow, M.D., and Victor Milstein, Ph.D., explore posttraumatic symptoms and dissociative phenomena as sequelae to incest. In Chapter 11, Bennett G. Braun, M.D., links the dissociative disorders to incest experiences, a theme elaborated further in David Spiegel, M.D.'s study of trauma, dissociation, and hypnosis in Chapter 12.

In Chapter 13, I discuss the vulnerability of those exploited incestuously to subsequent revictimization and illustrate this with a study of the extreme example of therapist-patient sexual misadventures. Finally, in Chapter 14, Judith Lewis Herman, M.D., offers a discussion and an overview.

A FINAL NOTE

Some readers may be puzzled by the frequency with which patients with dissociative disorders, especially multiple personality disorder, appear in illustrative vignettes. Gelinas (1983) was among the first to remark on the fact that dissociative symptoms are characteristic of incest victims. At the same point in time a large number of scientific investigators and clinicians were discovering that an incest history is commonplace in patients with severe and chronic dissociative disorders, especially multiple personality disorder. Consequently, many scientific investigators of dissociation become students of incest, and many experts within the field of incest develop expertise vis-à-vis the dissociative disorders. As a result of this, and because the phenomenology of multiple personality disorder often illustrates mental phenomena with striking clarity, a significant percentage of the contributors to *Incest-Related Syndromes of Adult Psychopathology* have used material from such patients for heuristic purposes.

REFERENCES

Armstrong L: Kiss Daddy Goodnight: A Speak-Out on Incest. New York, Pocket Books, 1983

Bass E, Davis L: The Courage to Heal: A Guide for Women Survivors of Sexual Abuse. New York, Harper & Row, 1988

Bass E, Thornton L: I Never Told Anyone: Writings by Women Survivors of Sexual Abuse. New York, Harper & Row, 1983

Beck JC, van der Kolk BA: Reports of childhood incest and current behavior of chronically hospitalized psychotic women. Am J Psychiatry 144:1474–1476, 1987

Courtois CA: Healing the Incest Wound. New York, WW Norton, 1988

DeYoung M: Case reports: the sexual exploitation of incest victims by helping professionals. Victimology 6:92–101, 1981

Donaldson MA, Gardner R: Diagnosis and treatment of traumatic stress among women after childhood incest, in Trauma and Its Wake: The Study and Treatment of Post-Traumatic Stress Disorder. Edited by Figley CR. New York, Brunner/Mazel, 1985, pp 356–377

Finkelhor D: Sexually Victimized Children. New York, Free Press, 1979

Finkelhor D: Child Sexual Abuse: New Theory and Research. New York, Free Press, 1984

Gelinas D: The persisting negative effects of incest. Psychiatry 46:312–332, 1983

Goodwin J: Sexual Abuse: Incest Victims and Their Families. Boston, Wright/ PSG, 1982

Goodwin J: Credibility problems in multiple personality disorder patients and abused children, in Childhood Antecedents of Multiple Personality. Edited by Kluft RP. Washington, DC, American Psychiatric Press, 1985, pp 1–19

Henderson D: Incest, in Comprehensive Textbook of Psychiatry, 2nd Edition.

Edited by Freedman A, Kaplan H, Sadock B. Baltimore, MD, Williams & Wilkins, 1975, pp 1530–1539

Herman JL: Father-Daughter Incest. Cambridge, MA, Harvard University Press, 1981

Herman JL, Schatzow E: Recovery and verification of memories of childhood sexual trauma. Psychoanalytic Psychology 4:1–14, 1987

Horowitz M: Stress Response Syndromes. Northvale, NJ, Jason Aronson, 1976

Hunter M: Abused Boys: The Neglected Victims of Sexual Abuse. Lexington, MA, Lexington Books, D.C. Heath & Co., 1990

Janoff-Bulman R: The aftermath of victimization: rebuilding shattered assumptions, in Trauma and Its Wake: The Study and Treatment of Post-Traumatic Stress Disorder. Edited by Figley CR. New York, Brunner/Mazel, 1985, pp 15–35

Kinsey A, Pomeroy W, Martin C, et al: Sexual Behavior in the Human Female. Philadelphia, PA, WB Saunders, 1953

Kluft RP (ed.): Treatment of victims of sexual abuse. Psychiatr Clin North Am 12:237–503

Landis C: Sex in Development. New York, Harper, 1940

Lew M: Victims No Longer: Men Recovering From Incest and Other Sexual Child Abuse. New York, Harper & Row, 1990

Lukianowicz N: Incest 1: paternal incest. Br J Psychiatry 120:301–313, 1972

Masson JM: The Assault on Truth: Freud's Suppression of the Seduction Theory. New York, Farrar, Straus, & Giroux, 1984

Putnam FW, Guroff J, Silberman EK, et al: The clinical phenomenology of multiple personality disorder: review of 100 recent cases. J Clin Psychiatry 47:285–293, 1986

Reinhart MA: Sexually abused boys. Child Abuse Negl 11:229–235, 1987

Rosenfeld A: Incidence of a history of incest among 18 female psychiatric patients. Am J Psychiatry 136:791–795, 1979

Russell DEH: The Secret Trauma: Incest in the Lives of Girls and Women. New York, Basic Books, 1986

Spencer J: Father-daughter incest. Child Welfare 57:581–590, 1978

Wyatt GE: The sexual abuse of Afro-American and white women in childhood. Child Abuse Negl 9:507–519, 1985

CHAPTER 2

On the Apparent Invisibility of Incest: A Personal Reflection on Things Known and Forgotten

Richard P. Kluft, M.D.

PROLOGUE

Incest is neither a pleasant nor a welcome subject. At many steps in the process of preparing this book, I had the opportunity to reflect on my own difficulty accepting and coming to grips with the phenomenon of incest, and acknowledging the dimensions of its prevalence and impact both among my own patient population and within our society as a whole. Again and again, I recalled how my ignorance did not become awareness, understanding, and knowledge without going through prolonged and re-current phases of skepticism, disbelief, and denial. I fought my increasing concern with incest and came to this field reluctantly. I experienced incest as a hideous and unspeakable act completely alien from my own personal life and experience, and reasoned that since I, to my best conscious knowledge, had had no exposure to incest until I encountered it in my patients' histories, and had never been taught about incest as an actual phenomenon (as opposed to incest fantasies) except to be told that it was vanishingly rare, I had no reason to reproach myself for either my lack of awareness or the difficulties that I encountered in assimilating my new insights.

I assumed that many readers of *Incest-Related Syndromes of Adult Psychopathology* might share the mental set toward incest described above and would have some degree of difficulty in grappling with a book that deals with material that appears so remote from their personal experience that they, as I, may have to engage in an uncomfortable struggle virtually to force themselves to contend with the problem of incest. With this in mind, I began to search for some way to bring the reader into the subject of the book in a less experience-remote fashion.

The approach that I have chosen is admittedly rather unconventional. I propose to share with you, the reader, a portion of a personal journey into my own past, a rather mundane and unremarkable past that I, as I began this book, thought was without a single exposure to incest prior to my beginning to treat incest victims in professional settings. I hope that these reflections will shed some light on why so many of us are so unfamiliar with incest, despite being surrounded by it. In sharing this journey, I have had to disguise and alter the vignettes I explore to protect the privacy of the people whose lives I discuss. I will not knowingly alter my best recollection of my own actions, however.

The method of my exploration is hardly novel. I am a psychoanalyst and, in the course of my own analysis in analytic training, became convinced, both intellectually and by experience, that internalizing the capacity to reflect on and understand one's own psyche is one of the best outcomes of a solid classical psychoanalysis. Since the formal termination of my own analysis nearly a decade ago, I have turned to self-analysis to explore issues of concern or of simple curiosity. As I worked on this book, I began to remember fragments of incidents from my childhood, adolescence, and early adult life that made it perfectly clear that I had had many exposures to incest, but had either repressed them or defended myself from unwelcome realizations by managing, in a variety of ways, to add up two and two without arriving at four. Despite overwhelming evidence to the contrary, I had sustained the untenable notion that I had grown up without exposure to incest and had managed to leave it uncorrected as I had gradually accumulated evidence to the contrary. My decision to begin a serious process of self-analysis was first stimulated by an experience in the late summer of 1987 and finally put into action in early October of the same year. What I will share is not the actual self-analytic process, but many of the incidents that I recalled along the way.

In the late summer of 1987, a colleague brought a young woman, an incest victim with multiple personality disorder, to my office for consultation. The patient had grown up in a town adjacent to my hometown, in a congested, polluted, and heavily industrialized part of New Jersey. As she talked about her life, I could visualize almost every place to which she referred. Granted, our perspectives were different. She had been "gang raped" (at the instigation of a cousin who himself had sexually abused her and who collected money from the boys who participated) in a park to which I, as a child, had gone with my parents to feed the ducks and, later, with my friends to play softball. I had been a participant in Boy Scout activities in the very campsite where she had been assaulted. I remember my physician father and his medical colleagues discussing the opening of a community mental health center in my hometown, the same center in which this patient alleged she had been molested by a therapist. Talking with this patient opened up long-buried memories. I found myself thinking of people and places that I had not thought about for decades. Much to my surprise, as I worked on this book, I found myself remembering incidents that related to its themes—incidents that I had long forgotten, and/or never recognized for what they were.

In early October, now a practicing mental health professional, I went to give a workshop near where I had spent many summers as a boy at the invitation of someone from my hometown. In the process, I visited what had been my grandparents' house, on a lake in New York State. This, too, triggered a flood of memories. Most regarded lost images of idyllic days fishing with my grandfather, which I was delighted to recover. However, to my astonishment, some, perhaps influenced by the workshop that I was about to give, bore directly on the themes of this book as well.

The following pages describe aspects of what I did not know I knew about incest and what I was exposed to, unknowingly, that bears on incest. They include nine vignettes of my own exposures to incest-related phenomena. I have omitted several others to avoid redundancy and withheld any that could not be disguised sufficiently. They are not represented as the epitome of clinical science, and the more academically inclined individual may find them a distraction. However, I offer them to you, the reader, as a bridge from the unfamiliar to the familiar. As noted, I omit my discoveries about my own individual dynamics; as any good analyst, I protect the confidentiality of the analysand.

Before deciding whether to include this chapter, I sent the entire first draft to nearly two dozen colleagues with expertise in the field of incest and used the vignettes in the course of dozens of scientific presentations. What I have found is that colleagues and professional audiences almost invariably respond by recalling or sharing similar experiences and feel that this type of illustration or sharing serves a valuable educational purpose.

Two final observations are in order. First, I deliberately chose to avoid casting these illustrations in the form of terse traditional case reports. Instead, I have been discursive. These events were not clinical; they were lived experiences. I have tried to convey a flavor of the affective and cognitive sets that made the incest component a minor or peripheral aspect of the experiences at the time they occurred. Second, some of my colleagues have urged me to make myself appear both more sophisticated and more attuned to contemporary values in these vignettes. With all due respect to their concerns for my representation of myself, I lived the 1950s and 1960s as a youngster, adolescent, and young adult with the values and mores of those decades and would not want to pretend otherwise. With regard to their recommendation that I depict myself as more sophisticated, I prefer to follow the style of my favorite author, Henry

Fielding, and find that events often stand out more clearly when a central figure is portrayed as rather naive, even, at times, depicted as an unwitting buffoon.

SCRATCH ONE GODDESS

I think that I was only 7 or 8 when I first saw her. My father and I had driven around the lake from my grandparents' place into town, and he had assigned me several errands to complete as he did his own. I wanted to get back as soon as possible because my grandfather had agreed to teach me to use his fly rod that afternoon, and it seemed that I had been begging him for years to initiate me into this manly pursuit, so much more aristocratic and demanding than the simple bait-casting that I had striven to master. I do not know if his agreement meant that I had reached a landmark of maturity, or if it was that I now could be trusted to undo any backlashes that I created, so I was a little less dangerous to the tackle.

After I stopped into Damgaard's Hardware to talk to Arnie, who always caught the biggest bass in the lake, one of my errands brought me into a small store, where a young girl about 10 or 11 was helping out at the cash register. Most of the businesses in town were family enterprises. I think I must have made a spectacle of myself, because I became immobilized. She was the most beautiful creature I had ever seen. Long dark hair, gold-fringed by the sunlight through a window behind her, beautiful fine features, large laughing eyes, and the first budding of her breasts— instantly, I was infatuated. I flattered myself that I "played it cool" after my initial reaction, but the facts that I stammered when I made my purchase, that I asked my father as we rode home when I would be old enough to go out with girls, and that my grandfather had to track me down to demonstrate fly fishing (instead of my pestering him) convince me that I had made a total fool of myself. Whenever there were errands to do in town, I became an eager volunteer instead of a reluctant draftee.

Over the years, catching a glimpse of the "goddess" (I could think of nothing else to call her) became a regular part of my summer routine. I never lacked an excuse to drop by her family's store. We never spoke except about the price of purchases, and I invariably stammered. She became an exceptionally beautiful girl. Even the hometown friends who occasionally visited me at the lake agreed that she was "incredible," and teased me about my crush on her. One even told her that I had a crush on her, and I was mortified to the point of near-homicidal rage.

By the time I was 12 or 13, however, the "goddess" had begun to change. The only way I have succeeded in describing it to myself is that she began to fade. Each year, I noticed it more. Although she grew even more beautiful, her posture began to slump. Her gestures, once animated, grew slack, and the life began to leave her eyes. Her smile, once warm and genuine, began to appear more forced and stiff. It no longer was a pleasure to look at her. Once I was in town to do some shopping and forgot to drop by. When not waiting on people in the store, she seemed distracted, sad, and in a world of her own. Once I noticed narrow scratches on one of her wrists. I assumed they were from one of the cats in the store. I told my friend Bill Hammerstein about how she had changed. He was the guy I had wanted to kill for telling her about my crush a few years before. Bill shrugged and, with the wisdom of mid-adolescence, remarked, "Well, scratch one goddess!"

For many years I was too involved with college and medical school to visit the lake very often. When I did, I did not see the "goddess." I was in my late 20s, married, and introducing my son to the lake and to fishing when I next heard of her. We were just beginning to drive home when our car lost power on the outskirts of the town. We were towed to the only garage that was open. I stayed with the car as the mechanic, a man in his late 50s, tried to set things right. We fell into conversation. He loved literature and fishing, and we spent an enjoyable hour or so talking as he located the problem and made the repairs. When he learned that I had spent part of my childhood nearby, he helped me update myself with the people I had known years ago. Most of my questions concerned the local "characters" and the men I remembered as heroes, the best fishermen.

Finally, I could not resist. I wanted to ask about the "goddess." To be subtle, and, out of respect to my wife who was within earshot, I asked about the store that the family had run, because I had seen that it had changed ownership. The mechanic looked at me kind of funny and said nothing. Curious, I asked what had happened. Finally, he sighed and said that the store had been sold when the man who ran it went to jail. "To jail! What for?" I asked. The mechanic looked uncomfortable, as if he might not speak. Very slowly and painfully, he told me that the man had been his customer for more than 20 years, and he had never heard a bad word about him. "But you never know about people, do you?" I guessed that we did not.

"They locked him up for what he did to his daughter. She got pregnant, and they said it was him who did it. You never know, do you?"

I had to ask, "What happened to the daughter? I sort of knew her a little when I was a kid."

"Oh, she went crazy. State hospital. A real good-looking kid. Do you remember?"

Did I remember? How could I not remember?

A quarter of an hour later, my wife, my son, and I were driving back to Philadelphia, where I was a resident in psychiatry. My wife noticed that I was distant. I told her that the mechanic had a wide knowledge of Dickens and Shakespeare, and that he had rekindled memories of what

I had left behind when I decided to go the medical school instead of graduate school in English. I told her about all the interesting characters that you encounter in small towns, and that Arnie Damgaard was still the only guy who could catch the really big bass in that lake—that had not changed since I was a boy. I babbled on until she fell asleep, thought a while about the "goddess," and then turned on the radio. To the best of my knowledge, I did not think about her again until October 1987.

In early October 1987, I drove back to the lake. My grandparents had been dead for years. The son whom I had helped hold his first fishing pole was now a college sophomore. I was now an "expert," in my old haunts, not to fish or do errands, but to give a workshop. That evening, my hosts would be having a small party to greet me, but, for this sun-drenched afternoon, I was alone at the lake. The lake was beautiful, mirroring the fall foliage that covered its far shore. I had chosen to visit the town first, because I knew that seeing my grandparents' old place, now no longer in the family, would tear me up. I wanted to be alone after that.

The town was deserted. All the old names on the stores had changed, except Damgaard's Hardware. A chalkboard in the window listed the 10 biggest bass of the season. Arnie Damgaard, who now would have to be 70 or more, still was the only guy who could catch the really big bass in that lake. The store where the "goddess" had worked was boarded up. Seeing that made me vaguely uncomfortable. I had been planning to stop for gas at the garage where my car had been fixed, but it too was boarded up. That triggered a deep well of hurt inside me; by the time I reached the house that had been such a haven for me, tears were streaming down my face, and I was wiping my eyes as I drove.

That brilliant and color-splashed fall day was full of tears—for the passage of years, for the loss of my grandparents, and for my loss of innocence. Tears for the burden of living now with the painful awareness of what I had been surrounded with, but never recognized or known in that earlier, happier time. I wept for the "goddess," who surely deserved better.

After an hour's drive through the wooded countryside on a magnificent autumn day, I arrived, rather drained, at my motel. I guess my composure was less than I thought. As I checked in, the rather worn and jaded woman at the desk looked hard at me and asked if I was OK.

"Yeah, sure," I lied.

AN EMPTY DESK IN MR. FINKLESTEIN'S ROOM

Having Greta in class meant congenial chaos. A big Scandinavian blond, she stood out among 30-some primarily Slavic, Polish, Puerto Rican, Italian, and Jewish kids. A recent immigrant, she was older than the rest of Mr. Finklestein's seventh-grade homeroom and was very well-developed. We boys could not stop staring at her, nor could the girls, but for other reasons. I first began to understand the expression, "If looks could kill." We boys would break her pencil point if she looked away, just to be able to see her make the trip to the pencil sharpener and watch her as her whole body moved as she turned the handle.

Greta was a big hit with the eighth-grade boys, but was already dating high-school seniors. One picked her up at every lunch recess in a pink and white '55 Chevy. The word was out that Greta was "fast." I had to dance with her in gym and found myself very confused by the way she held my hand and got real close. She appeared to find my confusion funny and teased me about my "love life."

As the year went on, the stories about Greta grew more extreme. She was absent more and more, and some kid said his big brother said Greta "went down." We did not know what that meant, but all nodded sagely. A few weeks later, Greta was called out of class to go the principal's office. We did not know what that meant, but it could not be good. She seemed very upset when she returned.

One day, my cousin Mokey Weiss, who was prematurely large, developed, and sexually aware, told me Greta was a whore. Others had told me the same, but I was so protected and naive that I did not understand most of the words and their implications. Mokey explained. He said that Greta "went down" for money, that her brother made her do it. Her brother said he had taught her how to have sex.

Toward the spring of the year, Greta rushed out of class to the girls' room. The girl who went after her told Mr. Finklestein that Greta had thrown up. I heard because my desk was near the teacher's. This happened for a few days in a single week. Greta was sent to the school nurse.

Later that same day, Mr. Finklestein was handed a note by the principal's secretary. He removed the personal articles from Greta's desk and handed them to her.

I never saw Greta again. It became known that she was pregnant. Her family moved out of town within the month.

I had never forgotten what I knew about Greta, but I had never recognized it for what it was. The fact of a seventh-grade classmate's becoming pregnant so dominated my recollection of the events that I had not "factored in" that Greta was not simply a "fast" or unfortunate girl—she was an incest victim, exploited and ruined by her own family.

YOU DON'T WANT TO KNOW WHAT SHE SAID

In my eighth-grade year, I sat near Maria. I was not yet 13, but Maria was 17. She had arrived from Puerto Rico about a year before, and her English was very poor. She was a warm and friendly girl, who understood and tolerated with good humor the puerile ribaldries of the boys in the class. We were superficially friendly, but our worlds had little in common. She socialized exclusively with the other Hispanic students and spoke English only when she had to.

In the spring of the year, Maria began to be tearful in class. She often folded her arms on the desk and put her head down on top of them. She stopped talking to me completely and seemed increasingly withdrawn.

I think it was in May, during a lunch recess, that I heard a commotion on the playground. Maria was screaming angrily, and two other Puerto Rican girls had their arms around her—it seemed as if they were at once consoling her and restraining her. It was a mystery to me. That afternoon, I asked Maria what was wrong. She just gave me an angry look and said something in Spanish that I did not understand, but made me recoil.

Later, I talked to my friend Carlos. I did not understand what was going on. I was worried about Maria and hurt by how she had turned on me. Carlos had been one of the first Puerto Rican kids in town, and we had been friends. When more Hispanic immigrants came, his family moved to a largely Spanish-speaking neighborhood and we had drifted apart. Carlos explained that Maria was very upset. When her father and mother had gone back to Puerto Rico for a while, she had stayed with her uncle. Her uncle had raped her, and she had moved out to live with a friend. Her period was overdue, and she was afraid that she was pregnant. I asked what was she screaming. Carlos gave a sinister grin. "You don't want to know what she said."

Toward the end of the summer, I ran into Maria at a carnival. She was not pregnant. She seemed in high spirits and showed me an engagement ring. She had gone to work so that she could support herself, met a man on her job, and they planned to marry. I wished her well. From time to time, I have seen her as I drive through my hometown. I have waved, but I do not think she recognized me.

As I think back, I realize that I had not really assimilated the full implications of what had happened and what I had been told. I had never forgotten what happened to Maria, but I suspect that I was too overwhelmed by what Carlos said to "put it all together."

THE GIRL FROM IPANEMA

"The Girl From Ipanema" was a hit song that summer, and I had wheels. That meant the Jersey shore every day I was not working, along with the two Bills, Hammerstein and Greenwald, and my other cousin, Shelly Weiss. Having staked out an optimal location (criterion 1: unobstructed girl-watching; criterion 2: sufficient room for Frisbee), the day could only go well. A bad day on the beach seemed inconceivable. One of the favorite intellectual pursuits of about four carloads of guys who often congregated in the same place for the same reasons was to select one young lady on the beach for the title of "The Girl From Ipanema," then to bribe a kid on the beach to so inform her of her selection by our august assemblage, and watch her reaction. I doubt that this would "fly" in the atmosphere of the present; but then, neither do high tailfins.

One girl kept on getting our votes early in the day, but left the beach rather early, so never got the accolade in person. We consoled ourselves that she would have been overwhelmed by the honor. One of the kids that we often employed, a bright 9-year-old named Joey, thought otherwise. "There's something weird about Liz," he said. We did not ask what he meant, but we took Joey seriously. He knew the beach and the people there better than anyone. His father sent the family to the shore for the whole summer and came down only on weekends. His mother did heaven knows what and deposited Joey, a season beach pass, a towel, and a few dollars when the lifeguards came on duty in the morning and picked him up around 6 o'clock. Joey roamed about all day and sooner or later nosed into everything.

In any case, one day Liz returned to the beach just as we were leaving. We were more uninhibited than usual because we had finally done what we often joked about doing—we had injected a watermelon full of vodka and consumed it down to the rind—and were feeling the effects of a full day of sun and watermelon. I do not remember who it was who started talking, but I think it was one of the Bills. He started to shout while Liz was several yards away. Liz was informed that she had received the "Girl From Ipanema Award," and the prize was his body. The other Bill chimed in and said that she was fortunate enough to win him as well.

Then something remarkable happened. Liz walked right through us as if she had not seen us. She showed no sign of having heard us. Some of us began to sing from the song, "Each day as she walks to the sea, she looks straight ahead, not at me," and collapsed in a mildly inebriated hilarity. We were incredibly impressed with ourselves.

The next time we were at the beach, Joey told us we had behaved like jerks. He was indignant. It reflected poorly on him. It crossed my mind to remind Joey about his saying Liz was weird. Joey said that Liz never went out with the college kids, only with the "hoods." Joey said that guys would get Liz into locker 83, and do stuff to her while their friends would watch through a hole in the locker with which it shared a common wall. We could not believe it, so Shelly, who knew one of the guys Joey mentioned, checked it out. He confirmed the story.

Twenty-two years later, I saw Liz again. I was visiting a patient on a locked psychiatric unit when I saw her walking up and down the hall, with the same apparent unawareness of the people around her. Now, I recognized this behavior as somnambulism and mentioned it to the staff. They told me that it was being regarded as a response to heavy doses of neuroleptics. Two years later, I was asked to consult on a suspected case of multiple personality disorder. I did not recognize the name on the referral as Liz's married name and was surprised to see her. I learned that she had married an abusive husband and had become a polysubstance addict. It was assumed that her unresponsive states were drug-related until it was found that they persisted even when she was drug-free.

Liz ultimately revealed that she was the victim of father-daughter incest and had, in dissociated states, been sexually exploited to an alarming degree. She had, in the personalities that I met, no recollection of her late adolescence. I elected to refer Liz to a colleague. How could I be sure, if I treated her, that some day a personality would not come out, give me a stern look, and say, "Weren't you one of the jerks who had too much watermelon?"

THE NIGHT TOMMY BLEW HIS COOL

On nights that we stayed in town, we often went down to "The Stand." It was the only concession on our town's little boardwalk, the informal headquarters where the teenagers and college kids home for the summer would congregate, plan parties, and take off into the night for any number of places. Drag races across the bridges from my hometown to another town down the coast were a big item. Another was going across still another bridge to Staten Island, a borough of New York City, where the drinking age was lower than in New Jersey.

We were deciding between Staten Island and cruising the main street of the town when we heard the loud squeal of brakes and shouted curses. A beefy red-faced guy, a big jock always in the papers, had jumped out of the Chevy convertible he had left in the middle of the street and was pushing his way through a crowd of kids, yelling "Tommy! Tommy! Where the f . . . are you?" He came up to Bill Greenwald, who was finishing a Coke. "Bill, have you seen Tommy?" He was frantic, breathing so fast he could hardly catch his breath.

"No," Bill said. "What's the problem?"

"I can't tell you."

"Is he in trouble?"

"I don't know. I think so. I've got to find him. He could—I can't say. Let's just say he blew his cool, OK?"

Bill offered to help. I did not know Tommy too well, so the whole thing was a mystery to me. I had gone to a private high school, while Bill had gone to the local high school and knew everyone. I knew he was close to Tommy, whom I knew only as a hulking defensive end about to go off to college in a week on a full football scholarship. I said I would help look. The guy who was looking for Tommy gave me a "Who's this nerd?" look. Bill told him I was OK and gave me the jock's seal of approval. "He played soccer on that shit team from Prep." Apparently, that made me kosher.

We agreed to drive through different areas. Some other guys would watch the bridges. We would get together in 2 hours. I asked Bill what was going on. He said he did not know, but he guessed it was about Tommy's girlfriend, Cheryl. I assumed he meant Tommy was depressed after a breakup and was likely to do something stupid.

Two hours later, we were back at The Stand. Somebody had found Tommy, who had gotten polluted and passed out. The big red-faced jock had taken him over to his place to sleep off a monumental drunk.

I did not get the rest of the picture for a couple of weeks. Bill finally learned about it and filled me in. Tommy was in love with Cheryl. He wanted to give her a ring before he went away to summer football practice. When he went to her house and gave her the ring, she broke into tears. For a couple of hours she sobbed and could say nothing. Tommy figured she might not have wanted to be committed to him and finally asked her if she was crying because she thought she was not sure, or if he was not good enough for her.

Instead, she said that she did not deserve him. She wanted him to go off to college and forget about her. She told him he should leave and never come back. Tommy insisted on an explanation and got loud. Finally, Cheryl said that her father did not want her to date boys any more, that she belonged to him. Tommy could not grasp what he was being told. It took a few minutes to sink in. Then he asked her if that meant that her father was having sex with her. She nodded yes. Tommy was silent for a few minutes and then started screaming. Cheryl's parents came down from upstairs, and Tommy did not remember what happened next. He remembered driving around aimlessly, getting a bottle somewhere, and drinking it all down. He was found in his car outside a junkyard.

The last I heard about this was 25 years ago from Bill Greenwald. On the way over to Staten Island one night the next summer, he said that Tommy had gotten it together, but would not come back to town, not even for vacations. He did not know about Cheryl.

I NEVER PAID FOR IT

Bill Hammerstein and I are at Princeton, long before coeducation. Occasionally, nonparty weekends on this then all-male campus prove tedious. However, one can take the tiny PJ & B (Princeton Junction and Back) railroad to the main rail corridor and head south to Philadelphia where Bill Greenwald can let us crash at Penn, or go north to the Big Apple and sleep on David White's floor at Columbia. Also, one can catch the Suburban Transit bus. That is why we are standing at the bus stop on Nassau Street on a raw Friday night that unconscionably falls between the football and basketball seasons.

As we wait, we recognize two other friends, Demchak and O'Hanlan, both football players. All of us are off to New York City. O'Hanlan is on his way to visit his girlfriend at Barnard. Demchak has no firm plans; he is just stir-crazy. Maybe O'Hanlan's girl can fix him up. She is trying, but he will not know for sure until he arrives and can call. What are our plans? It is the heyday of the dance called "The Twist," and we plan to check out the notorious Peppermint Lounge, where much of the craze originated. There is even a tune, "The Peppermint Twist," that gets a lot of play on party weekends.

Once in New York, Demchak finds that he has no date. The three of us arrive at the Peppermint Lounge and work our way through the line outside. The evening starts out with a bizarre "twist." Many couples in their late 20s through 40s have come to see the Peppermint Lounge, and many of the men will not dance. Soon, the three of us, who are real "two left feet" types, are being asked to dance by attractive and expensively dressed older women, who appear to think that we are "cool" or, conversely, have realized that their husbands will never dance, and are desperate. The evening passes rapidly and then Demchak has a great idea. "Gentlemen! May I have your attention? We are going to get laid!"

"Sure," says Bill. "Right," I say.

"No, I mean it. That girl over there is a pro." He nods toward an attractive woman in her early 30s, who is very much alone and appears to be on good terms with the musicians.

"You're full of it," I said, hoping to end the matter there. This is getting way over my head. I have only 5 dollars left, plus my ticket back to Princeton. I know Bill well enough to know that he is not at home with the idea either, but he takes a swaggering macho stance. Demchak nods and walks over to the woman. I tell Bill it's about to hit the fan—she is no pro, and she will scream bloody murder. Bill tells me Demchak is a legend and probably will turn out to be right. I wager my last 5 dollars. Demchak comes back to the table. "One hundred bucks for all three of us. She says it has been a slow night, and she already paid for a room around the corner."

How the hell do I get out of this? I am nearly broke and do not want to admit that, and I have not yet processed the whole idea of going to a prostitute. I would rather die than admit that. I do not think Bill has come to grips with this either, but he is faking great. I need inspiration.

"Well, gentlemen, what's it going to be?" Demchak wants an answer. "Gentlemen?" At Princeton, everyone is always a gentleman, so you needed to hear the inflection to understand that we were being challenged to prove our manhood.

I can barely believe the words that I hear myself say: "Demchak, I never paid for it yet and I'm not going to start now." An inspiration!

"Say WHAT?"

"I said that I never paid for it yet and I'm not going to start now." I get up. "I'm going to see who I can pick up."

"Bill?" asks Demchak.

"I feel the same as Rick."

"You guys are too much." He goes back to the woman, who hears him out and begins to howl with laughter. She points to me, Demchak nods, and she cackles hysterically. Soon Demchak and she leave. About half an hour later, they are back.

The woman asks me to dance. It is a slow dance, and she has mischief in mind, no doubt instigated by Demchak. "I wanted to meet the man who says he never paid for it. You must be real hot stuff." Bill dances by (the same Bill who embarrassed me in front of the "goddess"). His contribution? "Be gentle with him, Miss. He's a virgin."

The woman cannot stop laughing. It goes to hiccups. Soon we are sitting down, and I am spending my last 5 dollars, which I technically lost to Bill, to get her a drink. "You are a cherry," she says.

"Think what you like." I manage a crooked smile.

She laughs a while longer and sighs. "Well, my night's over. Buy a girl another drink?"

"I'd like to, but I'm broke." I borrow some money from Demchak. She and I get into a conversation. I find that she is very intelligent and finally I ask the classic, a version of "What's a nice girl like you doing in a place like this?"

"I drifted into it." For a while, she talked about trying to break into the theater, but this is an area I know well, and she cannot sustain the ruse. "The truth? I would have done anything to get away from home. You don't know what it's like. My father was an alcoholic. When he got drunk, my mother would throw him out of bed and he came to my room. You guess the rest. I had to get away from that pig. Even if it meant this. I keep trying to make it in a straight job, but it never works." We talk on and on.

After a while, Demchak and Bill tell me they want to take the last bus back. I agree. We say goodbye to the woman. She says to me, "So long, big spender." Demchak spills part of a drink on my head.

As we walk through the streets of Manhattan, Demchak revels in teasing me. Finally, at the Port Authority Bus Terminal, he waxes philosophic. "You are an English major and a pre-med. You will never be a poet. Great poets screw too many women, drink too much booze, and get syphilis. You don't screw women—you listen to them. You don't drink enough. You are afraid of VD. You will become a psychiatrist."

"The hell, you say!" I retort.

"Mark my words!" said Demchak.

YOU'LL NEVER MAKE IT AS A PIMP

The following summer I am traveling in Europe. Rome fascinates me, but I have a problem. At home, there is serious illness in the family. No one wants to inform me and bring me home, but with all the turmoil at home, something has been forgotten. I was to be sent the next installment of my funds in Rome. I have been checking in at the American Express office twice a day for a week. Nothing. A popular book that summer was Arthur Frommer's *Europe on Five Dollars a Day*. I am down to my last 12 dollars. I cannot reach anyone at home by phone, so I write a desperate letter, hoping that I will be sent some money within a week. My worst-case scenario is that my parents are staying an extra week at the lake and that they will wire me some money as soon as they get my message. Failing that, I will present myself at the American Embassy and, no doubt, receive a warm reception.

Meanwhile, I figure that I have to survive for a week without additional money. At 19, I take it as a challenge. I have a Eurailpass for unlimited first-class railroad travel. Ergo, I have lodgings. Each evening, I arrive to board a train early for a destination 4 to 6 hours distant. I claim an area, stretch out, and feign sleep until I do get to sleep. On arrival, I do the same on the next train back. I find a bakery near the railroad station in Rome that sells its day-old goods for nearly nothing. Each morning I purchase a supply of rolls and a bottle of water and explore the Eternal City.

One morning I am sitting in a small park near the railroad station. Not far away, several tour bus companies pick up passengers. I hear an Italian man trying to pick up an American girl. I see that he is very handsome, but having no luck. For one thing, he has gotten several English words confused and winds up saying very inappropriate things that do not serve his purpose. After he gives up, he notices me and shrugs, smiles. "Women! I'll never understood them."

"Understand," I say. We fall into conversation and soon I am offered a deal that appears to solve my immediate problems. Luciano wants to improve his English. He will pay me to talk with him and help him master colloquial American speech. However, if he does pick up a woman, the lesson is over for the day. The first day we talk 8 hours, and I can afford the luxury of a modest pension and a meal at a *tavola calda*. Luciano is a remarkably quick learner. The second day is the same. The third day Luciano picks up a very well-dressed American woman in her 40s and comes back smiling. Midway during the fourth day, the same thing occurs, but by late afternoon, Luciano is back, waving a bundle of money.

I am vaguely confused. This is a man who spends a day with a woman and comes back with money. On the fifth day, I finally express my confusion. Luciano laughs. "I did not think that you understood. Tonight, I will buy you dinner and explain. But for now—Ah! Bellissima!" and he is off.

That night, over Chianti, Luciano explains to me. He is apologetic. "At first, I did not think that you could be so naive, but then I realized that you are.

"I love women and I live off women. Women come to Rome with a dream—they will have an exciting time with a romantic Italian lover—and I provide that dream. Thanks to you, I do it better.

"I know that this is strange to you. But you have much to learn. Do not judge me too harshly."

I protest, but Luciano shakes his head. "I know you. Maybe better than you know yourself. You are not comfortable."

A big well-dressed man walks in with two beautiful women.

"Him you will like even less. He is a pimp. Those are two of his girls."

"How do you know?"

"He has some customers that want men. He asked me, but I said no. I am not a fag."

The big man tips his hat, Luciano nods, and the big man joins us. Luciano pours him some Chianti. They drink. The big man looks toward me and then at Luciano. Luciano introduces me as his English teacher and says it is alright to talk in front of me. The big man wonders if I could help his girls. I depreciate my talents.

Soon, the big man is talking freely. His own English is good, though thickly accented. He is proud of his prosperity and considers himself a bit of a philosopher. He decides to explain to me what he looks for in a woman he is considering to make one of his prostitutes.

"Beauty, yes. Sexual expertise, somewhat. That can be taught easier than you think. What is important above all is obedience. And how do you get obedience? You get obedience if you get women who have had sex with their fathers, their uncles, their brothers—you know, someone they love and fear to lose so that they do not dare to defy. Then you are nicer to the woman than they ever were, and more dangerous as well. They will do anything to keep you happy. That is how." He nods to the women and both smile. "Both those girls were had by their fathers. Now they make me rich and they are happy. And so, my young friend, Luciano no doubt has told you his secrets and I have told you mine. Now, what will you be—a gigolo or a pimp?"

This takes some thought. Up until then, it was grad school in English versus medical school. "Our young friend," says Lucinao, "looks more like a choir boy than a dashing man of the world. His ability to live off women, I doubt. His character is also a problem." Luciano lifts his glass in a mock salute: "You'll never make it as a pimp." The big man chuckles and raises his glass as well.

I had never forgotten this complex misadventure, but the shock of the experience and my confusion over my own naivete obscured from me the fact that I had been privy to a rather sophisticated discussion of the art of revictimizing incest victims. Only the then-inexplicable inclusion of scenes from my time in Rome waiting for mail at American Express among my free-associative exploration of what I had known and forgotten about incest led me to remember the conversation that night.

ANNIE DIED THE OTHER DAY

I had read a lot of e.e cummings' poetry, but somehow this poem had not made much of an impression until an incest victim showed it to me recently. The poem reminded me of another Annie, who has been dead for more than 20 years.

                                    22

          annie died the other day

          never was there such a lay—
          whom, among her dollies, dad
          first ("don't tell your mother") had;
          making annie slightly mad
          but very wonderful in bed
          —saints and satyrs, go your way

          youths and maidens: let us pray

Party weekends at Princeton were big events. Even the most "greasy grind," as the compulsive students were called, made heroic efforts to get a date. I had risen meteorically in Demchak's estimation since the night at the Peppermint Lounge, and the girl he was dating knew the girl I was dating. We decided to split Saturday night, half at the party at his club, half at the party at mine, where Bill Hammerstein also was a member. Princeton's clubs have changed a lot since the 1960s, but in that era they were the hub of the social happenings, and almost all the undergraduates joined a club midway through their sophomore year. All male and nonresidential, they were called "eating clubs"; most upper-classmen took their meals and partied there.

The weekend had started well. On Friday evening, my date and I were getting along famously. We had just come back from a late concert when disaster struck. She decided that we had to talk seriously.

Within 30 minutes: 1) she told me that she found herself liking me too much, that there was another boy that she thought that she loved and wanted to marry, and that if she stayed for the weekend, she was afraid "things would go too far," so she wanted to leave before things got "complicated"; 2) we had gathered her belongings from the place she was staying; 3) I had wished her good luck and many bouncing babies, and offered a chaste good-bye peck to her cheek as she boarded a bus; and 4) I was cursing a blue streak as I walked back to my dorm room, dateless on a major party weekend, and reasonably certain that God had taken a particular interest in promoting my displeasure. The thought of encountering Demchak and his date was mortifying.

I was unable to reach Demchak before Saturday night. Shouting to him from the stands as he beheaded Yale running backs would have been considered poor taste. At 6 o'clock Saturday, I dropped by his club and told him what had happened. To my surprise, there was no teasing. He already knew and had been looking for me. My date felt guilty and had talked to Demchak's date. The two of them had a friend who had no date that night and had never been to a Princeton weekend. A phone call was made and I had just 2 hours to kill before a girl named Judy would arrive at the same fateful bus stop. In the meantime, I went back to my club and climbed upstairs to the billiards room, my club's traditional refuge for the dateless.

I had just taken a few shots when I heard a female voice: "You're real good. Do you want to play?"

I turned around and found my challenger was a tall, beautiful blond woman, who wore a very low-cut black dress. It took me a few minutes to notice that she also wore rather thick glasses. She kept bending over even when she did not have to and seemed very conscious and deliberate about showing a lot of herself. I learned that her date was Jim Massengale, a very bookish engineering student. Jim had been talking about "Annie" for weeks. So this was Annie.

Jim had had too much to drink at the postgame party and was being sick. Annie had time to kill until he got himself together. Pretty soon, Annie asked me to help her with a shot and, as I helped her position herself, she started to rub against me. The message was clear, but there was no way that I would stand up Judy, and stealing someone's date, "bird-dogging" them, was gross and low behavior. When I did not respond, Annie got direct.

"I like you. We could go somewhere." She took my hand and started to bring it toward her breast.

"Annie, I'm flattered, but there's no way I'll bird-dog my friend, and I have a date coming." I disengaged my hand. Not a moment too soon, because there was Jim, looking green, but vertical.

Annie made as if to hug me and say good-bye, but she whispered in my ear, "You don't know what you're missing. I'm the best lay you'll ever have."

I told her that she probably was right, that I would regret not finishing the billiards. Within half an hour, right in front of Jim, Annie made a move on Ben Callison, my billiards opponent of the moment, and walked out with him. Jim was crushed, speechless. "But I thought I loved Annie and Annie said she loved me." Jim walked quietly to a chair and sat down, mute and immobile. He was still there an hour later when I returned to the club with Judy.

Judy and I got along fine, after an awkward start. After I had called her to confirm the date, Demchak had surreptitiously called her and "reminded" her that I was on the basketball team, which I was not. Already a few inches taller than I, Judy had arrived in very high heels. We spend a few minutes sizing one another up before we grasped that we had been had, and introduced ourselves. Judy was plain, but had a great sense of humor. Our sides were already splitting by the time we arrived at the club. Seeing Demchak before he saw us, I dropped to my knees and played Toulouse-Lautrec.

I wanted to check on Jim. He was still sitting immobile. I told Demchak and our dates what had happened. I was not surprised when Demchak insisted that we straighten out Jim before we started to party—his 'slab of beef' appearance was deceiving. It took an hour, but Demchak and Judy got Jim talking. Judy was supportive and warm, and Demchak worked on his pride, mobilizing his anger. Pretty soon, he was cursing, angry, and sobbing on Judy's shoulder. Demchak and his date moved on, but Judy and I spent the evening with Jim. I think that those two may have prevented a suicide attempt. Later in the evening, Ben and Annie made an appearance, conspicuously disarranged. Ben started to rib Jim, but Jim Hammerstein and I took him aside and told him what we thought of him. Judy was charming to Annie: "I'm pleased to meet you. I've never met a slut before."

Months passed. Judy fixed up Jim with a girl he eventually married. Judy and I were never more than friends, but saw a lot of one another.

The following summer, I was at the beach. Up came Annie. I told her that what she had done to Jim was cheap. She did not remember, she said. Annie told me that a lot of boys were crazy about her, found her irresistible, and that a few had attempted suicide when she dumped them. I told her that she was bad news. She began an involved monologue about how this one boy was still in a mental hospital over her.

"Annie, you're a sick bitch. Why are you telling me this junk?"

"I don't like it when a man says no. I'm the sexiest woman you'll ever meet. I can give a blow job that drives a man crazy; I can screw all night. . . ."

"Spare me the crap."

"You don't know what you are missing." Annie spent a long time detailing what she would be glad to do for me. I was really tempted. She was beautiful, and I had never heard of much of what she offered, but the whole thing was too sick. Finally, I told her to get lost.

Annie exploded at me. She was indignant. "I'm irresistible. I even turned my father on 'til he screwed me. He was the best. Go out with me tonight. You'll never regret it."

I gathered my things and moved near to a blanket occupied by a group of girls I knew vaguely. One was very intellectual and told me that I should not be hanging out with tramps, but should spend my time thinking and talking about serious topics. "Like, do you ever think about socialism?"

Thinking that that was the cleverest line I had heard for a while, I took her out. Son of a gun! She really wanted to talk about socialism!

Two years later, I was home from medical school. Shelly Weiss and I were in his family's store when we met a classmate of his who had become a state trooper. We talked about a mutual friend, a policeman, who had been hit by a car as he was ticketing another motorist. Then he said, "I think you knew Joe Pope."

I did. Joe was a fellow I had run into occasionally at the shore. He was with us that day when we injected the watermelon.

"He died last week." I was surprised. Joe was a good guy, my own age.

The state trooper had responded to the call. Apparently, Joe had been driving with a young lady who was attempting to perform a sex act at 60 miles per hour. He had lost control of the car and both were killed. My family saves newspapers. When I read the story, I found that the woman involved was Annie. My response was sorrow over Joe, good riddance to Annie.

It is only recently that I have begun to reflect on how Annie got to be the way she was. She was so aggressive with her sexuality, so hostile in the way that she used it, and hurt so many people that I knew (more than noted here) that I was without compassion for her. To me, she was a tempting plague, a menace to be avoided. I was not then aware that one possible outcome of early sexual abuse is a profound erotization. When she spoke of having seduced her father, I assumed it was a lie. Now, I wonder if Annie was erotized by incestuous experiences and, like many (primarily male) victims of sexual abuse, became a sexual abuser of others.

JEFFREY'S BASEMENT

Although this incident really occurred when I was rather young, it was the last that I recalled in my explorations. Perhaps I recalled it last because it was the most egregious that I had been exposed to, and hit closest to home.

Jeffrey's parents had been childhood friends of my parents. We never were close, but we were about the same age, only a grade or two apart, and grew up knowing one another. One day, when I was around 11, a bunch of us were playing poker at George Winters' house. The subject turned to sex. What was the sexual act really like? The reader must recall that this was a long time before cable television and X-rated movies. I had been told about sex in a way that left a lot to the imagination and had filled in the details inaccurately. So had many of my friends. George set us up. He asked everyone what he thought the sex act was. Luckily, we followed the model of our poker game, and I was to the dealer's right and spared the embarrassment of making a public disclosure of my ignorance.

Eddy Boone thought that it had something to do with the insertion of the middle finger into the vagina. Bill Greenwald said that that was trash, but was unable to express his idea. Tim Adamowicz gave some elaborate notion that sounded to me as if he were describing mutual urination. So far, Eddy seemed to have it and was confident in his knowledge. George could not contain himself and sprung his trap. "You're all wrong. What a bunch of fairies!"

Luckily, he did not ask us what that meant. Eddy stuck to his guns and defended the middle finger theory. George wanted to bet. Eddy put up a dollar, but there was a problem. Who was the authority who would settle things? George dropped the bomb: "I know what it is. I have pictures."

Somehow, George had found a pack of pornographic playing cards an uncle had brought back from Tijuana and surreptitiously absconded with a few. We all had to promise to cover our eyes while he retrieved them from a hiding place and suddenly, and irretrievably, we knew. "You can tell they are real Mexican cards," said George. "Why?" asked Eddy, who no longer was mourning the loss of his dollar and his theory. "Because the man still has his socks on."

"Oh." We were edified.

We were sworn to secrecy about the cards and asked if anyone else had seen them. Jeffrey had seen them.

"You mean 'free-show Jeffrey'?" Eddy asked. There were three Jeffries that we all knew. George nodded.

"Why do you call him 'free-show Jeffrey'?" someone asked.

Eddy thought he knew why, but his idea proved as accurate as his theory. Again, George swore us to secrecy. After school, Jeffrey, who was 14 or so, would get his 8-year-old sister Joyce to do a striptease for his friends in the basement and "let them touch her wherever they wanted to." In exchange for showing Jeffrey the cards, George had seen the "free show."

Over the years, I heard a lot about Jeffrey's basement, and each year the stories about the things Jeffrey would get Joyce to do for his friends became more lurid. Some of the boys involved spoke openly about Jeffrey and Joyce. One, who was so sexually preoccupied that many of us called him "Jerry the pervert," told me that I should have sex with my sister like Jeffrey did with Joyce. "She'll really know how to please a man."

From what I heard, Jeffrey involved his second sister after a while. Once, a few years later, we fell into conversation about it. I told him he was disgusting. He defended himself and finally, when I stuck to my guns, he punched me.

I still see Jeffrey sometimes when I return to my hometown, but we do not speak. Joyce has had a lot of psychiatric problems. She is in and out of the hospital a lot and has never married or been able to hold a job.

It is instructive to me that although I never had forgotten about Jeffrey and Joyce, I never fully allowed myself to grasp the implications of my knowledge, or to label what had occurred as what it was.

REFLECTIONS

Unfortunately, incest is a commonplace occurrence. Despite this, it has long been considered rare, and relatively few clinicians develop an index of suspicion for it and for the indirect expressions of its impact. By using some of my own life experiences, I have tried to demonstrate in a personal and subjective manner that many of us may have had far greater exposure to incest than we initially would have believed. The human mind is capable of defending itself from what it finds unacceptable and overwhelming. The pressure to deny the sordid realities of the widespread abuse of children in incest and any number of other forms of mistreatment is profoundly entrenched within ourselves and our society. The naivete I ascribe to myself in these vignettes is not so much a personal as a societal stance.

I found it disconcerting to realize how much I knew or could have known, but had forgotten, distorted, or otherwise failed to manage straightforwardly. Clearly, I was unprepared to convert the raw material of my experiences into an awareness of incest until many years had passed and I had both achieved some emotional distance from these events and acquired an intellectual scheme in which I could begin to organize and study my awarenesses and was motivated to do so. As I reread these vignettes, I am impressed with how minimal was my awareness of the implications of incest and with how infrequently I was sensitive to the plight of the incest victim, rather than to my own reactions and those of my friends. Certainly much of this had to do with my age at the time of these events, but much as well is due to the pressures we feel, as individuals and as a culture, to fail to recognize and address the issue of intrafamilial sexual abuse.

In the brushes with incest that touched me most closely, I am impressed that I blocked out what I had been told about the "goddess" for more than 18 years. Although I had hardly known her, she was important to me emotionally. I have no other choice but to assume that I found what I had been told intolerable and sequestered it in short order. The very next day after learning that she had been an incest victim, I was back at my residency, routinely maintaining a polite skepticism about patients' accounts of mistreatment and listening to lectures on the psychodynamics of patients' delusional accusations against those in their lives.

As clearly as I can recall, other aspects of the incidents with Greta and Maria were so arresting that it is only now that I am able to see their diverse manifestations as the result of their incestuous misuse. I was very naive and severely shocked. Or was I? I already had devised a way to live with an awareness and lack of awareness of what went on in "free-show Jeffrey's" basement. Also, I suppose that at the time I experienced Greta and Maria as too different from me for me to relate to them and their experiences. We tend to discount what we cannot believe happens to people like ourselves, and I guess that often, when it is undeniably close to home, as with Jeffrey's sister, we tend to dissociate the experience in some fashion.

In the situation with Tommy and Cheryl, I am embarrassed to reflect that I never gave much thought to Cheryl's plight. My concern was only for the impact of what Cheryl had said on Tommy who was, at best, a casual acquaintance. If he was a friend of Bill's, I would help—that was the "code." It is only now that I wonder what became of Cheryl and wonder why, out of a whole group of people, her plight received virtually no attention. Likewise with Annie. At the time, I had nothing but contempt for her and hated her for what she had done to a friend. At the Peppermint Lounge, I was too caught up in the adventure that Demchak had precipitated on me to reflect that I was joking around with a lovely and intelligent woman whose life was in a shambles, who was unable to remove herself from a masochistic and self-destructive life-style despite her charm and her intellectual assets, reduced to taking on nearly broke college students and other low-fee clients to make ends meet.

With Luciano and the big man, I was most aware of the picaresque aspect of my adventure and with my own guilt over my inadvertent complicity with Luciano. What I took from the big man's comments was the sense of entering into a forbidden world, both fascinating and repulsive, and a mortification over my own naivete. I did not respond to the bald statement that the best way to exploit a woman is to find one who had become inured to exploitation in the course of incest. It is only now that I fully realize all the implications of what he was saying to me.

With regard to Liz, "The Girl From Ipanema," by the time I came to learn that she had been an incest victim, I was already an experienced clinician. I did not block out any awareness of what I learned from her, but did not allow myself to make a full and affectively meaningful connection between her present circumstances and her behavior when I knew her because of my readily rekindled embarrassment over my own antics that summer long ago.

Almost every incest victim in these vignettes fared poorly. Of those whose fates I know, even remotely, perhaps only Maria survived relatively intact. The remainder spend years as prostitutes and/or terribly exploited individuals and/or chronic psychiatric patients. I do not regard this as a representative sample, simply as unsettling food for thought. Having evaluated more than 200 incest victims, I do not find their stories unusual any longer.

As you read the remainder of this book, you will meet individuals like those discussed above over and over, but they will be introduced in the more objective language of scientific discourse, or be registered as anonymous units in a cited series, points on a graph, and numbers on a chart. Perhaps this more personal journey, despite its inevitable shortcomings and imperfections, will provide you, the reader, with a less cognitive and distant way of entering into the areas of concern that the remainder of the book will approach in a more scholarly manner.

In writing this chapter I have taken pains to avoid the language of the clinic and the terminology of the scientific literature. Instead I have tried to illustrate the sort of experiences and reflections that emerge when one opens the Pandora's box of memory in the service of understanding one's countertransferential denial of the existence and the impact of incest. It is all too understandable that the human mind, even the mind of a trained psychiatrist, rebels at being confronted with incest. Despite Freud's difficulties with the issue of incest as a reality as opposed to incest fantasies, the corpus of his remarkable contributions bears witness to the power of incestuous concerns to arouse anxieties and to instigate complex symptoms and elaborate defensive constellations.

Incest provokes extreme countertransference difficulties. Sgroi et al. (1982) remarked that incest is a clinical situation in which the payoff for denial on the part of the clinician may equal or exceed the payoff for denial on the part of the victim. We tend to dismiss the incest victim's accounts all too often. We often become skeptical detectives rather than compassionate healers and approach the incest victim with incredulity. We make sure that incest is the province of the patient and is remote from our own experiences, and then we further detoxify the impact of the patient's account by wrapping ourselves in speculations that the incest may not have occurred. The "objectivity" of the clinician who takes an incredulous stance is not objective; it is a retreat from anxiety-provoking issues and candid exploration of countertransference concerns into the realm of wishful (or even magical) thinking.

Goodwin (1985) offered an eloquent observation:

> Incredulity can be understood as an intellectualized variant of derealization; and, like the dissociative defenses, incredulity is an effective way to gain distances from terrifying realities. Thus, physicians can be counted upon to routinely disbelieve child abuse accounts that are simply too horrible to be accepted without threatening their emotional homeostasis. (pp. 7–8)

This incredulity, which often occurs on a meta-level such that inquiry about incestuous experiences is rarely made in the taking of a routine clinical history, combats the anxieties that are raised when it is understood to be a commonplace phenomenon and has victimized people very much like ourselves and the members of our own families. It is emotionally easier for us to believe that such occurrences are infrequent or apocryphal or occur only to individuals who are very different from us. Our disbelief frees us from myriad anxieties about ourselves and our own lives and distances us from our own troublesome oedipal issues and conflicts, both in our roles as the children of our parents and as parents of our children.

When we avoid coming to grips with the powerful emotions that are raised by our work with incest patients, we can become deskilled in our clinical work with them. Since incest victims constitute a sizeable percentage of the patients with whom we work, neither we nor our patients can afford the luxury of our contertransferential problems in this area. To the extent that we do so, we impoverish our clinical skills and diminish ourselves as healers.

REFERENCES

Goodwin JM: Credibility problems in multiple personality disorder patients and abused children, in Childhhod Antecedents of Multiple Personality. Edited by Kluft RP. Washington, DC, American Psychiatric Press, 1985, pp 1–19

Sgroi S, Porter FS, Blick LC: Validation of child sexual abuse, in Handbook of Clinical Intervention in Child Sexual Abuse. Edited by Sgroi S. Lexington, MA, DC Heath, 1982, pp 39–79

CHAPTER 3

A Review of the Literature on the Long-Term Effects of Childhood Sexual Abuse

Diane H. Schetky, M.D.

This chapter is divided into two parts. The first part discusses the methodological problems encountered in doing long-term follow-up studies on childhood sexual abuse and reviews results of existing studies. Given the nature of many of these studies, it is not always possible to break down data by intrafamilial versus extrafamilial abuse, but such distinctions will be made where possible. The second part discusses several different perspectives on the victim-to-patient process, which attempts to link sexual abuse with ensuing psychopathology.

LONG-TERM STUDIES OF CHILDHOOD SEXUAL ABUSE

Research Problems

The major categories of research problems to be discussed below are problems of sampling, standardization, comparison groups, retrospection, pooling of cases, differentiating effects of abuse from conditions that predispose to it, and determining the source of trauma.

Sampling problems. The population one chooses to study inevitably will influence results to some degree. The choices are the general public, deviant populations, or victims followed from the time of abuse. Many of the larger retrospective studies on child sexual abuse (e.g., Finkelhor 1979; Fritz et al. 1981; Fromuth 1983; Landis 1956; Sedney and Brooks 1984) have been based on surveys of college students. The use of such populations introduces possible bias toward both higher-than-average IQ and socioeconomic status. Other researchers (e.g., Courtois 1979; Tsai et al. 1979) have solicited volunteers, which could create a bias toward normality or toward those factors associated with being a volunteer. A different approach was taken by Russell (1986), who drew her random sample from the San Francisco telephone directory. Letters were sent to the selected households; these were followed up with a visit to the household. When permitted, an interview by a well-trained individual matched for gender (and usually ethnicity) with the interviewee was undertaken.

Numerous surveys of sexual abuse have been done on deviant populations, such as psychiatric outpatients (Briere and Runtz 1988; Gelinas 1983; Herman 1981; Jacobson 1989; Meiselman 1978; Morrison 1989), psychiatric inpatients (Bryer et al. 1987; Carmen et al. 1984; Emslie and Rosenfeld 1983; Livingston 1987), drug addicts (Benward and Densen-Gerber 1975), prostitutes (James and Myerding 1977; Silbert and Pines 1981), and runaways (Reich and Guiterra 1979). Not surprisingly, histories of sexual abuse are frequent in these groups, but one must remember that they are not representative of the population at large.

Another approach is to follow up victims from the time of assault, as has been done in several studies (Adams-Tucker 1982; Anderson et al. 1981; Conte and Schuerman 1988; Friederich et al. 1986; Gomes-Schwartz et al. 1985; Peters 1979). It may be difficult to get adequate follow-up on these children, and among those followed sequentially, symptoms may not show up for many years. Further, treatment is presumably offered to such children, which introduces another variable for which it is difficult to obtain adequate controls.

Methods of obtaining follow-up information (i.e., telephone calls, questionnaires, or in-person interviews) may also affect results, as will the skills of the interviewer and the respondent's willingness and capacity to disclose. Using random-digit dialing, Wyatt (1985) sampled white and Afro-American women in Los Angeles County. Her interviewers received more training than those used by Russell (1986), and the interviews were much longer. Interestingly, however, her findings were comparable to those of Russell.

Very few studies differentiate according to race, ethnicity, or religion. It is possible that for some groups the stigma of sexual abuse is greater than for others and thus a factor in ensuing psychopathology. Indeed, Russell's (1986) data support this hypothesis. She noted that 83% of Latin victims reported extreme or considerable trauma as a result of incest versus 79% of Afro-American victims, 50% of Asian victims, and 49% of white victims. Wyatt (1985) also found that Afro-American women reported more long-lasting effects of childhood sexual abuse than did white women and that they tended to blame themselves for their victimization.

Standardization. Standardization is generally lacking in most outcome studies, and measurements of distress remain quite subjective. Measurements of adjustment, be they psychiatric diagnoses or psychological testing, may fail to pick up on problems such as mistrust or difficulties with intimacy. Finally, there is no consensus as to what constitutes a good outcome.

Comparison groups. Many of the existing outcome studies lack control or comparison groups. It becomes difficult to control for confounding independent variables (e.g., physical abuse) and risk factors, as will be seen in the presentation that follows. Moreover, when controls are used, one can never be entirely certain that they have not experienced sexual abuse, particularly when subjects are very young.

Retrospection. Studies of adult populations are almost all retrospective, which introduces the risks of the distortion of memories or their repression or both. However, some reassurance comes from the work by Herman and Schatzow (1987), which showed that a large percentage of women reporting sexual abuse were able to document it in the course of therapy.

Pooling of cases. No uniform definitions of sexual abuse exist for purposes of research. Some studies include as sexual abuse everything from exhibitionism to rape and incestuous intercourse, whereas others utilize more narrow inclusion criteria. Further, the age of the victim is likely to be a factor in the type of abuse. Thus when Gomes-Schwartz et al. (1985) concluded that sexual abuse seemed to have less effect on the very young child, one must ask whether it had to do with the age of the child or the fact that intercourse is (relatively) rarely attempted with a preschool child for whom the abuse may begin as "gentle molestation." Finally, many studies fail to differentiate regarding the relationship between the victim and the offender.

Differentiating effects of abuse from conditions that predispose to it. Factors that put a child at risk for sexual abuse include living in a rural setting, living without a natural father or mother, and having a mother employed outside of the home or a mother who is disabled or ill (Finkelhor 1986; Landis 1956; Maisch 1972; Meiselman 1978). The presence of a stepfather in the home greatly increases the likelihood of sexual abuse as does a natural father's lack of involvement with the socialization of his daughter (Finkelhor 1986; Parker and Parker 1986; Russell 1986, 1984). Several authors commented on ego impairment as a predisposing factor that probably adds to a child's neediness and difficulty avoiding an abusive situation (Browning and Boatman 1977; Gomes-Schwartz et al. 1985). Thus the child at risk for incest appears to be one with a poor relationship with at least one parent, lack of maternal protection, and probable underlying neediness and low self-esteem that may render her more vulnerable to sexual advances. Social isolation and poor peer relations may also increase the risk (Finkelhor 1986). It soon becomes apparent that this population is, in general, at risk for emotional problems given their life circumstances regardless of whether or not sexual abuse occurs.

Determining the source of trauma. It is also important to distinguish between the effects of sexual abuse and the traumatic events that may occur subsequently. Not uncommonly, these may include foster care, multiple interrogations and court proceedings, incarceration of the offender, dissolution of the family or alienation and lack of support in incestuous cases, moves, economic instability, and unsettling publicity.

Variables in Outcome Studies of Sexual Abuse

Having looked at some of the research problems, I will now consider what are the many variables in sexual abuse that need to be taken into consideration. Results are often contradictory and should be interpreted cautiously.

Duration of abuse. Tsai et al. (1979) compared 30 adult psychiatric patients seeking therapy for problems associated with childhood sexual abuse with a nonclinical group of 30 women sexually abused as children. They found that the patient group reported having endured the longest duration of sexual molestation. Russell (1986), studying a nonclinical population, also concluded that incestuous relations of long duration were the most damaging. Sierles et al. (1989) studied outpatient children who were incest victims and found a positive correlation between frequency and duration of sexual abuse and the pressure of a diagnosable psychiatric disorder. In contrast, Finkelhor (1979) could find no correlation, and Courtois (1979) found the longest lasting experiences to be the least traumatic.

Relationship to the offender. There is a consensus among researchers that sexual relations between father and daughter or stepfather and daughter are the most damaging. Beyond this, there does not seem to be much difference between other family members or persons outside of the family. The extent of the trauma in these cases may also have to do with the degree to which trust was violated.

Affective content.   Some clinicians believe that the child is better able to absolve herself from guilt when threats of physical assault are involved. Force is more likely to be used with the older female victim, whereas male victims are likely to experience rewards for their participation. Several authors correlated the use of force with more negative and lasting responses (Briere 1984; Finkelhor 1979; Fritz et al. 1981; Meiselman 1978; Russell 1986).

Type of sexual abuse.   Most studies agree that the more invasive the sexual abuse, the more traumatic it is (Bagley and Ramsey, in press; Friederich et al. 1986; Fritz et al. 1981; Gomes-Schwartz et al. 1985; Russell 1986). However, a few studies have shown no such correlation (Briere and Runtz 1984; Finkelhor 1979; Friederich 1988).

Sex of the victim.   Most studies to date have been done on females. Although about 10% of victims of sexual abuse are male, sexual abuse of males tends to be underreported, possibly because of the added stigma that the abuse is often homosexual. Finkelhor (1979) found homosexual abuse to be more upsetting to boys than girls. Friederich et al. (1986) found that 60% of the males in their sample had been abused by females and that they seemed to be less negative about the experience than were the girls studied. Boys were likely to view the experience as an initiation, whereas girls felt victimized. He also noted that girls were more likely than boys to be abused by persons in positions of authority.

Age of the victim.   Gomes-Schwartz et al. (1985) found that young children were less able than older ones to understand the sexual nature of the abusive experience, hence they believed they were less likely to show behavior changes. In contrast, the most affected group in their study was that composed of 7- to 13-year-olds. Incestuous experiences with an onset during the teen years are more likely to involve some degree of consent, and teens are felt to be better able intellectually to process the experience. Friederich et al. (1986) found that young children tend to internalize more than older children, who tend to externalize. In a prospective study of sexually abused children, Adams-Tucker (1982) found that emotional disturbances were more severe when the abuse began at an early age and was long standing. Finkelhor (1979), Anderson et al. (1981), and Russell (1986) found small tendencies for abuse that began at younger ages to be associated with more long-term trauma, but this fell short of achieving statistical significance.

Age difference between victim and offender.   Almost all studies agree that the greater the age difference between victim and offender, the greater the trauma is likely to be. Where there is an age differential, the offender is likely to be abusing power, the victim is not likely to be in a position to give informed consent to the relationship, and the victim is less able to say no to the offender.

Sex of the offender. Although increased attention is now being given to female offenders, very little has been written about the impact of abuse by females. Finkelhor (1979) noted that experiences with male offenders are more traumatic than those with females. Russell (1986) found that abuse by female perpetrators was low in her study and involved only 5% of incestuous cases and 4% of extrafamilial cases of sexual abuse. She concluded that such exploitations proved less serious and traumatic in the women she studied than did abuse by male perpetrators.

Parental variables. Gomes-Schwartz et al. (1985) and Adams-Tucker (1982) noted that the mother's response to the abuse is critical to the outcome. It is appreciated that a punitive response was associated with a worse outcome than a supportive response, but it is uncertain which type of response is most common.*

Treatment. Few of the adult victims in the retrospective studies had received treatment for childhood sexual abuse. Those who later sought treatment were likely to be more symptomatic than those who did not seek treatment (Herman et al. 1986). Obviously, for ethical reasons, it becomes difficult to control for treatment in prospective studies.

Summary of variables in outcome studies. Long-lasting negative effects of childhood sexual abuse appear to be correlated with abuse by a father or a stepfather, use of force, and being unsupported by a close adult. It is highly probable that sexual activity that is intrusive and of long duration is most disruptive. School-age children seem to be at greatest risk for developing behavioral problems related to the abuse, at least in short-term studies. Girls are more likely than boys to show acute distress following sexual abuse, but data are lacking on which to make adequate comparisons between male and female victims in terms of long-term effects and adjustments. Friederich (1988) reminds us of the need to view sexually abused children as a hetergeneous group. Each must be assessed

---

*Wyatt and Mickey (1988) conducted a retrospective study on 248 women and found that the outcome was not related to severity of abuse if the degree of support from parents and concerned others was held constant. Conte and Schuerman (1988) found parents' negative outlook on life was a significant variable in outcome. Friederich (1988) found that family conflict and cohesion were the primary independent variables for determining whether a child internalized or externalized his or her reactions.

within the context of the family unit. Family support remains a critical variable with regard to outcome.

Research on Long-Term Effects of Childhood Sexual Abuse

Having issued a caveat about the pitfalls of research on long-term effects of sexual abuse, I will now consider what some of the findings have been (Table 3-1).

Depression.   Depression, low self-esteem, and feelings of being damaged are commonly reported among adults who experienced childhood sexual abuse. The range of symptoms of depression among psychiatric patients who were victims of incest is from one-third to 100%, with most studies commenting on the high prevalence of these symptoms (Bagley and McDonald 1984; Briere and Runtz 1988; Courtois 1979; DeYoung 1982; Gelinas 1983; Herman et al. 1986; Jehu and Gazan 1983; Kaufman et al. 1954; Meiselman 1978; Murphy 1988; Russell 1986; Sedney and Brooks 1984; Stein et al. 1988). Sedney and Brooks noted a high incidence of depression among abused women who were not in treatment. A study of sexual and physical abuse histories in male psychiatric outpatients found a relationship between severity of adult psychiatric symptoms and a history of abuse. Among patients with a history of sexual abuse 14% had major affective disorders and 16% had anxiety or dysthymic disorders (Swett, Surrey, and Cohen 1990).

Psychiatric hospitalization.   Several studies point to an overrepresentation of victims of childhood sexual abuse on psychiatric inpatient units (Carmen et al. 1984; Emslie and Rosenfeld 1983; Sansonnet-Hayden et al.

Table 3-1.   Summary of research on long-term effects of childhood sexual abuse

---

Depression, low self-esteem
Psychiatric hospitalization
Substance abuse
Self-abuse
Somatization disorder
Eroticization
Learning difficulties
Posttraumatic stress disorder, anxiety
Dissociative disorders
Conversion reactions
Running away, prostitution
Revictimization
Impaired interpersonal relationships
Poor parenting

1987). Carmen et al. found that adult victims of sexual abuse tend to have longer stays than other patients, reflecting severity of illness and/or difficulties in treatment. Similar findings were reported by Sansonnet-Hayden et al. studying adolescents on an inpatient unit. They noted that sexually abused patients were more likely to present with major depression or conduct disorders than were nonabused patients.

Drugs and alcohol abuse.　Retrospective studies of sexually abused women not uncommonly find a history of substance abuse (Benward and Densen-Gerber 1975; Herman 1981; Peters 1979). Shearer et al. (1988) found a much higher incidence of substance abuse in male and female victims than controls in their non-clinical samples.). Several explanations exist for this, including the possibility that some victims may attempt to control their anxiety and intrusive thoughts related to the abuse through self-medication, and that drugs induce a chemical sort of latency, which victims of abuse failed to experience owing to premature sexual stimulation.

Self-abusive behavior.　Suicide attempts are a not uncommon sequel to sexual abuse. Studying a nonclinical population of women who had been sexually abused, Sedney and Brooks (1984) found that 16% had made suicide attempts versus 6% of controls. If one studies clinical populations of adults who have been sexually abused as children, the frequency of suicide attempts is much higher, with Briere and Runtz (1988) finding 51% versus 34% of controls, and Herman (1981) finding 38% versus 5% of controls. DeYoung (1982) reported 68% of her sample of adult incest victims had made attempts, 66% of them more than once. Maisch (1972) reported 33% in his clinical sample. Increased suicide attempts among adolescents who have been sexually abused have also been reported (Anderson 1981; Sansonnet-Hayden et al. 1987).

These findings are consistent with the high prevalence of depression, low self-esteem, and borderline personality disorder among this population. Psychodynamically, self-abuse may represent a perpetuation of the victim's tendency to internalize anger. Alternatively, as will be discussed later, some people may engage in abusive behavior (e.g., wrist-cutting) because it induces a sense of calm through stimulating the body's endorphins.

Borderline personality disorder.　The association between sexual abuse and borderline personality disorder has been noted by many authors (Herman et al. 1989; Horowitz and Braun 1984; Shearer et al. 1989) and will be discussed further by Stone in Chapter 9 of this volume.

Somatization disorder.　Two studies have reported an association between somatization disorder and a history of childhood sexual abuse (Coryell and Norten 1981; Livingston 1989; Morrison 1989). Walker et al. (1988) found that patients with chronic pelvic pain showed a higher prevalence of history of childhood and adult sexual abuse than a comparison group of women with specific gynecologic conditions.

Eroticization. Eroticization of sexually abused children has been described by Yates (1982), who noted that they can be quite sexually provocative, which unfortunately puts them at risk for revictimization. Friederich (1988) found that sexualization was a discriminatory variable between abused and nonabused children. These variables lose their discriminating ability for girls from ages 10 to 12, whereas boys remain sexualized through preadolescence (Friederich et al. 1990). Sexualized children are also difficult to contain in foster care because of their propensity to act sexually with other children. They also pose difficult problems to therapists.

Learning difficulties. Learning difficulties are a common occurrence among sexually victimized children (Fish-Murray et al. 1987; Gomes-Schwartz et al. 1985; Goodwin 1985; Kaufman et al. 1954; Sedney and Brooks 1984). Poor concentration, acting-out behaviors, anxiety, and social withdrawal all can impede performance. Gil et al. (1990) compared cognitive functioning with posttraumatic stress disorder, other psychiatric disorders, and controls. They found cognitive problems in both patient samples. They also found that premorbid intelligence had deteriorated significantly by the time of current testing. It is not clear to what extent these findings may be on an emotional or psychophysiologic basis, or reflect a combination of both factors.

Posttraumatic stress disorder and anxiety. Many studies document persistent anxieties and fears among victims of sexual abuse. Prevalence rates for both children and adults are close to 50% (Anderson et al. 1981; Briere 1984; Friederich et al. 1986; Gelinas 1983; Gomes-Schwartz et al. 1985; Peters 1979; Stein et al. 1988). Goodwin (1985) noted that symptoms of posttraumatic stress disorder occur in incest victims from preschool age to adulthood, but can easily be overlooked; hence, she stressed the need for clinicians to inquire about these symptoms. Two studies (Kiser et al. 1988; McLeer et al. 1988) described the onset of posttraumatic stress disorder in children following abuse and suggest that this is a common occurrence.

Dissociative disorders and conversion reactions. Dissociative disorders are marked by 1) disturbance in memory, such as amnesia, time loss, or intrusive recall; 2) disturbance in sense of identity involving fragmented sense of self and depersonalization; and 3) linkage of these events to a trauma. Hysterical seizures following incest have been described by Goodwin et al. (1979) and by Gross (1979). Dissociation (Briere and Runtz 1988) and its extreme, multiple personality disorder, are common sequelae of childhood sexual abuse and may serve as coping mechanisms. Almost all patients with multiple personality disorder have experienced severe abuse as children (Bowman et al. 1985; Braun and Sachs 1985; Goodwin 1987; Kluft 1985; Wilbur 1984). As many as 68% are reported to be incest victims (Putnam 1989). Often this diagnosis is missed because professionals fail to inquire about it or because such patients are labeled manipulative or borderline.

Running away, prostitution.   Several studies noted that about half of runaways have a history of sexual abuse (Herman 1981; Reich and Guiterra 1979). It is ironic to note that, in attempting to escape from abusive homes, many of these children, both male and female, end up being revictimized as prostitutes. Studies of prostitutes indicate that anywhere from 55% to 90% had experienced sexual abuse as children (Harlan et al. 1981; Cutter 1977; James and Myerding 1977; Silbert and Pines 1981).

One might wonder why an abused teen would put herself in this position. Often she is impelled by factors over which she has little control, including 1) her neediness, which renders her vulnerable to pimps; 2) her lack of marketable job skills; and 3) peer pressure to engage in prostitution, which may be presented to her as a fast way to get rich. On an unconscious level, the victimized teenager may be repeating her incestuous experience or even trying to get back at men. Similar dynamics may be at play for the victim of sexual abuse who is promiscuous. Many have learned to use sex in attempting to gratify their needs for affection and security.

Revictimization.   Revictimization may include repeated sexual abuse or entering into relationships with men in which the woman is physically or emotionally battered. Various studies showed this to be the pattern in about half of abused women (Briere 1984; Fritz et al. 1981; Russell 1986). Two studies of inpatients noted the pattern of revictimization among those who had been sexually abused (Bryer et al. 1987; Sansonnet-Hayden et al. 1987). More subtle forms of exploitation include allowing others to take advantage of them, and their not being able to assert themselves. (See Kluft, Chapter 13, this volume.)

Impaired interpersonal relationships and trust.   Difficulty in interpersonal relationships is a common complaint among incest victims seen in therapy who often complain about feeling detached, not being able to trust, and feeling hostile toward men (Briere 1984; Courtois 1979; Herman 1981; Herman et al. 1986; Kaufman et al. 1954; Lustig et al. 1966; Meiselman 1978). Sexual difficulties are common. Social skills may be impaired and separation-individuation is often discouraged in incestuous families (Sgroi 1982). Russell (1986) found that those women who were severely traumatized by incestuous abuse were more likely to be divorced or separated. She also found that if they were Catholic or Protestant, they were more likely than women who have never been sexually abused to defect from the religion of their upbringing.

Poor parenting. Clinicians are beginning to look at how sexually abused women function as parents. Goodwin et al. (1982) found in a study of abusive mothers that 24% of them had been incest victims. Gelinas (1983) noted that women who have been sexually abused tend to experience much ambivalence, have trouble setting limits, and feel overwhelmed. Studying parents whose parental rights had been terminated, Schetky et al. (1979) found that 37% of these mothers had been sexually abused as children.

Summary of research on long-term effects. There is considerable morbidity associated with a history of childhood sexual abuse. As noted, sexual abuse is often not an isolated trauma, and one must look at it in light of and in the context of those conditions that may have preceded it, bearing in mind as well the aftermath of sexual abuse. Despite the statistics, it should be remembered that some victims may recover with or without professional help. In Russell's (1986) study, which was based on the self-reports of 152 abused women, 22% felt that sexual abuse had no lasting effect on them, 27% felt it had little effect on them, 26% said it had some effect, and 25% said it had great effect on their lives. Because so many victims attempt to deal with abuse by denying its impact, one must question the validity of findings based on self-reports (see Kluft, Chapter 13, this volume).

THE VICTIM-TO-PATIENT PROCESS

Several theories exist to explain symptom formation in victims of sexual abuse. These include the traditional psychoanalytic model, the attempt to understand symptoms as accommodation to abuse, and a paradigm that views symptoms as secondary to the physiologic changes that occur as a result of trauma. All three models serve to enhance our understanding of symptom formation, and they may interact in a synergistic fashion.

Psychoanalytic Formulations

Freud's early studies. In 1896, Freud postulated in the "Etiology of Hysteria" that hysterical symptoms were based on early childhood sexual experiences and stated that:

> I therefore put forward the thesis that at the bottom of every case of hysteria there are *one or more occurrences of premature sexual experience*, occurrences which belong to the earliest years of childhood but which can be reproduced through the work of psychoanalysis in spite of the intervening decades. (p. 203)

He further speculated that:

> Injuries sustained by an organ which is as yet immature, or by a function which is in the process of developing, often cause more severe and lasting effects than they could do in mature years. Perhaps the abnormal reaction to sexual impressions which surprises us in hysterical subjects at the age of puberty is quite generally based on those experiences of this sort in childhood, in which case those experiences must be of a similar nature to one another and must be of an important kind. (p. 202)

Freud viewed symptom formation as arising from the repression of unacceptable thoughts or wishes. He cautioned that if the trauma was not put in historical context (i.e., understood), that the individual would be doomed to repeat it. This prophecy has certainly borne true in regard to the number of sexually abused children who have been revictimized. His psychoanalytic formulations have contributed to both the understanding of symptom formation in victims of sexual abuse and the therapeutic process with this population.

Fantasy versus reality.   Freud was apparently well aware of studies done by the 19th-century French physicians documenting the prevalence of child sexual abuse (see Masson 1985). Despite this, only a year after writing the "Etiology of Hysteria," he chose to renounce his seduction theory of neurosis. Rather than focus on real-life events and the adult's capacity for committing incest, Freud chose to pursue his patient's fantasies and explore the childhood desires that he believed were the cause of psychiatric illness. Given the prevalence of hysterical reactions in 19th-century Vienna, he apparently had difficulty accepting the idea that sexual perversions could be that prevalent or that so many fathers could have such inclinations. The medical community, which was initially offended by Freud's seduction theory, readily embraced his new position. As noted by Anna Freud, "keeping up the seduction theory would mean to abandon the Oedipus complex and with it the whole importance of phantasy life, conscious or unconscious phantasy. In fact, I think there would have been no psychoanalysis afterwards" (quoted in Masson 1985, p. 113). Thus what became a giant step forward for psychoanalysis became a major step backward for women, children, and the ability of physicians to recognize sexual abuse. I realize that my interpretation of this crucial issue in the history of the study of incest may be perceived as unsettling or even offensive to many. However, I must emphasize that my focus here is neither to disparage nor pay tribute to Freud and his monumental contributions, but to offer a perspective on the impact of his stance on incest for the future study of this subject.

Ferenczi: "The Terrible Truth." In contrast to Freud and his followers, psychoanalyst Sandor Ferenczi remained convinced that his patients' reports of sexual abuse were "the terrible truth." In an eloquent paper entitled "Confusion of Tongues Between Adults and the Child," first presented in 1932, Ferenczi (1949) described the effects of sexual abuse on the psyche. He noted the child's need to remain silent, the child's total submission to the aggressor at the expense of the self, and the child's attempts to deal with the trauma through dissociation and even identification with the aggressor. Sadly, Ferenczi was ridiculed by his colleagues, who accused him of being paranoid, said that his patients' accounts were mere fairy tales, and suppressed the publication of his paper. Thus the matter of child sexual abuse was to remain repressed in psychoanalytic circles until Ferenczi's paper was finally published in 1949.

Symptoms as Accommodation to Sexual Abuse

Sexual Abuse Accommodation Syndrome. Several authors continued where Ferenczi left off, looking at symptoms as the child's attempt to accommodate to sexual abuse. Summit (1983) described the "Child Sexual Abuse Accommodation Syndrome" as a model to help the clinician understand the child's position and the dynamics that surround incestuous abuse. The five components of the syndrome are 1) secrecy; 2) helplessness; 3) entrapment and accommodation; 4) delayed, conflicted, and unconvincing disclosure; and 5) retraction. Summit stated that "However gentle or menacing the intimidation may be, the secrecy makes it clear to the child that this is something bad and dangerous. The secrecy is both the source of fear and the promise of safety" (p. 181). Secrecy also confers with it the power to destroy the family and the responsibility to hold the family together; hence the child's tendency to delay disclosure, or to retract following disclosure.

Helplessness ensues from the power the adult as an authority holds over the child. Given her status as child, the youthful victim is incapable of giving informed consent to sexual activity with an adult. The conditions of informed consent require that a truly willing participant be informed as to the consequences of the proposed activities and free to say yes or no. Obviously she cannot do this if she is emotionally and physically dependent on her abuser.

Because the child in an ongoing incestuous relationship cannot escape, she must learn to accept the situation in order to survive. If the young child cannot trust and believe her parent is good, she is left with existential despair. She may employ various strategies to preserve the image of the good parent, including 1) denying that the abuse is occurring; 2) dissociation (i.e., surrendering her body but not her mind); and 3) blaming herself rather than her parent. She may also rationalize that she is protecting others by sacrificing herself.

The pathological fixation of defenses.   Rieker and Carmen (1986) elaborated on how the mechanisms the child uses to cope with abuse become pathologic when they persist into adult life and invade other areas of functioning. They noted that loyalty to family demands sacrifice of self, and, because of this, victims often grow into adulthood without having been children or ever knowing their own feelings as separate from parental needs. This leaves them devoid of a sense of self or self-protective mechanisms. This, in turn, renders them more vulnerable to abuse and exploitation from outside the family. The accommodation also demands that the child alter her reality testing and adjust to a world where "abusive behavior is acceptable but telling the truth about it is sinful" (p. 369). The child's perceptions become undermined when they are not validated; this leads to a loss of self-confidence and impaired reality testing.

As an example, one teenager continued to doubt herself years after an incestuous relationship with an uncle for which she blamed herself, saying, "I shouldn't have believed him [that he was just checking her glands]; I should have known better." By age 13, she was demonstrating many features of borderline personality. Her older sister, who had also been abused as a young teen, showed classic symptoms of posttraumatic stress disorder and harbored much guilt for not having protected her younger sisters. At the time of the abuse, she believed that by going along with her uncle's demands, she was sparing her younger sisters. The youngest sister, who had been 6 at the time of the abuse, proceeded to develop eroticized behavior and the symptoms of a conduct disorder. This family demonstrates the multiplicity of symptoms that can result from the same type of trauma and the roles that development and personality have to play in determining which symptoms will emerge. The sex of the victim will also affect how the abuse is handled. It has been noted that females tend to suppress their anger or turn it inward, whereas male victims may direct their anger toward others or identify with the abuser.

Traumatogenic aspects of sexual abuse.   To summarize, the traumatic aspects of sexual abuse include exploitation, violation of trust, premature sexualization, and a damaged sense of self. Added to this is often the loss of childhood and the loss of normal parenting. The child turns to her father for affection but can only receive it on his terms, which are sexual and totally disregard her developmental needs. At no point does she experience normal fathering; rather she feels (and in fact is) continually exploited. Further, her mother is often unavailable to her emotionally and fails to protect her. The development of diverse symptoms may help the child accommodate to this dysfunctional environment while she is trapped within it. However, as noted, too often this symptomatic adaptation persists into adult life, rendering the victim dysfunctional.

Neurophysiologic Changes Associated With Trauma

Depletion of catecholamines.   Research suggests that posttraumatic stress disorder may be biologically based (van der Kolk and Breenberg 1987). Hyperarousal of the nervous system has been measured in Vietnam veterans suffering from posttraumatic stress disorder as well as in infants separated from their caretakers. It is postulated that an unresponsive or abusive early environment can stimulate the emergence of hyperarousal states that have long-term effects on the child's ability to modulate anxiety and aggression. Parallels have been drawn between animal responses to inescapable shock and human responses to overwhelming trauma. In both, there is a depletion of catecholamines, postulated to result in psychological constriction and numbing. The symptoms of hyperarousal seem to follow an outpouring of these neurotransmitters after a period of depletion. It is speculated that the period of depletion renders the brain hypersusceptible to these neurotransmitters and that stimuli reminiscent of the initial trauma may induce a similar physiologic response. Consistent with this hypothesis is the fact that catecholamines are shown to have a positive effect on memory (Gold and Zornetzer 1983). Thus, in response to stress and the outpouring of these neurotransmitters, a traumatized individual may reexperience the initial trauma in the form of flashbacks and nightmares. The model of state-dependent memory may prove relevant here. In some cases, there may be a delay of years between the initial trauma and its being relived through symptoms. Thus a child who seems to have survived child sexual abuse may not become symptomatic until puberty, or when she marries, or when she has a child.

Endogenous opioids.   There may also be a physiologic basis for the numbing and constriction that often follows trauma. Prolonged stress in animals seems to activate brain opiate receptors, and their bodies respond by producing opioid-like substances termed *endorphins* that mediate stress and inhibit pain (Maier et al. 1980). These substances have also been found to be elevated in humans following surgery (Cohen et al. 1982), marathon running and extreme stress (Bortz et al. 1981; Colt et al. 1981), and self-mutilation (van der Kolk and Greenberg 1987). It is speculated that endorphins may have a calming action and perhaps even antidepressant and antiaggression properties. Some individuals may deliberately reexpose themselves to trauma as a way of self-medicating painful or overwhelming affects. This could explain why some patients deliberately engage in risk-taking behaviors or self-abusive behaviors (e.g., wrist cutting). Although these findings are preliminary, their implications for understanding and treating victims of trauma are profound.

SUMMARY

In this chapter, I have explored the many difficulties faced by researchers investigating the long-term effects of sexual abuse. Despite the varied approaches to studying the aftereffects of childhood sexual abuse, there is considerable consensus regarding the symptomatology seen in adult female survivors of sexual abuse who did not receive treatment as children. Further more sophisticated research is needed that will control for problematic variables and look at the outcome for sexually abused children who receive treatment. We also must, along the lines of Conte and Schuerman's (1988) and Friederich's (1988) studies, investigate the efficacy of various treatment modalities. Attention needs to be given to male victims of child sexual abuse and to the issue of female perpetrators. It is hoped that this chapter will stimulate more research into the short- and long-term effects of childhood sexual abuse and that future research may overcome some of the flaws in existing research protocols.

REFERENCES

Adams-Tucker C: Proximate effects of sexual abuse in childhood: a report of 28 children. Am J Psychiatry 139:1252–1256, 1982

Anderson L: Notes on the linkage between the sexually abused child and the suicidal adolescent. J Adolesc 4:157–162, 1981

Anderson SC, Bach CM, Griffith S: Psychosocial sequelae in intrafamilial victims of sexual assault and abuse. Paper presented at the Third International Conference on Child Abuse and Neglect, Amsterdam, The Netherlands, April 1981

Bagley C, McDonald M: Adult mental health sequelae of child sexual abuse, physical abuse, and neglect in maternally separated children. Canadian Journal of Community Mental Health 3:15–26, 1984

Bagley C, Ramsey R: Sexual abuse in childhood: psychosocial outcomes and implications for social work practice. Social Work and Human Sexuality 5:33–42, 1986

Beck JC, van der Kolk B: Reports of childhood incest and current behavior of chronically hospitalized psychotic women. Am J Psychiatry 144:1474–1476, 1987

Benward J, Densen-Gerber J: Incest as a causative factor in anti-social behavior: an exploratory study. Contemporary Drug Problems 33:323–340, 1975

Bortz WM, Angevin P, Mefford IN, et al: Catacholamines, dopamine, and endorphin levels during extreme exercise. N Engl J Med 305:466–469, 1981

Bowman E, Blix S, Coons P: Multiple personality in adolescence: relationship to incestual experiences. Journal of the American Academy of Child Psychiatry 24:109–114, 1985

Braun BG, Sachs RG: The development of multiple personality disorder: predisposing, precipitating, and perpetuating factors, in Childhood Antecedents of Multiple Personality. Edited by Kluft RP. Washington, DC, American Psychiatric Press, 1985, pp 37–64

Briere J, Runtz M: Post sexual abuse trauma, in Lasting Effects of Child Sexual Abuse. Edited by Wyatt GE, Powell GJ. Newbury Park, CA, Sage Publications, 1988, pp 85–100

Browning DH, Boatman B: Incest: children at risk. Am J Psychiatry 134:69–72, 1977

Bryer J, Nelson B, Miller J, et al: Childhood abuse as a factor in adult psychiatric illness. Am J Psychiatry 144:1426–1430, 1987

Carmen E, Rieker P, Mills T: Victims of violence and psychiatric illness. Am J Psychiatry 141:378–383, 1984

Cohen MR, Pichas D, Dubois M, et al: Stress induced plasma beta endorphin immunoreactivity may predict postoperative morphine usage. Psychiatry Res 6:7–12, 1982

Colt EW, Wardlaw SL, Frantz AG: The effect of running on plasma beta endorphin. Life Sci 28:1637–1640, 1981

Conte JR, Schuerman JR: The effects of sexual abuse on children: a multidimensional view, in Lasting Effects of Child Sexual Abuse. Edited by Wyatt GE, Powell GJ. Newbury Park, CA, Sage Publications, 1988, pp 157–169

Coryell W, Norten SG: Briquet's syndrome (somatization disorder) and primary depression: comparison of background and outcome. Compr Psychiatry 22:249–256, 1981

Courtois C: The incest experience and its aftermath. Victimology: An International Journal 4:337–347, 1979

Cutter L: Female Offenders. Lexington, MA, Lexington Books, 1977

DeYoung M: The Sexual Victimization of Children. Jefferson, NC, McFarland & Co, 1982

Emslie G, Rosenfeld A: Incest reported by children and adolescents hospitalized for severe psychiatric problems. Am J Psychiatry 140:708–711, 1983

Ferenczi S: Confusion of tongues between adults and the child: the language of tenderness and the language of passion. Int J Psychoanal 30:225–230, 1949

Finkelhor D: Sexually Victimized Children. New York, Free Press, 1979

Finkelhor D: A Sourcebook on Child Sexual Abuse. Beverly Hills, CA, Sage, 1986

Fish-Murray CC, Koby EV, van der Kolk BA: Evolving ideas: the effect of abuse on children's thought, in Psychological Trauma. Edited by van der Kolk BA. Washington, DC, American Psychiatric Press, 1987, pp 89–110

Freud S: The etiology of hysteria (1896), in The Standard Edition of the Complete Psychological Works of Sigmund Freud. Edited and translated by Strachey J. London, Hogarth, 1962. Original work published in 1896.

Friederich WN: Behavior problems in sexually abused children, in Lasting Effects of Child Sexual Abuse. Edited by Wyatt GE, Powell GJ. Newbury Park, CA, Sage Publications, 1988, pp 171–192

Friederich WN, Urgquiza AJ, Beilke RA: Behavioral problems in sexually abused young children. J Pediatr Psychol 11:47–56, 1986

Friederich WN, Graubsch P, Koverola C, et al: The Child Sexual Behavior Inventory: a comparison of normals and clinical populations. Paper presented at the 1990 Symposium on Child Victimization, Atlanta, April, 1990

Fritz GS, Stoll K, Wagner NA: A comparison of males and females who were sexually molested as children. Sex Marital Ther 7:54–59, 1981

Fromuth M: The long term psychological impact of childhood sexual abuse. Unpublished doctoral dissertation, Auburn University, Auburn, IL, 1983

Gelinas D: Persistent negative effects of incest. Psychiatry 46:312–331, 1983

Gil T, Calev A, Greenberg D, et al: Cognitive functioning in post-traumatic stress disorder. J Traumatic Stress 3(1):29–45, 1990

Gold PE, Zornetzer SF: The mnemon and its juices: neuromodulation of memory processes. Behav Neural Biol 38:151–189, 1983

Gomes-Schwartz B, Horowitz J, Sauzier M: Severity of emotional disturbance among sexually abused preschool, school age, and adolescent children. Hosp Community Psychiatry 5:503–508, 1985

Goodwin J: Post-traumatic stress symptoms in incest victims, in Post-Traumatic Stress Disorder in Children. Edited by Eth S, Pynoos RS. Washington, DC, American Psychiatric Press, 1985, pp 155–168

Goodwin J: Recognizing dissociative symptoms in abused children, in Incest Victims and Their Families, 2nd Edition. Edited by Goodwin J. Boston, MA, Wright/PSG, 1987

Goodwin J, Bergman R, Simms M: Hysterical seizures: a sequel to incest. Am J Orthopsychiatry 49:698–703, 1979

Goodwin J, McCarthy T, DiVasto P: Physical and sexual abuse of the children of adult incest victims, in Sexual Abuse: Incest Victims and Their Families. Edited by Goodwin J. Boston, MA, Wright/PSG, 1982, pp 139–154

Gross M: Incestuous rape: a cause for hysterical seizures in four adolescent girls. Am J Orthopsychiatry 49:704–708, 1979

Harlan S, Rogers L, Slattery B: Male and female adolescent prostitutes (Huckleberry House Sexual Minority Youth Services Project). Washington, DC, Youth Development Bureau, U.S. Department of Human Services, 1981

Herman J: Father-Daughter Incest. Cambridge, MA, Harvard University Press, 1981

Herman J, Schatzow E: Recovery and verification of memories of childhood sexual trauma. Psychoanalytic Psychology 4:1–14, 1987

Herman J, Russell D, Trocki K: Long term effects of incestuous abuse in childhood. Am J Psychiatry 143:1293–1296, 1986

Herman JL, Perry JC, van der Kolk BA: Childhood trauma in borderline personality disorder. Am J Psychiatry 146:490–495, 1989

Horowitz RP, Braun BG: Are multiple personalities borderline? Psychiatr Clin North Am 7:69–87, 1984

Jacobson A: Physical and sexual assault histories among psychiatric outpatients. Am J Psychiatry 146:755–758, 1989

James J, Myerding J: Early sexual experience and prostitution. Am J Psychiatry 134:1381–1385, 1977

Jehu D, Gazan M: Psychological adjustment of women who were sexually victimized in childhood or adolescence. Canadian Journal of Community Mental Health 2:71–78, 1983

Kaufman L, Peck A, Tagiuri C: The family constellation and overt incestuous relations between father and daughter. Am J Orthopsychiatry 24:266–279, 1954

Kiser L, Ackerman B, Brown E, et al: Post traumatic stress disorder in young children: a reaction to purported sexual abuse. J Am Acad Child Adolesc Psychiatry 27:645–649, 1988

Kluft RP: Childhood Antecedents of Multiple Personality. Washington, DC, American Psychiatric Press, 1985

Landis J: Experiences of 500 children with adult sexual deviants. Psychiatr Q (suppl) 30:91–109, 1956

Livingston R: Sexually and physically abused children. J Am Acad Child Adolesc Psychiatry 26:413–415, 1987

Lustig N, Dresser J, Spellman S, et al: Incest. Arch Gen Psychiatry 14:312–340, 1966

Maier SF, Davies E, Grau JW: Opiate antagonists and long term analgesis reaction induced by inescapable shock in rats. J Comp Physiol 94:1172–1183, 1980

Maisch J: Incest. New York, Stein & Day, 1972

Masson JM: The Assault on Truth: Freud's Suppression of the Seduction Theory. New York, Penguin, 1985

McLeer S, Deblinger E, Atkins M, et al: Post traumatic stress disorder in sexually abused children. J Am Acad Child Adolesc Psychiatry 27:650–654, 1988

Meiselman K: Incest: A Psychological Study of Causes and Effects With Treatment Recommendations. San Francisco, CA, Jossey-Bass, 1978

Morrison J: Childhood histories of women with somatization disorder. Am J Psychiatry 146:239–241, 1989

Murphy S: Current psychological functioning of child sexual abuse survivors. J Interpersonal Violence 3:55–79, 1988

Parker H, Parker S: Father-daughter sexual abuse: an emerging perspective. Am J Orthopsychiatry 56:531–549, 1986

Peters JJ: Children who were victims of sexual assault and the psychology of offenders. Am J Psychother 30:398–421, 1979

Putnum FW: The Diagnosis and Treatment of Multiple Personality Disorder. New York, Guilford Press, 1989

Reich J, Guiterra S: Escape/aggression incidence in sexually abused juvenile delinquents. Criminal Justice and Behavior 6:239–243, 1979

Rieker P, Carmen E: The victim to patient process: the disconfirmation and transformation of abuse. Am J Orthopsychiatry 56:360–370, 1986

Russell D: The prevalence and seriousness of incestuous abuse by stepfathers versus biological fathers. Child Abuse Negl 8:15–22, 1984

Russell D: The Secret Trauma: Incest in the Lives of Girls and Women. New York, Basic Books, 1986

Sansonnet-Hayden H, Haley G, Marriage K, et al: Sexual abuse and psychopathology in hospitalized adolescents. Journal of the American Academy of Child Psychiatry 26:753–757, 1987

Schetky DH, Angel R, Morrison C, et al: Parents who fail: a study of 51 cases of termination of parental rights. Journal of the American Academy of Child Psychiatry 18:366–383, 1979

Sedney MA, Brooks B: Factors associated with a history of childhood sexual experience in a nonclinical female population. Journal of the American Academy of Child Psychiatry 23:215–218, 1984

Sgroi S: Handbook of Clinical Intervention in Child Sexual Abuse. Lexington, MA, Lexington Books, 1982

Shearer SL, Peters CP, Quaztman MS, et al: Frequency of childhood sexual and physical abuse histories in adult female borderline patients. Am J Psychiatry 147:214–216, 1990

Silbert M, Pines A: Sexual abuse as an antecedent to prostitution. Child Abuse Negl 5:407–411, 1981

Sirles EA, Smith JA, Kusame H: Psychiatric status of intrafamilial child sexual abuse victims. J Am Acad Child Adolesc Psychiatry 27:650–654, 1988

Stew J, Golding J, Siegel J, et al: Long-term psychological effects of child sexual abuse, in Lasting Effects of Child Sexual Abuse. Edited by Wyatt GE, Powell GJ. Newbury Park, CA, Sage Publications 1988, pp 135–154

Summit RC: The child sexual abuse accommodation syndrome. Child Abuse Negl 7:117–193, 1983

Tsai M, Feldman-Summers S, Edgar M: Childhood molestation: variables related to differential impacts on psychosexual functioning in adult women. J Abnorm Psychol 88:407–417, 1979

van der Kolk BA, Greenberg MS: The psychobiology of the trauma response: hyperarousal, constriction, and addiction to traumatic reexposure, in Psychological Trauma. Edited by van der Kolk BA. Washington, DC, American Psychiatric Press, 1987, pp 63–87

Walker E, Katon W, Harrop G, et al: Relationship of chronic pelvic pain to psychiatric diagnoses and childhood sexual abuse. Am J Psychiatry 145:75–80, 1988

Wilbur C: Multiple personality and child abuse. Psychiatr Clin North Am 7:3–8, 1984

Wyatt G: The sexual abuse of Afro-American and white women in childhood. Child Abuse Negl 9:507–519, 1985

Wyatt GE, Mickey MR: Mediating factors to outcomes for children, in Lasting Effects of Child Sexual Abuse. Edited by Wyatt GE, Powell GJ. Newbury Park, CA, Sage Publications, 1988, pp 211–226

Yates A: Children eroticized by incest. Am J Psychiatry 139:482–485, 1982

CHAPTER 4

Applying to Adult Incest Victims What We Have Learned From Victimized Children

Jean M. Goodwin, M.D., M.P.H.

Since the mid-1970s, the legal, medical, and social redefinition of incest as child abuse has led to geometric annual increases in the numbers of child incest victims reported to protective service agencies (Goodwin 1987). This increase has led to similarly geometric increases in our knowledge about the epidemiology, natural history, and effective treatment of incestuous abuse. In this chapter, I will explore the implications of these new data for the treatment of adults who disclose a history of prior incest in psychotherapy. This exploration is not merely academic. Incest is not merely an incidental finding in an otherwise unremarkable psychotherapy. The delayed effects of incest have a remarkable capacity to obscure diagnostic clarity and lead to a series of unsuccessful psychotherapeutic encounters. Furthermore, the incest victim almost invariably has, at the core of her difficulties, a posttraumatic state. A therapy that fails to identify and address the impact of the incest trauma is unlikely to achieve optimal results.

Our profession has been slow to acknowledge the importance of actual incest as a determinant of psychopathology. As recently as 1975 a major psychiatric textbook described incest as a rare disorder, occurring with an incidence of one per million population (Henderson 1975). These were the same figures Freud was working from nearly a century ago. Freud decided that it was statistically impossible for all his hysterical patients to be actual incest victims and that some must be reporting incest fantasies as if they were actual occurrences (Goodwin 1982; Masson 1984).

Current surveys indicate that these earlier figures were gross underestimates. Sixteen percent of women in the general population have experienced sexual contact with a relative and 1% to 4% have experienced father-daughter incest (Goodwin et al. 1982; Russell 1984). In psychiatric populations the prevalence is higher, with 22% to 35% of adult female psychiatric inpatients reporting incest experiences in childhood with fathers, stepfathers, mothers, grandfathers, brothers, or uncles (Bryer et al. 1987; Goodwin et al., in press). Psychiatrists, psychologists, and family counselors encounter these problems frequently; more than half have treated one or more incest victims within the past year (Attias and Goodwin 1985).

Male victims are less well studied. In his survey of New England college students, Finkelhor (1979) found that 19% of the women and 9% of the men reported a sexual assault in childhood; this would predict that at least one-third of child sexual abuse victims would be male. Greater reluctance in men to report probably accounts for their lower representation in most series (10% to 25%) (Goodwin 1982; Rogers and Terry 1984). There is considerable anecdotal evidence that in the most severely disturbed families all children—both male and female—are sexually and/or otherwise abused, often by multiple family members—both male and female (Goodwin 1985b).

In the past 10 years certain evaluation and treatment strategies have become routine for child incest victims (Goodwin 1988a; MacFarlane et al. 1986; Sgroi 1982). In the initial phase this routine includes 1) a complete physical examination, 2) investigation to document abuse and to detect other victims, 3) legally mandated reporting to protective services and in some jurisdictions to law enforcement, 4) interview and evaluation of the alleged abuser and other family members, and 5) assessment of the child for posttraumatic symptoms.

Treatment for child victims tends to be similarly organized around the same five axes: 1) structuring adequate physical care, which sometimes requires placement of the child away from the abuser or both parents; 2) individual and group treatment of abused and/or neglected siblings; 3) guidance and support for family members as they progress through various legal interventions; 4) individual, group, behavioral, couples', and family therapy to rehabilitate the sexually abusive parent and to improve parental and family functioning; and 5) individual and group treatment to decrease posttraumatic and other symptoms in the victim.

Even in child victims this ideal model is not always followed, as the following examples illustrate for each of the five problem axes. 1) When confronted by a hypothetical case in which a 9-year-old retracts under pressure a detailed account of long-term oral sex with her father, 75% of pediatricians would recommend that the child be physically examined and screened for gonorrhea and other venereal diseases. Only 50% of psychologists, psychiatrists, and counselors recommended physical examination, although all recommended psychological testing for the child (Attias and Goodwin 1985). 2) In this same survey, professionals in all categories tended to underestimate the 30% to 40% likelihood that if this child were abused, her siblings would have been also (Herman 1981; Tormes 1968). 3) Professionals often try to avoid the legal ramifications of incest. In 1978, 58% of pediatricians surveyed stated that they would not report to protective services a confirmed case (James et al. 1978). 4) Parents, especially fathers, often flee, avoid, or legally resist evaluation and treatment (Ryan 1986). 5) Child victims who fail to appear for appointments or who continue to function without major behavior problems may not be referred for treatment or even systematically evaluated for posttraumatic symptoms (Adams-Tucker 1984). As many as 43% of children seen in an emergency room for sexual assault do not reappear for follow-up (Byrne and Valdiserri 1982).

When an adult victim discloses prior incest, the approach to substantiation is even less systematic. Such disclosures typically occur in the middle phase of a treatment begun because of another chief complaint. Westermeyer (1978) found that fewer than 25% of adult incest survivors disclosed early in treatment. The therapist may not even conceptualize an investigation phase for the disclosure. A generation ago, the understanding of such disclosures as "fantasies" focused treatment on internal rather than external realities and made investigation irrelevant (Goodwin 1985a; Masson 1984).

However, the importance of ascertaining the realities of the abusive incidents is attested by the high proportion of adult victims who question the authenticity of their own often fragmented or derealized memories and set as a treatment goal either the verification of those memories or some sort of confrontation or acknowledgment of those memories from the abuser or other family members. Herman and Schatzow (1987) found that three out of four patients (of 53 women incest survivors) were able to validate their memories by obtaining corroborating evidence from other sources. Nevertheless, with the adult victim, the therapist typically does not 1) require a physical examination, 2) interview siblings, 3) consider possible legal obligations, or 4) evaluate the parents. However, 5) posttraumatic symptoms are targeted here much as they are in a child victim, although the powerful tool of group therapy is less often used (Tsai and Wagner 1978).

This review offers clinical examples illustrating how adult victims can benefit from more careful attention to the five problem areas that have been identified as important in child victims. This five-problem model will be applied systematically to assessment and treatment planning for adults. Particular attention will be paid to the recognition of severe posttraumatic symptoms in adult victims whose untreated multiple impairments may have been misinterpreted as a borderline or antisocial personality disorder or even as psychosis (Beck and van der Kolk 1987). The more symptomatic and regressed adult victims have concerns about bodily sensations and intactness, concrete realities, punishment, and family members who may still be caretakers or abusers. These issues may respond to approaches developed for children, who operate at similar cognitive-developmental levels (Lane and Schwartz 1987).

As noted in a classic article by Gelinas (1983) and as discussed in-depth by numerous contributors to a symposium on treating the victims of sexual abuse (Kluft 1989), incest victims often present with a complex clinical picture that disguises the fact that their problem is essentially posttraumatic and that they will not recover unless their psychotherapy addresses their victimization as a central factor in their psychopathology.

APPLYING THE FIVE-POINT MODEL TO TREATING THE ADULT INCEST VICTIM

In the introduction I described the clinical dilemmas that occur when an adult patient discloses prior incest midway in a treatment begun for another reason. Should the therapist proceed, focusing on already identified dynamic conflicts? Or should the therapist halt the treatment and reassess? In this section, I propose the five-point scheme used in child victims as a model for the reassessment of adults (Table 4-1).

Inquiry is indicated about bodily sensations, physical pain, and physiologic indicators of fear occurring during disclosure in the psychotherapy session. Review of physical problems in adulthood may reveal patterns

Table 4-1. A five-point intervention model for child and adult incest victims

Child	Adult
Physical examination	Somatic symptoms
Establish physical safety	Pediatric and medical records
	Query if contacts with family remain abusive
Interview siblings	Interview collaterals
Identify other victims	Use documents to reconstruct
Report to protective services	Query if children endangered
Explain legal system	Other legal questions
Evaluate abuser	Explore character of abuser
Restore family functioning	Understand family functioning
Screen for posttraumatic symptoms	Screen for posttraumatic symptoms
Link symptoms with abuse	Link symptoms with abuse

of pelvic pain, headache, or somatization disorder, which are common in incest victims (Goodwin et al. 1988; Walker et al. 1988). Exploration of physical symptoms may uncover fantasies and fears about death and body damage as well as physical details of the prior abuse. Review of past pediatric records is always indicated. This can reveal hospitalizations in infancy that were related to unrecognized neglect or abuse.

For example, one patient, whose sexual abuse had not been reported, had been treated for multiple vaginal infections by her pediatrician. In adulthood, she had undergone multiple gynecologic surgeries; like the original pediatrician, no doctor had been able to discover her "real problem." In another case, a brother's death certificate confirmed the patient's uncertain memory that he had been beaten to death. In yet another case, an emerging memory of a concealed incest pregnancy resulting in a deformed stillborn infant led to consultation with a geneticist who was able to identify the genetic syndrome. Some abused children develop hysterical conversion symptoms or chronic somatic complaints such as headache or stomachache (Goodwin 1989; McFarlane, Waterman, Conerly, et al. 1986); these also may have led to prior treatment and documentation of family problems.

Informal investigation is often undertaken by the adult incest victim, especially if amnesia obscures her own memories. Siblings are often the first collateral informants to be interviewed. Sometimes siblings are found to have been sexually abused by the same alleged perpetrator, by family members other than the identified abuser, or even by the identified "victim." Siblings may have witnessed elements of the sexual abuse; for example, when a 12-year-old incest victim refused her father for the first time, she heard him go into the next bed and sodomize her brother.

School and neighborhood friends of the identified victim may also have been approached sexually by the abuser. Peers are sometimes told about the abuse by the victim, long before adults are consulted. These kinds of witness data can be useful, especially if the credibility of the victim is in question (DeJong 1985). In one case in which the victim had been completely amnesic for the incest for many years, a family servant was able to describe the induced abortion that had terminated the patient's forgotten incest pregnancy.

Revisiting the former family home or reviewing old photo albums can clarify fragmentary memories. If entire years are lost to amnesia, I recommend that the patient make a notebook for the lost years, including photographs, old report cards, and information gained from family members, neighbors, and friends.

Legal complications are still possible, even if the disclosure comes from an adult victim (MacFarlane and Korbin 1983). Younger siblings, nieces and nephews, or the adult's own children may continue to be at risk from her abuser or other victims in the family. Potential abusers include the victim herself, who may have been driven to disclosure by her impulses to abuse or neglect her own child (Goodwin et al. 1982). Protective service referrals may be necessary.

Other legal involvements may arise. I have treated victims who have been able with treatment to mobilize the family to have the incestuous father civilly committed for psychiatric treatment. In cases where amnesia has deprived the victim of memory of the event, adults still have 3 years, in most jurisdictions, after recovering the memory to initiate a civil suit against the parent for damages caused; even if a parent is dead, the estate may be liable. The therapist is most helpful if aware of these potential legal entanglements.

Some adult incest victims pursue a role of family caretaker, remaining concerned and involved with the abuser and his pathology and with other dysfunctional family members. Therapists narrowly focused on increasing autonomy and assertiveness may try to discourage such involvement. An absolute ban on contact with the family may be necessary when physical or sexual abuse has continued into adulthood or when emotional abuse remains so severe as to trigger suicidality or other severe symptoms.

However, multiple motives may contribute to the wish for continued involvement with the family: 1) the (sometimes unconscious) perception of the severity of the parent's pathology and realistic concerns about suicide or psychosis; 2) an attempt to use adult skills to see the family as it really is so that development can proceed; 3) a realization that confrontation of the feared father is a direct way to challenge the entire array of fears and phobias related to victimization; and 4) an unconscious realization that many of the symptoms reflect an identification with the aggressor and an internalization of his actions, feelings, and thought patterns. In reality a child needs a parent just as desperately as he or she needs a self; reconstruction of a serviceable parent is a critical step in completing interrupted developmental tasks from childhood. The realization that parents are not fixable may unleash painful and terrible grief.

The techniques of individual family therapy (Friedman 1971, 1987) are useful in exploring these issues. Sibling group sessions can also be helpful. Parents thought to be hostile and unapproachable can sometimes cooperate if approached in a nonthreatening way for historical information.

Confrontation and "apology" sessions with the abuser or with the nonprotective mother can be very useful but require extensive preparation of both parties (Trepper 1986). The victim needs to explore her fantasies that the "apology" will occur in such a complete and perfect way that she can believe that the parent never abused her at all. Similarly, the abuser needs to understand all the ways he can admit what he did without really admitting that he did it and that it was seriously wrong and harmful.

The victim's fears of the abuser cannot be overestimated. Many victims are extremely adept at concealing their fearfulness in a face-to-face interview. However, underneath her mask of impassivity, the victim's internal terror can be reactivated by a letter, a photograph, or a gift. Confrontation at times must be approached gradually through a process akin to systematic desensitization. Use of one-way mirrors or videotape can allow physical distance during confrontation (Dale et al. 1986).

Even if the abuser is unwilling to talk with the victim or therapist, collateral sources can often be used to document his previous patterns of sexual, physical, and emotional violence. In one case, military records revealed a court martial for pedophilia. In another case, family members had witnessed the father holding a rifle to the mother's head and threatening to kill the entire family and then himself. Hospital records and police reports may document spousal violence or rape, previous investigations for child sexual abuse in previous marriages, psychiatric treatment for paranoia, or alcohol or substance abuse. Job and financial records may reveal patterns of instability and habitual deception. School records may document paternal overinvolvement with the child, jealous rage reactions, or a pattern of intimidation of teachers by the father.

These fathers may appear on the surface as the exemplary, "endogamic," involved fathers described in the older literature on incest (Lustig et al., 1966; Weinberg 1955). It is only with more detailed history taking that their involvement is understood as rooted in feelings and fantasies of persecution and grandiosity rather than in an adult capacity to parent (Goodwin 1985c). Clarification of the nature and motivation of the perpetrator is an important aspect of the "search for meaning" that more than 80% of victims pursue (Silver et al. 1983). It is also important for victims who have defended themselves by "identifying" with the aggressor but who may not be aware of the abusive components of their own behaviors.

An example is Oedipus, who explores his own guilt self-excoriatingly through three plays by Sophocles. Oedipus gives very little attention to his abusive father, Laius, who had tried to kill Oedipus both in infancy and adolescence, who had "set up" Oedipus for incest, and who had previously sexually abused another boy. Perhaps if Oedipus had put more effort into understanding Laius, he might have gained more control of the destructive ways in which he interacted with his own children, none of whom survived to adulthood (Goodwin 1989).

RECOGNIZING POSTTRAUMATIC SYMPTOMS

Various studies report that 20% to 100% of sexually abused children are acutely symptomatic at the time of the allegation (Adams-Tucker 1981; Bagley 1984; Conte and Schuerman 1987; DeYoung 1982; Gomes-Schwartz et al. 1985; Maisch 1972; Mrazek and Kempe 1981). Some children present with severe psychosis or characterological problems that seem to predate the sexual abuse; these may reflect constitutional factors or the result of neglect, emotional abuse, or battering that interfered with development in earlier years of life (Emslie and Rosenfeld 1983). Some children are completely asymptomatic (MacFarlane et al. 1986).

The most commonly seen symptoms, each found in 10% to 33% of sexually abused children (Conte and Schuerman 1987), include: 1) emotional upset and fears, 2) regression in behavior and abandonment of former activities, 3) repressed and overt anger, 4) recurrent nightmares, and 5) low self-esteem with depression. In previous publications (Goodwin 1985d; Goodwin et al. 1988), the mnemonic "FEARS" has been used to designate these five types of common sequelae: 1) fears, 2) ego constriction, 3) anger dyscontrol, 4) repetitions (in nightmares or flashbacks), and 5) sadness with sleep disturbance (Table 4-2).

These symptoms constitute the five cardinal signs of posttraumatic stress disorder originally described by Kardiner (1959) in shell-shocked combat veterans. In studies of adults these five types of symptoms are each found in more than half of incest victims entering treatment (Donaldson and Gardner 1985; Herman et al. 1986; Lindberg and Dystad 1985; Sedney and Brooks 1984). The higher frequency of symptomatology in these adult groups may result from the exclusion of possibly less-damaged victims abused by nonfamily members or from the fact that it is the more symptomatic survivors who seek treatment; however, data from victims not in treatment also document the occurrence of symptoms at higher frequen-

Table 4-2.   Moderate and severe posttraumatic symptoms in adult incest victims

Moderate		Severe	
Symptoms	%	Symptoms	%
Fears		Fugues	
Hyperalert	76	Dissociative symptoms	24
Nervous	63	Multiple personality	8–10
Ego constriction		Ego fragmentation	
Sexual inhibitions	61–94	Borderline personality	17
Social inhibitions	61	Multiple personality	8–10
Anger dyscontrol		Antisocial acting-out	
Continuing anger	70	Alcohol, substance abuse	12–31
Afraid of anger	65		
Repetition		Reenactments	
Flashbacks	80	Rape or other crime victimization	20–46
Nightmares	70		
Sleep disturbance		Somatization	
Nightmares	70	Medical problems	23
Sadness		Suicidality	
Guilt	100	Suicidal thoughts	46–48
Depression	66	Suicidal attempts	21–24

cies than found in child populations (Herman et al. 1986; Sedney and Brooks 1984; Silver et al. 1983).

One might conceptualize an incubation period for the development of post-incest symptoms, mediated in part by the increased demands in adulthood for intimacy, caretaking, and integration, areas of functioning particularly vulnerable to the developmental impacts of child abuse. Adult incest victims complain of being hyperalert (76%) and nervous (63%); of having inhibitions around sexuality (61% to 94%) (Donaldson and Gardner 1985; Lindberg and Dystad 1985) and socialization (61%) (Donaldson and Gardner 1985); of experiencing continuing anger about the incest (70%) (Donaldson and Gardner 1985); flashbacks (80%) and nightmares (70%) (Donaldson and Gardner 1985); guilt (100%) (Lindberg and Dystad 1985); and depression (66%) (Sedney and Brooks 1984).

Because the five elements of the syndrome can appear in many guises and degrees of severity at different developmental stages, I will review each in some detail.

F stands for fears and anxiety. Phobias are found and may encompass all men or may focus on a particular feature of the abuse, such as the room where incest occurred. Fears about sexuality are common with most symptomatic adult incest victims reporting sexual dysfunction (Donaldson and Gardner 1985; Lindberg and Dystad 1985; Meiselman 1981). Dysfunction can be pervasive, such as avoidance of all kissing in a patient where oral sexual abuse had been prominent, or avoidance of all penile contact in victims who maintain the capacity for satisfying sexual experience with females. Sometimes the fears are more circumscribed and can be gotten around by avoiding certain specific sexual practices.

Easy startle is characteristic of posttraumatic stress disorder. One incest victim blacked her roommate's eye when approached suddenly. Adolescent and adult victims may take fear for granted when it becomes chronic and may lose sight of the connection between incest-related fears and such coping strategies as alcohol or drug abuse or keeping the lights on all night.

Certain factors are predictable: female victims will have worries about pregnancy; male victims will have concerns about being made homosexual. All victims at some level assume that the abuser's threats about disclosure will "come true" if they break their pledge of secrecy; thus anxiety and fears will increase as disclosures are made in treatment.

E stands for "ego constriction," the phrase Kardiner (1959) used to describe the "numbing" processes used by the victim to avoid overwhelming anxiety. In young children, the constriction appears as loss of recently acquired developmental gains, such as exploration or toilet training in a toddler or adaptive school performance in an older child. Parents or teachers may be able to pinpoint a time when the child changed or "faded," which coincides with the onset of sexual abuse. Difficulty concentrating and learning problems are reported by 23% to 35% of adult victims, and 61% describe themselves as emotionally isolated (Donaldson and Gardner 1985; Sedney and Brooks 1984).

A stands for "anger dyscontrol." Mildly affected victims often have difficulty expressing anger, masking it with compliance and perfectionism, which are nonetheless punctuated by angry outbursts usually more terrifying to the victim herself than to her targets. Seventy percent of adult victims say they are still angry about the incest; 65% say they are afraid of their anger (Donaldson and Gardner 1985); and 64% report displacing anger onto their current sexual partner (Meiselman 1981). Tantrums in young children or "hysterical" outbursts in older children manifest these problems in expression of anger.

R stands for "repetition," usually reflected, in mild cases, in repetitive thoughts, feelings, or images of the events. "Flashbacks" to incest during sexual activity are characteristic. Eighty percent of adult victims report flashbacks (Donaldson and Gardner 1985). Places, odors, or anniversaries may trigger perceptual reliving of traumatic events. Phobias and "numbing" often reflect strategies for avoiding flashbacks.

S reminds the evaluator of the importance of "sleep disturbance" in posttraumatic stress disorder and also stands for "sadness." Repetitive posttraumatic nightmares are an important feature of posttraumatic stress disorder. In very young children, frequent night terrors are an indicator of abuse. Posttraumatic nightmares may incorporate specific elements of the sexual abuse experience (e.g., the image of a large penis; the sensation of being crushed; the color of the childhood bedclothes) and are accompanied by physiologic arousal or awakening. Having trouble sleeping or nightmares are reported by 60% to 82% of adult incest victims (Donaldson and Gardner 1985; Lindberg and Dystad 1985; Sedney and Brooks, 1984). Incest victims and other victims of posttraumatic stress disorder usually have some vegetative signs of depression, such as crying spells, insomnia, appetite disturbance, or morbid self-reproach. Two-thirds of incest victims say they are depressed (Sedney and Brooks 1984); 84% say they lack self-confidence (Donaldson and Gardner 1985); and 100% report guilt (Lindberg and Dystad 1985). Antidepressant medication is helpful in some patients with posttraumatic stress disorder (van der Kolk 1987).

SCREENING FOR SEVERE POSTTRAUMATIC SYMPTOMS

In a small percentage of victims, symptoms are quite severe and potentially disabling. Severe symptoms have been associated with 1) the presence of a parental perpetrator, 2) long duration of abuse, 3) serious threat or violence associated with the abuse (Herman et al. 1986), and 4) the degree of family disruption (Goodwin et al. 1983).

Severe symptoms have been described previously in child victims but at relatively low frequencies. In 318 children sexually abused within the past 6 months (Conte and Schuerman 1987), severe symptoms included: 1) daydreaming with memory loss (14%); 2) body-image problems (8%); 3) problems with police (3%) and drugs or alcohol (2%); 4) age-inappropriate sexual behavior (7%) and self-endangering behaviors (5%); and 5) suicidal thoughts (6%), psychosomatic complaints (10%), and eating disorders (1%).

Adult incest victims report a higher frequency of severe symptoms. Dissociative symptoms are reported in 33% (Lindberg and Dystad 1985), and 8% are diagnosed as having multiple personality disorder (Cole 1985; Goodwin, in press). Borderline personality disorder is the diagnosis in 17% (Herman and Schatzow 1984). Alcohol and substance abuse are found in 12% to 31% of adult victim samples (Donaldson and Gardner 1985; Goodwin et al., in press; Herman and Schatzow 1984; Sedney and Brooks 1984). Rape or other crime victimization is found in 20% to 46% (Cole 1985; DeYoung 1983; Miller et al. 1978; Sedney and Brooks 1984). Suicidal thoughts are reported by 46% to 48% (Donaldson and Gardner 1985; Lindberg and Dystad 1985), with 21% to 24% having made prior attempts (Herman and Schatzow 1987; Lindberg and Dystad 1985). Finally, medical problems are reported by 23% (Donaldson and Gardner 1985).

A modified "FEARS" mnemonic describes this severe symptom pattern. Preliminary data (Goodwin et al. 1988) indicate that all victims with the severe FEARS syndrome also have the moderate posttraumatic FEARS symptoms.

In the severe syndrome, *F* represents "*fugue* and other dissociative symptoms." When anxiety becomes too intense to experience, fugues, amnesia, depersonalization, and derealization can help distance and insulate the victim from the fear-provoking situation. As many as two-thirds of victims will have patchy memories for the abuse (Herman and Schatzow 1987). Runaways with fugue-like qualities are seen in adolescent victims (Goodwin et al. 1979). Although many victims use dissociative strategies in emergency situations, in the severe cases, dissociation becomes habitual and uncontrolled.

The utility of dissociative defenses in combating fears and phobias is illustrated by data from incest victims with multiple personality disorder (Coons and Milstein 1986; Saltman and Solomon 1982; Wilbur 1984). Here, one can see in the various alters the spectrum of adaptations open to a sexually abused child: 1) alters who deny the abuse and maintain a childlike asexual innocence; 2) alters who rebel against hypocritical authority by rule breaking and open, sometimes violent, defiance; 3) alters who become sexual experts and use sexual expertise to advantage in promiscuity, prostitution, or satisfying marital sex; 4) alters who exonerate the perpetrator by taking on all the guilt and abandoning themselves to suicidal regret and self-blame; and 5) alters who feel chosen, special, and above society's rules.

"*E*go fragmentation" replaces ego constriction in severely affected victims who may fragment completely into multiple personalities or more complexly into the "part-object/part-self" representations seen in borderline personality disorder. Abuse in childhood is reported in 97% to 99% of patients with multiple personality disorder (Putnam et al. 1986). Preliminary surveys indicate that 75% of patients with borderline personality disorder have sexual abuse histories (Herman and van der Kolk 1987). It is intriguing to try to conceptualize the alternating idealizing and devaluing relationships that characterize the borderline patient as related to difficulties integrating the "public," often "perfect" parent with the secretly abusive parent known only to the child (Miller 1984; Nadelson 1976; Shengold 1979).

A in the severe syndrome represents "antisocial acting-out." Rather than struggling to repress and control anger, these victims often simply act on angry impulses. Such actions may include paraphiliac sexual activities, prostitution, or repeated family violence in adulthood (e.g., spousal or child abuse). Antisocial actions may coincide with severe alcohol or drug addiction. Burgess et al. (1987) found that almost 10% of 66 children involved in a pornography ring had been convicted of a crime within 2 years of disclosure. Six became involved in prostitution. The antisocial behaviors were associated with psychodynamic patterns of identification with the aggressor.

R signifies the "reenactments" that occur in these victims in addition to the predominantly sensory repetitions seen in less severe cases. Repetitive reenactments include experiencing multiple rapes and choosing multiple mates who are physically abusive or multiple mates who incestuously abuse the victim's children (in some cases at exactly the same age that mother was when she was incestuously victimized). Incest also may be reenacted in a therapeutic relationship in the form of therapist-patient sex. In one sample, 30% of adult incest victims described having been abused by a therapist (DeYoung 1983); in another sample 46% had been raped at least once since the original incest (Donaldson and Gardner 1985).

For the severe syndrome, S refers to "suicidality" and "somatization." Patients who present with multiple suicidal attempts or self-mutilations should be screened both for prior incest and the other manifestations of both the moderate and severe "FEARS" syndromes, especially dissociative symptoms. There is some evidence that suicidality and somatic symptoms tend to cluster together and to be associated with greater severity of child abuse (Goodwin et al. 1988). In a study of 50 women treated in an adult incest victims' group, 10% were diagnosed as having multiple personality disorder (Goodwin, in press). All five with multiple personality disorder had multiple prior suicide attempts, severe multimodal abuse in their childhoods, and prior psychiatric hospitalization. Three had lost custody of their own children because of abuse and neglect. All had prominent somatic symptoms, including two with Briquet's syndrome and one with Munchausen's syndrome (Goodwin 1988b). Somatic symptoms could often be interpreted as somatic memories of the sexual abuse. When somatization is a part of a severe syndrome, close cooperation between psychotherapist and general physician may be necessary.

COMPARING MODERATE AND SEVERE "FEARS" SYNDROME

Two European fairy tales allow us to compare and contrast the moderate and severe syndromes (Table 4-3). The first tale, "Thousandfurs," is currently available (Grimm and Grimm 1977). The second, "Manekine," is a more obscure Hungarian tale (Cox 1892; Goodwin 1982). Both fairy tales describe similar situations: a beautiful beloved mother dies leaving her grieving daughter and her widowed husband, the king, who vows that he will never remarry. Later, however, he becomes aware of the beauty of his daughter and asks for the hand of the princess. It is at this point that the two stories diverge, making visible the differences in the two syndromes and their divergent family origins and interpersonal implications.

In "Thousandfurs," the princess bargains and negotiates with her father. She asks for a dress as beautiful as the sun, then for a dress as beautiful as the moon, and finally a dress as beautiful as the stars. She is amazed and dismayed each time when her father actually meets her demands. This re-framing of "taking bribes" as "staving off" the abuse is often

Table 4-3.   Moderate and severe posttraumatic symptoms in two fairy
tale princesses

	Thousandfurs	Manekine

F	Fears father and men
	Flees but with planning and
	   control
		Fugues using mannequin to bear
		   pain
		Flees losing part of herself

E	Ego constricted by beast-suit
	Disguises true self as a beast and
	   scullery maid
		Ego fragmented; functions lost
		Objects are viewed as all-good or
		   all-bad

A	Hostile testing of the prince
	Image of self as wild beast
	   indicates fear of her own anger
		Abuse: Child death
		Arrests: Repeated trouble with
		   the law

R	Repeats with the prince the
	   running away and bargaining
	   that she tried with father
		Reenacts abandoment,
		   multilation, burning at the
		   stake, being cast adrift

S	Sadness appears as unresolved
	   grief at mother's death
		Self-multilation
		Somatic symptoms: conversion
		   losses of speech and use of
		   hand

welcomed by victims who have experienced similar moments but still view their actions as shameful rather than as representing active coping. Finally, she asks for a thing that she knows is impossible—a coat made of the furs of a thousand animals. To her horror, her father meets even this last most difficult demand.

The princess, however, is resourceful. She dons the coat of a thousand furs and, in this disguise, she escapes to the forest. As it happens, a neighboring prince is hunting in the forest and his hunting dogs tree the strange animal with the unique fur coat. When I read this story to incest victims, they almost uniformly misunderstand this section of the story and assume that the person who captures Thousandfurs in the forest is actually her father, the king. This error can be the beginning of a discussion about the persistence of the perception of the incest father, as omnipotently manipulative and ultimately inescapable. It also opens for scrutiny the impact of the incest relationship on the victim's current marriage. Nonabused children of all ages, however, are not confused at this point and realize—as Thousandfurs is put to work in the kitchen while the prince plans a series of balls—that this story is going to be one of those "Cinderella" fairy tales that always have a happy ending.

Thousandfurs sneaks out of the scullery to each of the prince's three balls, each time wearing a different one of her spectacular dresses. The prince pursues her each time, but always finds himself ending up back in the kitchen, confronting that mysterious many-furred beast. Thousandfurs tests and bargains with the prince much as she had done with her father. Once she is certain that he will not be as intrusive and destructive as her father, she lets him pull off her beast-suit, her coat of a thousand furs. Moments similar to this occur often in psychotherapy with incest victims as the restricting defenses that they used to control their fear and anger and flashbacks are lifted off momentarily, revealing the beautiful princess underneath.

In contrast, the "Manekine" story begins on a much grimmer note. In this story, the king becomes terribly melancholic at the death of his wife. Playing chess with his daughter is the only amusement that distracts him. One day, as they are playing chess, he reaches over, takes his daughter's hand, and asks for her hand in marriage. She, in turn, reaches across, pulls his sword from its scabbard, and cuts off the hand that her father is holding. He immediately sends her to the dungeons, commanding that she be burned at the stake.

Already we see the contrasts with the Thousandfurs family. This is a family in which aggression rapidly escalates to mutilation, incarceration, death threats, and extreme violence. Impulsive action, not negotiation, is the rule here. Emotional upset has gone out of control and become melancholy, a psychiatric disorder.

Fortunately, the court jester knows the way to avoid the death sentence. He helps Manekine make a mannequin of herself. Possibly he realizes that, given the nature of the parent-child relationship, the father will not be able to tell the difference between a mannequin and his own daughter. The jester helps Manekine to escape. She has now taken on the name of the mannequin that was burned, and to some extent its persona as she escapes in a rudderless boat and is washed up on the shores of a new land. Like the mannequin, she has now lost the power of speech. It is as if it were the real princess who was burned; only the mannequin was feelingless enough to survive.

Despite this new handicap, the king of the country in which she has landed immediately falls in love with her and marries her. Unfortunately, he is called away to a crusade and Manekine is left with her wicked mother-in-law, who immediately conspires against her. When Manekine's baby is born, the mother-in-law writes the king saying that the baby is deformed and this means that Manekine is a witch who must be burned at the stake forthwith. Thus the fairy tale princess experiences an exact reenactment of her childhood trauma. Manekine, however, is quite experienced in being burned at the stake, and she makes mannequins of herself and her baby and escapes again in a rudderless boat. This time, she is cast up on a shore near Rome, where she becomes a beggar, but she is so poor that her baby starves to death.

Time passes. One day she is sitting at a fountain in Rome and overhears the conversation of two wealthy men dining on a porch above her. These two have had to come to Rome to do penance, one for a great wrong he did to his daughter, and the other for a great wrong he did to his wife. As they speak, Manekine suddenly realizes that one is her father and that the other is her husband. At that moment of realization, her severed arm appears from out of the waters of the fountain and reattaches itself to her body. Her child, too, appears lifting up his arms to her as he stands laughing in the fountain.

Most people like this story because it offers some hope for those victims of parental abuse who are most broken and hopeless. The story also illustrates many of the features of the severe syndrome. For these victims, ego changes are drastic, involving, not a constriction due to heightened defensive activity, but an actual splitting off and loss of ego functions, exemplified by Manekine's loss of her hand and loss of speech. Here, the self is not merely cloaked in a disguise as in Thousandfurs, but a false self, a mannequin, is constructed to bear the brunt of the pain.

This is similar to the process seen in patients with childhood multiple personality disorder where the child designs alternate selves that are pain-immune and "not bothered" by the abuse. Manekine cannot assert herself well enough to bargain as Thousandfurs did. She continues to protect herself from abuse, but in a way that can be interpreted as mere mis-behavior and thus strengthens her persecutors' case against her rather than effectively challenging them.

The final scene in this story can be seen as parallel to scenes from family or group therapy in which the men who have hurt the incest victim are forced at last to confront themselves and each other. This is a process that proves enormously healing for Manekine. I have noted the reenactments in the story involving repeated accusations and flights. There is also a reenactment in the near fatal abuse of her own child. In a previous study (Goodwin et al. 1982), we showed frequency of prior incest to be significantly higher in mothers whose children are abused than in women in the general population.

Manekine's cutting off her hand is an apt image for the self-mutilation and suicidality found so universally in the severe syndrome. Victims attack themselves in part to make themselves less sexually attractive in the eyes of the abuser, and in part to make visible the injury that the abuser insists must be kept secret and invisible.

Eating disorders function in a similar way. The self-starvation or the self-mutilation is often kept as secret as was the original abuse, allowing for complex reenactments of the old ambivalence about keeping the abuse secret versus asking for help. These behaviors may also represent dissociated memories of the abuse. For example, victims with bulimia may experience eating and regurgitation as a repetition of the sensations they underwent while performing fellatio (Goodwin et al. 1988).

Somatization is represented in this story through Manekine's beliefs that she cannot function because her hand has been severed, that she cannot speak, and that she cannot enjoy her child because he has died of hunger. Severely symptomatic victims tend to misinterpret their difficulties as resulting from physical illnesses or injuries rather than from the interpersonal injury of incest. Three-quarters of patients with multiple personality disorder have Briquet's syndrome or somatization disorder (Bliss 1986). Munchausen's syndrome and other somatic disorders such as psychogenic pain have been reported in victims of extreme child abuse (Goodwin 1989).

Does Manekine have a multiple personality disorder? The startlingly sudden healing process that occurs at the end of the story is not that dissimilar from the startling improvement that can occur when a fragmented incest victim reintegrates a split-off part of the self. However, had the story continued, one might have seen equally startling regression in Manekine, reappearing under stress, as very regressed fragments regained control (Kluft 1986).

CONCLUSION

Especially with severely symptomatic adult victims, treatment may need to focus on 1) physical sensations and symptoms and the achievement of physical safety; 2) concrete investigative data-gathering from collateral informants and records; 3) questions of right and wrong, of legal punishment and/or retribution; 4) evaluation of the perpetrator and other family members; and 5) the systematic identification of posttraumatic symptoms and the connection of these symptoms with specific traumatic events in childhood. The telling or reading of fairy tales is one of the many techniques that can be equally useful in child and adult incest victims.

REFERENCES

Adams-Tucker C: Proximate effects of sexual abuse in childhood: a report on 28 children. Am J Psychiatry 139:1251–1256, 1981

Adams-Tucker C: The unmet psychiatric needs of sexually abused youths: referrals from a child protection agency and clinical evaluations. Journal of the American Academy of Child Psychiatry 23:659–667, 1984

Attias R, Goodwin J: Knowledge and management strategies in incest cases: a survey of physicians, psychologists, and family counselors. Child Abuse Negl 9:527–533, 1985

Bagley C: Mental health and the in-family sexual abuse of children and adolescents. Canada's Mental Health 17–23, 1984

Beck J, van der Kolk B: Reports of childhood incest and current behavior of chronically hospitalized psychotic women. Am J Psychiatry 144:1474–1476, 1987

Bliss E: Multiple Personality, Allied Disorders and Hypnosis. New York, Oxford University Press, 1986

Bryer JB, Nelson BA, Miller JB, et al: Childhood sexual and physical abuse as factors in adult psychiatric illness. Am J Psychiatry 144:1426–1430, 1987

Burgess AW, Hartman CR, McCormack A: Abused to abuser: antecedents of socially deviant behaviors. Am J Psychiatry 144:1431–1436, 1987

Byrne JP, Valdiserri EV: Victims of childhood sexual abuse: a followup study of a noncompliant population. Hosp Community Psychiatry 33:938–939, 1982

Cole C: A group design for adult female survivors of childhood incest. Women and Therapy 4:71–82, 1985

Conte J, Schuerman JR: Factors associated with an increased impact of sexual abuse. Child Abuse Negl 11:201–211, 1987

Coons P, Milstein V: Psychosexual disturbances in multiple personality: characteristics, etiology and treatment. J Clin Psychiatry 47:106–110, 1986

Cox MR: Cinderella: Three Hundred Forty-five Variants of Cinderella, Catskin, and Cap o' Rushes. London, Folk-Lore Society, 1892

Dale P, Waters J, Davies M, et al: The towers of silence: creative and destructive issues for therapeutic teams dealing with sexual abuse. Journal of Family Therapy 8:1–25, 1986

DeJong AR: The medical evaluation of sexual abuse in children. Hosp Community Psychiatry 36:509–512, 1985.

DeYoung M: The Sexual Victimization of Children. London, MacFarland, 1982

DeYoung M: Case reports: the sexual exploitation of victims by helping professionals. Victimology 6:92–98, 1983

Donaldson MA, Gardner R: Diagnosis and treatment of traumatic stress among women after childhood incest, in Trauma and Its Wake: The Study and

Treatment of Post-Traumatic Stress Disorder. Edited by Figley C. New York, Brunner/Mazel, 1985, pp 356–367

Emslie GT, Rosenfeld AA: Incest reported by children and adolescents hospitalized for severe psychiatric problems. Am J Psychiatry 140:708–711, 1983

Finkelhor D: Sexually Victimized Children. New York, Free Press, 1979

Friedman EH: The birthday party: an experiment in obtaining change in one's own extended family. Fam Process 10:345–359, 1971

Friedman EH: The birthday party revisited: family therapy and the problem of change, in The Therapist's Own Family. Edited by Titleman P. Northvale, NJ, Jason Aronson, 1987, pp 163–188

Gelinas DL: The persisting negative effects of incest. Psychiatry 46:312–322, 1983

Gomes-Schwartz B, Horowitz JM, Sauzier M: Severity of emotional distress among sexually abused preschool, school-age, and adolescent children. Hosp Community Psychiatry 36:503–508, 1985

Goodwin J (ed): Sexual Abuse: Incest Victims and Their Families. Boston, MA, Wright/PSG, 1982

Goodwin J: Credibility problems in multiple personalities and abused children, in Childhood Antecedents of Multiple Personality. Edited by Kluft R. Washington, DC, American Psychiatric Press, 1985a, pp 1–20

Goodwin J: Family violence: principles of intervention and prevention. Hosp Community Psychiatry 36:1074–1079, 1985b

Goodwin J: Persecution and grandiosity in incest fathers, in Psychiatry: The State of the Art, Vol 6. Edited by Pichot P, Berner P, Wolf R, et al. New York, Plenum, 1985c, pp 309–322

Goodwin J: Post-traumatic symptoms in incest victims, in Post-Traumatic Stress Disorder in Children. Edited by Eth S, Pynoos RS. Washington, DC, American Psychiatric Press, 1985d, pp 155–168

Goodwin J: Developmental impacts of incest, in Handbook of Child Psychiatry, Vol 5. Edited by Noshpitz J, Berlin I, Call J, et al. New York, Basic Books, 1987, pp 103–110

Goodwin J: Evaluation and treatment for incest families: a problem-oriented approach, in Modern Perspectives in Psychosocial Pathology. Edited by Howells JG. New York, Brunner/Mazel, 1988a, pp 43–57

Goodwin J: Munchausen's syndrome as a dissociative disorder. Dissociation 1:54–60, 1988b

Goodwin J: Sexual Abuse: Incest Victims and Their Families, 2nd Edition. Edited by Goodwin J. Chicago, Year Book Medical, 1989

Goodwin J: Recognizing multiple personality disorder in adult incest victims. Victimology (in press)

Goodwin J, Simms M, Bergman R: Hysterical seizures in adolescent incest victims. Am J Orthopsychiatry 49:704–708, 1979

Goodwin JM, McCarty T, DiVasto P: Physical and sexual abuse of the children of adult incest victims, in Sexual Abuse: Incest Victims and Their Families. Edited by Goodwin J. Boston, MA, Wright/PSG, 1982, pp 139–154

Goodwin J, Cormier L, Owen J: Grandfather-Granddaughter incest: a trigenerational view. Child Abuse Negl 7:163–170, 1983

Goodwin J, Cheeves K, Connell V: Defining a syndrome of severe symptoms in survivors of extreme incestuous abuse. Dissociation 1:11–16, 1988

Goodwin J, Attias R, McCarty T, et al: Routine questioning about childhood sexual abuse in psychiatry inpatients. Victimology (in press)

Grimm J, Grimm W: Grimms' Tales for Young and Old (1819). Translated by Mannheim R. New York, Doubleday, 1977

Henderson DJ: Incest, in Comprehensive Textbook of Psychiatry, 2nd Edition. Edited by Freedman AH, Kaplan HI, Sadock BJ. Baltimore, MD, Williams & Wilkins, 1975, pp 1530–1538

Herman J: Father-Daughter Incest. Cambridge, MA, Harvard University Press, 1981

Herman J, Schatzow E: Time-limited group therapy for women with a history of incest. Int J Group Psychother 34:605–616, 1984

Herman J, Schatzow E: Recovery and verification of memories of childhood trauma. Psychoanalytic Psychology 4:1–14, 1987

Herman J, van der Kolk B: Traumatic Antecedents of Borderline Personality Disorder, in Psychological Trauma. Edited by van der Kolk B. Washington, DC, American Psychiatric Press, 1987, pp 111–126

Herman J, Russell D, Trocki K: Long-term effects of incestuous abuse in childhood. Am J Psychiatry 143:1293–1296, 1986

James J, Womack W, Strauss F: Physician reporting of sexual abuse of children. JAMA 240:1145–1146, 1978

Kardiner A: The traumatic neuroses of war, in American Handbook of Psychiatry, Vol 1. Edited by Arieti S. New York, Basic Books, 1959, pp 245–257

Kluft R: Personality unification in multiple personality disorder: a follow-up study, in Treatment of Multiple Personality Disorder. Edited by Braun B. Washington, DC, American Psychiatric Press, 1986, pp 29–60

Kluft RP (ed): Treatment of victims of sexual abuse. Psychiatr Clin North Am 12, Whole No 2, 1989

Lane RD, Schwartz G: Levels of emotional awareness: a cognitive-developmental theory and its application to psychopathology. Am J Psychiatry 144:133–143, 1987

Lindberg FH, Dystad LJ: Post-traumatic stress disorder in women who experienced childhood incest. Child Abuse Negl 9:329–334, 1985

Lustig N, Dresser J, Spellman SW: Incest: a family group survival pattern. Arch Gen Psychiatry 14:31–40, 1966

MacFarlane K, Korbin J: Confronting the incest secret long after the fact: a family study of multiple victimization with strategies for intervention. Child Abuse Negl 7:225–240, 1983

MacFarlane K, Waterman J, Conerly S, et al: Sexual Abuse of Children: Evaluation and Treatment. New York, Guilford, 1986

Maisch H: Incest. New York, Stein & Day, 1972

Masson JM: The Assault on Truth. New York, Farrar, Strauss & Giroux, 1984

Meiselman K: Incest: A Psychological Study. San Francisco, CA, Jossey-Bass, 1981

Miller A: Thou Shalt Not Be Aware: Society's Betrayal of the Child. New York, Farrar, Straus, & Giroux, 1984

Miller J, Moeller D, Kaufman A, et al: Recidivism among sexual assault victims. Am J Psychiatry 135:1103–1104, 1978

Mrazek PB, Kempe CH: Sexually Abused Children and Their Families. New York, Pergamon, 1981

Nadelson T: Victim, victimizer: interaction in the psychotherapy of borderline patients. International Journal of Psychoanalytic Psychotherapy 5:115–119, 1976

Putnam FW, Guroff JJ, Silberman EK, et al: The clinical phenomenology of multiple personality disorder: review of 100 recent cases. J Clin Psychiatry 47:285–293, 1986

Rogers CM, Terry T: Clinical intervention with boy victims of sexual abuse, in Victims of Sexual Aggression: Treatment of Children, Women and Men. Edited by Stuart IR, Greer JG. New York, Van Nostrand Reinhold, 1984, pp 91–104

Russell D: Sexual Exploitation: Rape, Child Sexual Abuse, and Workplace Harassment. Beverly Hills, CA, Sage, 1984

Ryan T: Problems, errors, and opportunities in the treatment of father-daughter incest. Journal of Interpersonal Violence 1:113–124, 1986

Saltman V, Solomon RS: Incest and multiple personality. Psychol Rep 50:1127–1141, 1982

Sedney MA, Brooks B: Factors associated with a history of childhood sexual experiences in a nonclinical female population. Journal of the American Academy of Child Psychiatry 23:215–218, 1984

Sgroi SM: A Handbook of Clinical Intervention in Child Sexual Abuse. Lexington, MA, Lexington Books, 1982

Shengold LL: Child abuse and deprivation: soul murder. J Am Psychoanal Assoc 27:533–559, 1979

Silver RL, Boon C, Stones MH: Searching for meaning in misfortune: making sense of incest. Journal of Social Issues 39:81–102, 1983

Tormes Y: Child Victims of Incest. Englewood, CO, American Humane Association, 1968

Trepper TS: The apology session, in Treating Incest: a Multi-Modal Perspective. Edited by Trepper TS, Barrett MJ. New York, Haworth Press, 1986, pp 93–102

Tsai M, Wagner NN: Therapy groups for women sexually molested as children. Arch Sex Behav 7:417–427, 1978

van der Kolk BA: Psychological Trauma. Washington, DC, American Psychiatric Press, 1987

Walker E, Katon W, Harrop-Griffiths J, et al: Relationship of chronic pelvic pain to psychiatric diagnoses and childhood sexual abuse. Am J Psychiatry 145:75–80, 1988

Weinberg S: Incest Behavior. New York, Citadel, 1955

Westermeyer J: Incest in psychiatric practice: a description of patients and incestuous relationships. J Clin Psychiatry 39:643–648, 1978

Wilbur C: Multiple personality and child abuse: an overview. Psychiatr Clin North Am 7:3–8, 1984

CHAPTER 5

Somatoform Disorders in Victims of Incest and Child Abuse

Richard J. Loewenstein, M.D.

According to DSM-III-R (American Psychiatric Association 1987), somatoform disorders are characterized by "physical symptoms suggesting physical disorder . . . for which there are no demonstrable organic findings or known physiologic mechanisms, and for which there is positive evidence, or a strong presumption, that the symptoms are linked to psychological factors or conflicts" (p. 255). The DSM-III-R somatoform disorders include conversion disorder, somatization disorder, somatoform pain disorder, hypochondriasis, body dysmorphic disorder, and undifferentiated somatoform disorder.

Somatoform disorders and somatization symptoms represent extraordinarily complex problems in psychiatric medicine (Barsky and Klerman 1983; Ford 1983). Surveys estimate that in any one week as many as 60% to 80% of the normal population will suffer somatic symptoms, frequently without discoverable organic cause (Cassem 1987; Kellner 1985). Many psychiatric syndromes such as affective disorders, anxiety disorders, psychotic disorders, and dissociative disorders may have somatic symptoms as a significant part of their clinical presentation (Barsky and Klerman 1983; Bliss 1986; Cassem 1987; Ford 1983, 1986; Putnam et al. 1986). Somatoform disorders skirt the border of factitious and malingered con-

I gratefully acknowledge the assistance of Anne M. Fredenburg, Barbara Y. Jobson, Margaret A. Long, and Evelyn D.F. Nicholson of the Kubie Library at Sheppard Pratt Hospital, without whose assistance this chapter would never have been completed. Carole Harris and the staff of PDS also provided invaluable assistance.

ditions on the one hand, and that of misdiagnosed medical illness on the other (Ey 1982; Ford 1983). The latter has been reported as the actual etiology of symptoms in 40% to 60% of adult and child patients in some series of apparent somatoform disorder (Dubowitz and Hersov 1976; Ford and Folks 1985; Goodyer 1981; Lazare 1981; Slater 1965; Slater and Glithero 1961; Stefansson et al. 1976).

Somatoform disorders in DSM-III (American Psychiatric Association 1980) and DSM-III-R encompass some of the diagnostic categories that have evolved from the classic concept of hysteria (Merskey 1979). In DSM-III and DSM-III-R, hysteria has been transformed into the somatoform disorders, the dissociative disorders (psychogenic amnesia, fugue, and multiple personality disorder), two of the personality disorders (histrionic and borderline personality disorders), and even posttraumatic stress disorder—since, particularly in males, traumatic and war neuroses were another aspect of classic hysteria (Ellenberger 1970; Freud 1893; Kretschmer 1960).

There are a number of different subliteratures on somatization with divergent sets of implicit and/or explicit theoretical presumptions and clinical preoccupations. Psychoanalytic writers are relatively uninterested in the phenomenology of somatoform disorders and are more concerned with explication of the intrapsychic dynamics of individuals with characterological difficulties thought to be associated with these symptoms (Kernberg 1975; Krohn 1978; Lazare 1971). Those of the Washington University "school," on the other hand—who have promulgated the diagnosis of "chronic hysteria" or Briquet's syndrome—are primarily concerned with an apsychological typology of the symptoms and associated features of the "disease of hysteria" (Cleghorn 1969; Guze 1967). Psychiatric authors working in the medical setting are more focused on problems of somatoform symptoms in relation to medical illness and "illness behavior" (Dubowitz and Hersov 1976; Ford 1983, 1986; Leigh 1983). Military psychiatrists finding somatoform symptoms in combat settings have another set of clinical and theoretical concerns (Jones and Hales 1987; Kardiner 1941; Kubie 1943).

There are also several subpopulations being studied in the literature on somatoform disorders. This is probably true even *within* specific somatoform disorder diagnoses, especially conversion disorder and somatoform pain disorder (Coryell 1980; Ford 1983; Guze 1967; Katon et al. 1985; Roy 1982b; Stefansson et al. 1976). Thus simple unifying explanations of all somatization phenomena are unlikely. Many authors suggest a "multidimensional approach" to somatization "in which there are both separate and simultaneous biologic, psychodynamic, sociocultural, and behavioral explanations" (Lazare 1981, p. 746).

Among the most profound controversies concerning classic hysteria is that of its relationship to disordered sexuality, particularly female sexuality (Chodoff 1982; Cleghorn 1969; Veith 1965, 1977). This question has been a part of the medical literature since the Egyptian papryi and the writings of Hippocrates (Chodoff 1982; Ellenberger 1970; Veith 1965, 1977). One aspect of this controversy is the disagreement in the psychiatric and psychoanalytic literatures concerning the frequency and importance of *actual* childhood sexual experiences—primarily incest and extrafamilial childhood sexual abuse—in the development of somatization and psychopathology in general (Ellenberger 1970; Ferenczi 1933; Freud 1896a, 1896b, 1896c, 1925; Garcia 1987; Goodwin 1985; Jones 1953; Krohn 1978; Krystal 1978; Masson 1983; Morrant 1985; Peters 1976; van der Kolk 1986). There are, however, a large number of studies and clinical case reports with data bearing on aspects of this question.

In this chapter, I will review the literature on conversion disorder, somatization disorder/Briquet's syndrome, somatoform pain disorder, and hypochondriasis in children and adults, with specific attention to the problem of childhood sexual abuse as a factor in development of these conditions. Then I will review the outcome literature on the short- and long-term consquences of childhood sexual abuse as it pertains to the development of somatization. Where relevant, I will discuss the literature on dissociative disorders and posttraumatic stress disorder. I will not review the literature on body dysmorphic disorder, since this relatively rare condition is reported to occur in a very different population from that of the other somatoform disorders and has not been described in the literature in association with child abuse (Cassem 1987; Ford 1983).

In this chapter, the terms *somatization* and *somatoform* will be used relatively interchangeably. For convenience in discussing the pre-DSM-III literature, *hysteria* and *hysterical* will be used as roughly synonymous with these terms as well. *Briquet's syndrome* will be used to identify the condition also known as *chronic hysteria* in the pre-DSM-III literature. Diagnostic criteria for DSM-III-R somatoform disorders are found in the Appendix to this chapter.

HISTORICAL REVIEW: BRIQUET AND FREUD

The writings of Briquet and Freud form the basis for two of the most important, and divergent, literatures on somatization: the phenomenological descriptive and the psychoanalytic, respectively (e.g., Cloninger 1986; Krohn 1978). Although the methodology and patient samples described by Briquet and Freud are not strictly comparable with those in the modern literature, it is important to detail their views concerning the relationship of childhood mistreatment and hysteria.

Briquet

Briquet's *Treatise on Hysteria* (1859) is a comprehensive investigation of 430 patients with hysteria seen over a 10-year period, including cases in children, in males, and in relatives of the index cases (Mai and Merskey 1980, 1981). Briquet attempted to dispute the prevailing view that hysteria was caused by sexual continence. He also attempted to show that the disorder was unrelated to pathology of the female reproductive system.

Briquet believed that hysteria was most frequently caused by the impact on the nervous system of a variety of life's sufferings, primarily marital and family woes and losses. The largest subgroup of his sample, about 27%, were thought to have had this etiology in the genesis of their hysterical symptoms. Severe chronic mistreatment by parents or by a spouse and losses of significant people headed the list of these family problems. Another 14% of his patients were said to have become ill after a traumatically induced panic caused by events such as witnessing a fire or seeing a sibling jump from a high window. A number of other cases were thought to have been precipitated by stresses such as rape, "abuse of coitus," illegitimate pregnancy, unhappy marriage, or difficulty with in-laws (Mai and Merskey 1980).

In 87 cases of hysteria in children under the age of 12, Briquet stated that one-third had been "habitually maltreated or held constantly in fear or had been directed harshly by their parents" (Mai and Merskey 1980, p. 1402 [translation of Briquet 1859, p. 112]). Another 10% of the childhood cases were thought to have been caused by other frightening experiences. Briquet also reported that one-third of his sample had been in "poor health during childhood" with "migraine, abdominal pain, disturbances of appetite, chronic malaise, etc."; another 40% had had "poor health" after puberty (Mai and Merskey 1980, p. 1402). Although some of these patients may have had chronic medical illnesses, modern writings on abused children frequently describe them as having similar symptoms.

To study the relation of hysteria to sexual activity, Briquet acquired data computing the prevalence of hysteria in nuns, house servants, and prostitutes—both from the street and the bordellos. He declared that hysteria in nuns was extremely rare but that 104 of 197 prostitutes (53%) had hysteria and another 29 (15%) were "impressionable" (i.e., had intense "nervous reactions" bordering on hysteria). One-third of the servants also had hysteria, which was ascribed to their tumultuous and traumatic lives.

One must be cautious in comparing these findings to those in modern samples. However, in modern reports, between 45% and 69% of prostitutes report histories of childhood sexual abuse, although in one study 37% of a matched nonprostitute comparison group had also been abused (Browne and Finkelhor 1986; James and Meyerding 1977; Silbert and Pines 1981; Steele and Alexander 1981).

Freud

According to Freud's (1925) autobiographical study, he did not investigate the presence of childhood sexual trauma in most of the cases originally reported in *Studies in Hysteria* (Breuer and Freud 1893–1895). He reported in a 1924 footnote to the latter work, however, that, in the case of "Katharina," hysterical symptoms developed in response to sexual advances by the patient's father. Anna O, the most celebrated of the patients in *Studies in Hysteria*, was described by Ellenberger (1970) as having a "magnetic illness" (i.e., a dissociative disorder). Jones (1953), Freud's biographer, reported that she had a "double personality" and noted the clinical similarity between Anna O and Sally Beauchamp, Morton Prince's (1905) most famous case of multiple personality disorder described in *The Dissociation of a Personality*.

Anna O's symptoms are also suggestive of a modern diagnosis of multiple personality disorder (Kluft 1987a; Loewenstein 1989), a condition now thought to be almost invariably associated with a history of severe childhood trauma (Kluft 1987b; Putnam 1985; Putnam et al. 1986). Unfortunately, little early childhood history is given in the case study, although it is stated that Anna O was "passionately fond" of her father (Breuer and Freud 1893–1895, p. 22). One can only speculate about possible early traumatic experiences that may have predisposed Anna O to the development of a symptomatic dissociative disorder at the time of her father's death.

In Freud's (1893, 1896a, 1896b, 1896c) subsequent papers on hysteria, he developed the idea that the distal etiology of hysterical symptoms could be traced back to early childhood sexual traumas occurring long before the emergence of active symptoms. The actual development of symptoms was related to the effect of unconscious memories of the traumatic experiences operating "in a deferred fashion as though they were fresh experiences" (Freud 1896b, p. 167).

Freud initially reported the "complete psychoanalysis" of 13 cases (1896b, 1896c) and later 18 cases (1896a) of severe hysteria refractory to all other treatment, including institutional treatment in several cases. Six of the 18 cases were male. Many of Freud's general clinical observations are concordant with those reported in the modern literature on adult sequelae of childhood sexual abuse and trauma (Goodwin 1982; Herman 1981). He minimized, however, the possibility of immediately harmful physical and psychological effects of the seduction on the child. This was primarily because, at the time these papers were written, Freud lacked a substantive theory of psychosexual development and childhood mental life (Garcia 1987).

Freud (1896a, 1896b) postulated that the underlying cause of hysteria was sexual abuse beginning before the age of 8, primarily "grave sexual injuries" perpetrated by "close relative(s)," especially siblings; teachers, governesses, servants, and strangers were also reported as abusers. Fathers as perpetrators were apparently only specifically mentioned in letters to Fleiss, Freud's confidant of the time (1896b [p. 164, editors footnote]; Freud 1954). Freud (1896b) also described victimized boys who later became abusers of girls, primarily their younger sisters.

Freud (1896a) discussed a variety of sexual abuse experiences suffered by his patients, including single episodes of molestation as well as complex ongoing sexual relationships between adults or older siblings and young children. He reported independent confirmation of the childhood sexual abuse in two cases. He described the powerlessness and helplessness of the child against the abusing adult.

With respect to conversion symptoms, Freud (1896a, 1896b) posited a specific relationship between the adult's hysterical physical symptoms and repressed memories of the physical sensations related to the childhood sexual experiences. A hysterical outcome was thought to be related to a "passive" experience of the sexual abuse (Freud 1896a, 1896b, 1986c). Freud (1896a) also stated that some obsessional neuroses may be due to sexual abuse in childhood, resulting from active enjoyment or guilt over aggressive sexual behavior in childhood. These latter cases probably would not meet modern criteria for obsessive-compulsive disorder, however. The one case that is described in some detail appears to involve a repetitive, dissociated reenactment of an episode of molestation, not true obsessive-compulsive symptoms. Freud (1896a) also described a history of childhood sexual abuse in a chronic case of paranoia. In contrast to Briquet, who did not specifically mention sexual abuse in the etiology of hysteria, Freud does not consider other forms of childhood mistreatment in its genesis.

Subsequently, Freud relinquished the "seduction theory." He decided that many of his patients' reports of childhood sexual abuse were the product of fantasies related to what became known as the Oedipus complex (Freud 1896b, 1914, 1917, 1925, 1933). Freud (1896b [p. 168, footnote 2, added 1924]) later stated, however, that "seduction retains a certain aetiological importance" in the development of hysteria (see also Freud 1925; Garcia 1987; Greenacre 1967; Jones 1953). Also in his later writings, Freud continued periodically to point out the noxious effects of seduction on psychosexual development (e.g., Freud 1905a, 1905b, 1918, 1931; Garcia 1987). Generally, however, Freud (1917, 1933) consigned to fantasy accusations by girls of seduction by their fathers.

The disavowal of the seduction theory is said to have led Freud to develop fully his theories of an intrapsychic mental life: infantile sexuality; psychosexual development; the Oedipus complex; and the importance of unconscious conflicts, fantasy, and subjective experience in human psychology (Anthony 1982; Freud, 1905b, 1925; Garcia 1987; Greenacre 1967;

Jones 1953; Krohn 1978; Krystal 1978; Morrant 1985). Even in its original form, however, the seduction theory centered not so much on the actual effects of the childhood seduction itself in the production of hysterical and obsessional symptoms but rather on the intrapsychic conflicts over later emergence of repressed memories of the seduction (Anthony 1982; Garcia 1987; Krohn 1978).

After this, the concept of trauma remained important for Freud and his followers, but a specific interest in child abuse was essentially abandoned (Ferenczi 1933; Furst 1967; Krystal 1978; Masson 1983; Rothstein 1986). Because of the central importance of infantile sexuality, the Oedipus complex, and other intrapsychic phenomena in psychoanalytic theory, and because of the way Freud arrived at these ideas, many psychoanalytic writers tend to take a polarized position implying that belief in childhood "seduction" means rejection of the other tenets of psychoanalytic theory (e.g., Greenacre 1967; Jones 1953). Of course, there is no logical necessity for an either-or approach. A different solution would be to consider the *impact* of childhood sexual abuse and other forms of severe psychic trauma in childhood on psychosexual development, fantasy, defensive formation, ego development, unconscious mental life, and so on. A small number of psychoanalytic authors have written papers from this latter point of view (e.g., Ferenczi 1933; Freud 1981; Galdston 1981; Kluft 1987a; Krystal 1978; Marmer 1980; Rothstein 1986; Shengold 1979; Terr 1983), and, as noted above, Freud did continue to describe seduction as a factor in the development of certain forms of psychopathology.

After discarding the seduction theory, Freud (1905a) wrote one additional major clinical study of hysteria: the Dora case. No history of an early seduction was described in the case report. From childhood on, however, the patient was deeply enmeshed in her parents' marital conflicts and the liaisons of her seductive, syphilitic father; his mistress, Frau K; and the latter's husband, Herr K. Between the ages of 6 and 8, Dora suffered from a vaginal discharge (leucorrhea) and enuresis, which recurred after she had achieved several years of nocturnal continence. Vaginal discharge as well as regression in bladder control have frequently been described in modern reports on sexually abused children (Goodwin 1982). Freud, on the other hand, ascribed these problems to masturbation ending at about age 8 when Dora's first hysterical symptoms appeared.

When Dora was 14, Herr K made sexual advances toward her. Two years later, he again attempted to seduce her. During childhood and adolescence, Dora had always shared a bed with Frau K during visits, and the two had engaged in extensive intimate discussions of sexual matters and the Ks' marital problems. In discussing Dora's hysterical symptoms, Freud focused primarily on Dora's unconscious conflicts over erotic and romantic feelings toward Herr K and the relation of these to conflictual feelings toward her parents. Modern commentators have focused more on Dora's developmentally inappropriate sexual overstimulation in her deceit-filled, chaotic family (Erikson 1962; Slipp 1977). These writers have particularly noted Dora's role as "erotic barter" (Erikson 1962, p. 456) between her father and Herr K. We would now consider Herr K's behavior a clear-cut attempt at sexual exploitation of an adolescent girl— implicitly sanctioned by her own father—in which Herr K may well have consciously attempted to capitalize on Dora's psychological vulnerability related to the family problems with which he was intimately acquainted. Modern studies describe a relationship between sexual exploitation and abuse and emergence of conversion symptoms in adolescents (LaBarbera and Dozier 1980; see also this chapter, below), although, to be sure, Dora had already had hysterical symptoms beginning earlier in childhood.

Later Writers

Childhood sexual and physical abuse continued to be reported in association with hysteria, although usually without systematic comment. For example, in a paper on 219 cases of hysteria, Schilder (1939) described 9 in some detail and 6 others very briefly. Of these 15 patients, 5 reported histories of severe childhood physical abuse, 1 with associated neglect. One patient reported repeated incest. Two patients had slept with a parent into adolescence. One of these, a patient with "repeated amnesia attacks" (p. 1398) stated she would be "crucified" before admitting incest with her father with whom she had slept alone until she was 19. In two cases, Schilder described that the hysterical attacks recreated specific episodes of reported physical abuse. Schilder gave no systematic discussion concerning the child abuse, although commentary is made on the oedipal attachment of the hysterical women to their fathers.

THE MODERN LITERATURE

Conversion Disorder

The modern view of somatization has tended to separate conversion symptoms from somatization disorder, somatoform pain disorder, and hysterical/histrionic personality disorder (Chodoff and Lyons 1958; Coryell 1980; Ford 1983, 1986; Guze 1967; Lazare 1981). Several reports have strongly suggested that conversion symptoms can occur in the context of virtually any psychiatric diagnosis, medical illness, or personality configuration, not just in patients with histrionic (hysterical) personality disorder. The latter diagnosis is thought to occur in only a minority of patients with conversion disorder (Chodoff and Lyons 1958; Ford 1983, 1986; Guze et al. 1971; Lazare 1981; Lewis and Berman 1965; Meares and Horvath

1972; Perley and Guze 1962; Rangell 1959; Slater 1965; Stefansson et al. 1976; Zeigler et al. 1960). A variety of biologic, psychological, developmental, interpersonal, and cultural factors are said to bear on the development of conversion symptoms (Ford 1983; Lazare 1981).

Conversion disorder in DSM-III and DSM-III-R is defined primarily in terms of "pseudoneurologic" symptoms such as paralysis or pseudoseizures (Ford and Folks 1985). Many of the early papers on conversion are difficult to evaluate from the perspective of DSM-III and DSM-III-R diagnoses, since the articles appear to describe heterogeneous samples of patients with conversion disorder, somatization disorder, somatoform pain disorder, as well as conversion disorder superimposed on acute or chronic medical illness (Coryell 1980).

Conversion Disorder and Child Abuse

In a retrospective chart review study of 57 patients with "conversion hysteria" diagnosed by psychiatrists, internists, and neurologists in a general medical hospital, Lewis and Berman (1965) unexpectedly found that 25% of the female patients reported or strongly implied histories of incest. Male and adolescent patients with conversion symptoms also described neglect, abuse, and sexual overstimulation and confusion in their families of origin. No systematic attempt had been made by the investigators to uncover histories of child abuse.

A series of case reports have described a specific relationship between hysterical pseudoseizures and incest, incest rape, and sexual trauma, primarily in adolescent girls (Goodwin et al. 1979; Gross 1979; LaBarbera and Dozier 1980; Liske and Forster 1964; Standage 1975). Goodwin et al., who reported independent confirmation of incest in her six pseudoseizure patients, estimated that at least 10% of pseudoseizure cases are related to incest. The two earlier reports on pseudoseizures (Liske and Forster 1964; Standage 1976) made no systematic attempt to look at child abuse as a variable, although patients with incest histories were described in each series.

Roy (1982b) described clinical features of nonepileptics and epileptics with pseudoseizures compared to epileptics without pseudoseizures. Organic brain disease was more common in pseudoseizure patients from medical and neurologic hospitals as compared with those from psychiatric settings. Both pseudoseizure groups were said to have a higher prevalence of depression, suicide attempts, sexual problems, somatic preoccupations, anxiety, and family history of psychiatric disorder. These symptoms have considerable overlap with those commonly described in adults with histories of childhood sexual abuse (Browne and Finkelhor 1986; Gelinas 1983; Goodwin 1982; Meiselman 1978; Steele and Alexander 1981). Of course, these symptoms may also be found among patients with other nontraumatically induced psychiatric disorders, such as the affective disorders.

Davies (1979) described a high percentage of abnormal electroencephalograms, low IQ, and "neuropsychiatric findings" in a sample of incest survivors. He felt that neurologic impairment might increase the vulnerability of some children to incest. Several methodological problems limit the generalizability of this study. Nonetheless, taking the study at face value, one could infer that incest or other forms of child abuse might be a factor in the development of pseudoseizures in some neurologic patients as well as in the neurologically normal adolescents described above.

Mogielnicki et al. (1977) described three cases of adults who developed conversion or somatoform symptoms in the context of anxiety that *they* themselves would become abusive to their children. Goodwin and Geil (1982) described another similar case. Antecedent history of abuse in these adults was not detailed, however.

Somatization Disorder and Briquet's Syndrome

The DSM-III and DSM-III-R diagnosis of somatization disorder developed from the earlier concept of Briquet's syndrome. More recent studies show reasonably good concordance between the two diagnoses (Cloninger et al. 1986; DeSouza and Othmer 1984). The disorder is described as a lifelong, chronic condition primarily affecting females. It is characterized by dramatically described polysymptomatic physical complaints without medical explanation; sexual problems and marital maladjustment; a feeling of chronic or recurrent ill health; conversion symptoms; and associated anxiety and depression (Arkonac and Guze 1963; Bohman et al. 1984; Cassem 1987; Cloninger and Guze 1970a, 1970b; Cloninger et al. 1975, 1984, 1986; Coryell 1980; Farley et al. 1968; Ford 1983, 1986; Goodwin and Guze 1979; Guze 1964, 1967; Guze et al. 1967, 1971, 1972; Kroll et al. 1979; Lilienfeld et al. 1986; Meares and Horvath 1972; Monson and Smith 1983; Oxman et al. 1985; Perley and Guze 1962; Purtell et al. 1951; Robins et al. 1952; Sigvardsson et al. 1984; Smith et al. 1986; Woerner and Guze 1968; Woodruff et al. 1971).

Studies have shown that female relatives of patients with Briquet's syndrome received the diagnosis of Briquet's syndrome more frequently than controls (Arkonac and Guze 1963; Cloninger et al. 1975; Coryell 1980; Guze 1967; Guze et al. 1967, 1971). Male relatives and spouses of these patients more often met criteria for alcoholism and/or antisocial personality disorder (Arkonac and Guze 1963; Cloninger et al. 1975; Guze et al. 1967, 1971; Lilienfeld et al. 1986; Woerner and Guze 1968).

Some authors consider Briquet's syndrome and antisocial personality disorder to be expressions of the same underlying pathology in females and males, respectively (Cloninger and Guze 1970a; Warner 1978). Guze (1964) described male criminals with antisocial personality disorder who had conversion and somatization symptoms. Female patients with criminal backgrounds and/or antisocial personality disorder also commonly received a diagnosis of Briquet's syndrome. Briquet's syndrome patients were often described as displaying antisocial behavior (Cloninger and Guze 1970a, 1970b; Cloninger et al. 1975; Guze et al. 1971; Lilienfeld et al. 1986; Martin et al. 1979; Robins 1966).

Few attempts have been made to look at child abuse in patients with somatization disorder, or, even when reported, to consider abuse as a variable relevant to the development of symptoms in these patients. For example, Cloninger and Guze (1970a, 1970b) studied the background of 66 convicted female felons; 41% of the sample received a diagnosis of Briquet's syndrome and 26% were diagnosed with both Briquet's syndrome and antisocial personality disorder.

These patients described paternal neglect in 29% of their families and maternal neglect in 9%. They reported cruelty or physical abuse by 14% of their fathers and by 12% of their mothers; 14% of the sample reported incest and 6% paternal incest rape. Incest histories were about equally divided between the patients with antisocial personality and those without. Alcoholism was highly prevalent in the families of origin of these women as well. About one-quarter of the sample described a history of prostitution. Of the women, 14% had been legally declared "unfit mothers," and about half of those declared unfit had also been convicted of child abuse. No mention is made by the authors if the child abuse histories were pursued as part of their structured interview protocol, were discovered because of the extensive record review that was part of the study, or were simply volunteered by the subjects (Cloninger and Guze 1970a, 1970b).

Amazingly, 7.5% of the patients in this sample "spontaneously described themselves [to the investigators] as having a 'split personality' or a 'multiple personality' " (Cloninger and Guze 1970a, p. 557). No additional comment is made about this finding, however. Bliss (1986) speculated that the percentage of dissociative disorder patients in this study would have been even higher if an attempt had been made to find the more common covert presentations of multiple personality disorder and dissociation (Kluft 1985).

Zoccolillo and Cloninger (1985) reported on a chart review study of 50 lower-class women meeting criteria for both Briquet's syndrome and somatization disorder. They were compared to a control sample of nonsomatizing female psychiatric patients—suffering primarily from nonpsychotic affective disorders—matched specifically for race and age but who differed little from the subjects on other demographic variables. Somatizers were three times as likely to be "poor parents," defined as "being reported for child abuse to the authorities, losing custody of a child through court proceedings . . . or giving a child to another person to rear" (p. 444). Somatizers were twice as likely to have had children with severe conduct disturbances, although both groups had children with "severe behavioral disturbances." Several children of the somatizers had disappeared or died under mysterious circumstances. No data are provided on the somatizers' own child abuse histories, although a considerable body of scholarly and clinical research supports the notion that child abuse is a multigenerational phenomenon and that child abusers frequently have histories themselves of being abused in childhood (Finkelhor 1984; Goodwin 1982; Goodwin et al. 1981; Groth 1979; Krugman 1986; Steele and Alexander 1981).

Morrison (1989) reported on 60 women with somatization disorder diagnosed by DSM-III criteria who were compared with 31 women with primary affective disorder. With respect to sexual history, significantly more somatization disorder patients (about 55%) reported being sexually abused before the age of 18 as compared with controls (16%). Mean age of molestation was about 9–10 years old for the both groups. Intrafamilial sexual abuse accounted for about 36% of the molestation experiences for the somatization disorder group as compared with 12% of controls. Somatization disorder patients also were significantly more likely to report anorgasmia. Otherwise, there were no significant differences between the two groups' sexual histories. Three of the molested somatization disorder patients also met criteria for multiple personality disorder.

There are other more indirect findings that suggest a possible relationship between somatization disorder and childhood sexual abuse. For example, there is considerable demographic overlap between somatization disorder patients and many incest victims. Both are frequently associated with multiproblem families, where poverty, alcoholism, drug abuse, and multigenerational child abuse are common—although it is well-recognized that these are hardly the only families where child abuse occurs. Long-term effects of childhood sexual abuse in these patients must be separated from those of the overall pathology of their upbringing, including other kinds of abuse, however (Finkelhor 1984; Ford 1986; Goodwin 1982; Goodwin et al. 1981; Mrazek and Mrazek 1981; Steele and Alexander 1981).

Other findings in incest victims also have been noted in patients with somatization disorder. Poor self-identity and sexual problems are among the most consistent long-term findings in the outcome literature on incest (Bagley and Ramsay 1986; Browne and Finkelhor 1985; Gelinas 1983; Jehu and Gazan 1983). In a linguistic analysis of the speech of 11 somatization disorder patients compared to depressed, paranoid, and medically ill controls, Oxman et al. (1985) unexpectedly found that somatizers manifested "a confused, negative self-identity" (p. 1150) in their utterances when compared with the other groups. With respect to sexual difficulties,

Goodwin and Guze (1979) considered sexual problems and menstrual difficulties so ubiquitous in somatization disorder patients that they doubt the diagnosis if these symptoms are not present (see also Cassem 1987).

Studies of adoptees have tried to distinguish environmental from genetic factors in the etiology of somatization (Bohman et al. 1984; Cloninger et al. 1975, 1984; Sigvardsson et al. 1984). Bohman et al., Cloninger et al. (1984), and Sigvardsson et al. reported on somatization in 859 women adopted at birth by nonrelatives. They were compared with a sample of nonadopted controls. Complete medical and psychiatric records were gathered from the registry of the Swedish National Health Insurance Board. Two groups of chronic somatizers were characterized among the adoptees. In one of these, alcohol abuse in the adoptive father was one of the only environmental factors associated with development of somatization problems. Alcoholism has frequently been cited as a significant factor in the backgrounds of adults who abuse children (Finkelhor 1984; Goodwin 1982; Meiselman 1978). This latter group of somatizing women was not, however, the one thought to be most similar clinically to Briquet's syndrome patients (Bohman et al. 1984).

Studies have also suggested that attention-deficit disorder (hyperactivity) in children is associated with parental antisocial personality disorder and Briquet's syndrome (Cantwell 1972; Cloninger 1986). Fish-Murray et al. (1986) described four cases of apparent attention-deficit disorder in children who had been abused and were exhibiting symptoms of a posttraumatic stress disorder. The authors noted an overlap between diagnostic criteria for attention-deficit disorder and posttraumatic stress disorder. Hyperactivity has also been reported in case descriptions of severely sexually abused boys (Dixon et al. 1978). In a retrospective study of 124 children, Heffron et al. (1987) found that a history of physical abuse was more prevalent in boys and girls with hyperactivity with or without attention-deficit disorder as compared with children without hyperactivity. Learning and school problems also have frequently been described in abused children (Browne and Finkelhor 1986; Goodwin 1982; Mrazek and Mrazek 1981). Thus child abuse may be an important unstudied variable in the familial association of antisocial personality, somatization disorder, and apparent hyperactivity/attention-deficit disorder.

Dissociative Symptoms in Patients With Somatization Disorder

Amnesia is among the symptoms listed in the diagnostic criteria for both Briquet's syndrome and somatization disorder (American Psychiatric Association 1987; Feighner et al. 1972; Guze et al. 1972). Psychogenic amnesia is also a dissociative symptom and a dissociative disorder according to DSM-III and DSM-III-R. Many studies reported that dissociation is strongly correlated with an antecedent history of trauma and/or abuse both in children and adults (Eth and Pynoos 1985; Putnam 1985; Spiegel 1984; van der Kolk 1986).

In a validation study of a shortened screening test for somatization disorder, Othmer and DeSouza (1985) reported that 49% of patients with somatization disorder reported amnesia. Amnesia and "burning in [the] sex organs" were two of the seven symptoms that best discriminated the somatization group from the control group. As will be discussed below, chronic pelvic pain is also associated with a history of incest.

In the historical literature, Ellenberger (1970) reported that Blanche Wittman, "la reine des hysteriques"—Charcot's most famous patient in his public demonstrations of grand hysterical phenomena—left La Salpetriere and was studied independently by Jules Janet, Pierre's brother. Janet discovered an unsuspected dual personality in the patient with an alter who reported complete co-consciousness even for experiences in deep hypnosis. Ultimately, Blanche underwent yet a third change in character, denied her whole prior history, and died of a painful cancer after many years of work in the radiology laboratory of La Salpetriere. She was said never again to have shown any hysterical symptoms (Ellenberger 1970).

Guze (1964) reported that among 13 male criminals diagnosed with conversion disorder, 3 had amnesia as their presenting conversion symptom. Two of these 3 accounted for 12 of the 18 psychiatric admissions in the group. In a case report of a male with Briquet's syndrome (Kaminsky and Slavney 1976), the patient was noted to have had an extensive history of fugues, episodic memory loss, periods of "fabricated life history," severe headaches, treatment unresponsiveness, and lability of mood and character traits—for example, appearing fussy and controlled at one time and dramatic and disorganized at another. Family background was said to have been "tumultuous" but abuse was not noted specifically (Kaminsky and Slavney 1976). As noted above, Cloninger and Guze (1970a) stated that 7.5% of their sample of female criminals—almost half of whom also met criteria for Briquet's syndrome—reported the presence of multiple personalities. Also, three (5%) of the 60 somatization disorder patients reported on by Morrison (1989) met criteria for multiple personality disorder.

Bliss (1986) reported that 42% of 33 patients meeting criteria for Briquet's syndrome also met DSM-III criteria for multiple personality disorder. Of 21 patients originally diagnosed as having multiple personality disorder by DSM-III criteria, 76% also met criteria for Briquet's syndrome. Putnam et al. (1986) and Loewenstein et al. (1986) reported extensive histories of chronic somatization and conversion symptoms in samples of both female and male patients with multiple personality disorder. Headache was the most common somatization symptom in both males and females. The males had a higher percentage of pseudoseizures.

All of the males and 97% of the females in these studies reported childhood histories of severe abuse or trauma.

Somatoform Pain Disorder

Chronic pain syndromes are a heterogeneous group of complex conditions that affect a diverse group of patients (Cassem 1987; Ford 1983, 1986; Katon et al. 1985). Several reports described a relationship between certain forms of somatoform pain disorder and prior sexual abuse (Gross et al. 1980–1981; Haber and Sitley 1987; Harrop-Griffiths et al. 1987; Walker et al. 1988). Gross et al. conducted an in-depth, uncontrolled study of 25 women with chronic pelvic pain who had essentially normal gynecologic examinations. The authors reported surprise at finding that 36% of their patients revealed a history of incest, generally involving "intercourse or prolonged sexual contact . . . for as long as eight years" (p. 88). Several patients had incestuous relationships beginning before the age of 5. Six of nine patients who received a diagnosis of borderline personality disorder reported histories of incest. The other incest victims were diagnosed with a "severe hysterical character disorder" (p. 88).

Walker et al. (1988), also reported in Harrop-Griffiths et al. (1987), investigated 25 chronic pelvic pain patients who had little gynecologic disease, comparing them to 30 pain-free women undergoing tubal ligation or a fertility workup. No difference in gynecologic pathology was found by laparoscopy between chronic pain patients and controls. A diagnostic interview was performed including the Diagnostic Interview Schedule (Robins et al. 1981) and a structured interview inquiring about childhood sexual abuse. Of the chronic pain patients, 64% had been sexually abused before the age of 14 compared to 23% of controls, the latter figure approximating the prevalence of childhood sexual abuse previously reported in community samples (Russell 1983, 1986). The abused group was more likely to have suffered from adult victimization as well.

Chronic pelvic pain patients had a significantly greater number of other somatization symptoms than controls (7.0 compared to 1.7, respectively) on the somatization disorder section of the Diagnostic Interview Schedule, although only one patient met full criteria for somatization disorder. In particular, nonpelvic abdominal pain and discomfort were present in about 50% of the chronic pelvic pain patients. Chronic pelvic pain and sexual abuse were significantly associated with sexual dysfunction and a current or lifetime history of depression. The association between depression and chronic pelvic pain was significant only among sexual abuse victims (Walker et al. 1988).

Draijer (1989) conducted a long-term epidemiologic study of 1,054 Dutch women. Six percent had been sexually abused before the age of 16. The abused group had significantly more pelvic pain, dysmenorrhea, headaches, and other somatic problems as compared with the nonabused women. Draijer (1989) also cites other Dutch studies that show a higher prevalence of incest and/or rape in women with chronic pelvic pain.

In two separate studies looking specifically at histories of child abuse in women presenting to a university pain service, Haber and Sitley (1987) found physical and sexual abuse histories in 53% of 181 subjects in the first study and 52% of 84 women in the second. Abdominal pain and headaches were more common in the abused groups when compared to pain patients without abuse histories. Abdominal pain accounted for 75% of the sexual abuse cases. Major depression by DSM-III criteria was more common in the nonabused group. The abused group was also significantly younger, leading the authors to conclude that abused women may develop chronic complaints and utilize medical services more at a younger age. Walker et al. (1988), whose chronic pain group also was significantly younger than controls, implied as well that chronic somatization problems in adult survivors of childhood sexual abuse may lead to overutilization of medical resources.

Hypochondriasis

Hypochondriasis has a different historical configuration from hysteria. At one time it was thought to be a prototypically male disorder—the antithesis of hysteria—related to problems not of the uterus but of the hypochondria, an area beneath the ribs holding the viscera (Ford 1983; Kenyon 1976; Sigvardsson et al. 1984; Veith 1965). Much debate in the modern literature concerns the rigorous definition of hypochondriasis as a primary disorder so that it can be studied systematically (Barsky and Klerman 1983; Kellner 1985; Kenyon 1976; Sigvardsson et al. 1984). In general, however, the clinical presentation and family background of patients with hypochondriasis are described as quite different from those of patients with somatization disorder (Cassem 1987; Ford 1983). Hypochondriasis patients are said to be equally divided between males and females, for example. They are commonly described as obsessional and focused on detail, whereas somatization disorder patients are usually described as global, vague, and dramatic in their cognitive style (Cassem 1987; Ford 1983). Hypochondriasis patients are reported to come from overprotective but emotionally distant families where ill relatives were often present and emotional support was given primarily to those in the family who were physically ill (Cassem 1987; Ford 1983, 1986; Kellner 1985). Childhood sexual abuse or physical abuse has not been noted frequently in the histories of patients with hypochondriasis in any of the major studies or reviews of the subject (Barsky and Klerman 1983; Ford 1981, 1986; Kellner 1985; Kenyon 1976).

One form of child abuse could possibly be associated with the development of hypochondriasis, however: the syndrome of Munchausen by proxy. This is a condition in which the parent reports or induces factitious symptoms of medical illness in his or her child (Cassem 1987; Ford 1983; Hosch 1987; Jones et al. 1986; Libow and Schreier 1986; Meadow 1977, 1984; Orenstein and Wasserman 1986). Severe psychological morbidity, physical morbidity, and even death have been reported in children abused in this way (Jones et al. 1986; Meadow 1984). In many instances, the Munchausen-by-proxy syndrome goes on for years with a parent and child extensively involved with the medical system (Jones et al. 1986; Meadow 1984; Orenstein and Wasserman 1986).

Meadow (1984) described several adults who had been raised as Munchausen-by-proxy children with factitious epilepsy. They were said to persist in their "illness behavior" into adulthood, visiting physicians insistent on a workup of their nonexistent disease. It is unclear if Meadow viewed these individuals as having a factitious disorder or a form of hypochondriasis. In any event, this abuse-related somatoform condition might present as apparent primary hypochondriasis in adult patients. It is also possible that some chronically somatizing patients with histories of childhood sexual abuse might receive a diagnosis of hypochondriasis as they come into repeated contact with the medical system.

Somatoform Disorders in Childhood

Somatoform symptoms are thought to be a relatively common way that children and adolescents communicate psychological distress relating to many developmental, interpersonal, and family problems (Anthony 1982; Dubowitz and Hersov 1976; Goodyer 1981; Herzog and Jellinek 1987; Richtsmeier and Waters 1984). As in adults, somatization in children is likely to be a reflection of a number of different underlying processes and occurs in a number of clinical contexts (Anthony 1982). One large sample of normal adolescents found that 11% of boys and 15% of girls reported substantial numbers of physical symptoms (Garrick et al. 1988). The presence of excessive physical symptoms in these adolescents was significantly correlated with disturbances of self-concept as measured by a variety of scales (Garrick et al. 1988). No attempt was made to correlate these findings with histories of abuse in these children, however.

Conversion Disorder and Somatization Disorder in Childhood

Procter (1958) described 25 cases of conversion and "dissociative reactions" in 191 unselected admissions to the child psychiatric unit of the University of North Carolina Medical School. Sexual themes were prominent in some of the symptoms: a 10-year-old boy with tic-like pelvic thrusting who requested circumcision; another boy with recurrent dissociative reactions who ran down the ward in a trance-like state, holding his testicles and screaming. No specific case material is presented in detail, but Procter noted the frequent coexistence of a highly repressive fundamentalist religious culture in many families, combined with incestuous sexual overstimulation, such as children sleeping with parents of the opposite sex into adulthood. Child abuse was not specifically discussed, however.

Hardwick and Fitzpatrick (1981) described development of pseudocyesis in a 15-year-old girl. She herself denied a history of incest, but her symptoms began in the context of the death of her older sister's handicapped child. This child was reportedly the product of an incestuous pregnancy with the patient's violent, brutal alcoholic father. Possible pseudoseizures or amnesia episodes ("blackouts") were also noted in this patient. Royal and Goodwin (1982) also reported two cases of pseudocyesis occurring in adolescent incest victims.

Volkmar et al. (1984) described a retrospective study of 30 children with conversion disorder compared to a control group with adjustment disorder. Twenty-one children in the conversion group were thought to have "sexual stressors" prior to symptom onset, a proportion significantly higher than that found in controls. In "a majority" of these cases, molestation or sexual overstimulation by a relative represented the sexual stressor. Unfortunately, most patients terminated treatment when the sexual issues became the focus. No further details were given concerning the sexual stressors. The authors recommended more systematic prospective studies concerning sexually stressful events in the development of conversion symptoms in children and adolescents. They also suggested that clinicians seeing children with conversion disorders actively seek data on sexually traumatic experiences.

Livingston and Martin-Cannici (1985) reported on five children, ranging in age from 6 to 12, who met Research Diagnostic Criteria (RDC) (Spitzer et al. 1978) that was slightly modified and slightly modified DSM-III criteria (Feighner et al. 1972) for Briquet's syndrome and for somatization disorder, respectively. One 11-year-old-girl described having "another self whose name was a variant of hers and who 'does the bad things' " (p. 605). Another child, who had been chronically symptomatic for several years, reportedly first developed somatoform symptoms after seeing a man expose himself. Her mother was alcoholic and her father had engaged in antisocial activities. Child abuse histories were not reported by the authors.

Kreichman (1987) described 12 sibling pairs, each of whom developed a somatoform disorder. More than half of the children reported "sexually stressful events ranging from problematic sexual encounters and situations to sexual abuse, incest, and rape" (p. 228). Such events were reported by 75% of the girls and about a third of the boys, but the boys were thought to be underreporting sexual stresses. None of the children was thought to meet full criteria for posttraumatic stress disorder. The families of these children were seen as highly disturbed, with the mothers having severe personality disorders or somatization disorder and the fathers having alcoholism and antisocial traits. The author stressed the role of the somatoform symptoms in both concealing and revealing important family secrets, full disclosure of which tended to cause crises and withdrawal from treatment.

SOMATOFORM SYMPTOMS AS AN OUTCOME OF CHILDHOOD SEXUAL ABUSE

Somatoform symptoms are routinely reported as a sequela of childhood sexual abuse in a large number of case reports as well as in more systematic studies in the literature. Somatoform symptoms have been described in children shortly after the abuse experience as well as in adults many years after cessation of the sexual abuse (Adams-Tucker 1982; Browne and Finkelhor 1986; Dixon et al. 1978; Finkelhor 1987; Gelinas 1983; Goodwin 1982; Herman 1981; Meiselman 1978; Steele and Alexander 1981).

Reviewers of the child sexual abuse literature have pointed to methodological problems in many studies, including lack of uniformity in the definition of incest, difficulty in comparing data between clinical and nonclinical samples, problems in devising appropriate control groups, and variable use of standardized meausres (Browne and Finkelhor 1986; Meiselman 1978; Mrazek and Mrazek 1981; Schetky, Chapter 3, this volume). Somatization itself has infrequently been studied directly in the literature on the outcomes of childhood sexual abuse, probably because other behavioral and psychological disturbances seem more pressing than the somatic complaints of these patients.

Adults

Meiselman (1978) described 58 female psychotherapy patients who reported incest experiences and compared them to a control group. The sample was drawn from a large urban prepaid group health plan with a diverse social class and ethnic makeup. At intake, 52% of the incest victims reported physical problems among their chief complaints, as compared with 30% of the controls. It was not noted, however, whether the physical problems were thought to have a bona fide medical basis.

Donaldson and Gardner (1985) reported an uncontrolled study of the symptoms of posttraumatic stress disorder in 26 adult women with a history of incest. A "history of quasi-medical complaints" was found in 23% of the women, ranking behind only suicidal behavior and alcohol abuse in the list of their prior psychiatric symptomatology.

In a prospective study of 66 female psychiatric patients, Bryer et al. (1987) found that 59% reported a history of physical abuse, sexual abuse, or both before the age of 16. Abuse had occurred primarily within the family. On the SCL-90-R (Derogatis 1983), the somatization score was significantly higher for all three abused groups compared to the nonabused group. A similar trend was noted on the somatoform subscale of the Millon Clinical Multiaxial Inventory (Millon 1983).

Herman and Schatzow (1987) stated that somatoform disorders such as conversion disorder are more common in incest victims who utilize dissociative defenses. The authors presented data showing that amnesia and dissociation of abuse experiences tend to occur more often in patients who have been more violently or intrusively abused. Systematic data on somatization was not presented, however, although a case of a patient with pseudoseizures was described.

King (1986) reported on somatic dysfunction in 60 women with a history of incest. Somatic symptoms as rated by the Wahler Physical Symptoms Inventory (Wahler 1968) were significantly related to the invasiveness of the abuse. Those reporting intercourse and penetration had the highest scores on the inventory. Subjects reporting penetration without actual intercourse had the highest levels of total physical complaints.

Children

Kaufman et al. (1954) reported on incest in 11 girls ages 10 to 17 whose fathers had been incarcerated because of the child abuse. Four had somatic complaints such as abdominal distress and "generalized aches and pains." Several of the girls were thought to seek out painful medical procedures as a form of punishment. An 11-year-old patient oscillated between hypermaturity, severe rage reactions, and regression to an apparent 3-year-old state asking for her "mummy."

Lewis and Sarrel (1969) described the outcome of incest and other sexually traumatic experiences in childhood, relating trauma to developmental stages from infancy through adolescence. The cases came from patients seen in psychiatric treatment or consultation. Abdominal pain, psychogenic vomiting, and other somatic symptoms were described in many of the patients. One little girl with a history of abuse had undergone invasive medical procedures for abdominal pain without an organic cause having been found.

Frederick (1986) reported on 15 cases of posttraumatic stress disorder in preadolescent and adolescent boys sexually victimized by two male physicians. Subjects were studied in-depth with a variety of standardized measures. The author also summarized his data from other studies of sexually abused children with posttraumatic stress disorder. He reported "psychophysiological disturbances," including headaches, abdominal pain, and enuresis in his sample. He noted that somatization disorder can be found in victims of childhood molestation but provided no systematic data about this.

Gomes-Schwartz et al. (1985), reporting on behavioral and psychological problems in 112 children from preschool age to adolescence who had been sexually abused, described negative findings with respect to somatization. Most children were victims of repeated intrafamilial abuse and most had had intercourse, oral-genital contact, or other sorts of penetration, although a considerable range of sexual abuse experiences were noted in the children. Abused children were compared on the Louisville Behavior Checklist (Miller 1981) to a normal population and to a "clinical sample" of disturbed children receiving psychiatric services. In two groups of abused children ages 4 to 6 and 7 to 13 years old, respectively, "somatic behavior" on the inventory was not significantly different from the normal controls but was significantly *less* than for the clinical sample. Ratings for many other behavioral abnormalities were significantly higher in the abused group compared to the normal controls, but many were less severe compared to the clinical sample.

There are also many case reports in both the child-adolescent and adult literatures describing somatoform disorders in patients with a prior history of incest. Generally, these include patients meeting criteria for conversion disorder and somatoform pain disorder. Common somatoform symptoms included paralysis, gait disturbance, pseudoseizures, headache, abdominal pain, and pelvic pain (e.g., Dixon et al. 1978; Goodwin 1982; Krieger et al. 1980; Mrazek and Kempe 1981; Peters 1976; Weeks 1976).

DISCUSSION

A large number of studies from diverse sources going back over a century indicate a relationship between a history of childhood abuse—primarily sexual abuse—and somatoform disorders. The literature on this issue, however, is a mixture of case reports, uncontrolled and controlled studies, and retrospective and prospective accounts with differing methodologies.

The development of the somatoform disorders is a complex process. All child abuse victims probably do not develop a somatoform disorder, and it is highly unlikely that every patient with a somatoform disorder has had a history of child abuse. In addition, in somatizing patients from highly disturbed, globally abusive families, the effects of sexual abuse per se must be differentiated from those of other factors. On the other hand, in most studies where childhood sexual abuse was reported in association with somatization, no systematic effort had been made to elicit a history of abuse. Since the uncovering of child abuse generally requires active, and often longitudinal, inquiries by the investigator (Goodwin 1982; Goodwin et al. 1981; Herman 1981), these studies may well have underreported the prevalence of abuse. The prospective controlled studies using standardized inventories and more structured history taking about child abuse do show a higher prevalence of histories of abuse as well as a significant relationship between adult somatization and reported antecedent abuse (Bryer et al. 1987; Draijer 1989; Haber and Sitley 1987; Harrop-Griffiths et al. 1987; Walker et al. 1988). One controlled study in children, however, did not demonstrate a significant difference in somatization in a population of abused children compared with controls, at least on the behavioral checklist used (Gomes-Schwartz et al. 1985).

From a clinical perspective, this review supports the importance of acquiring data on child abuse in all patients presenting with somatoform disorders. Many recent reports support Freud's early idea that, in a number of patients, somatoform symptoms represent disguised symbolic communication ultimately related to memories of prior childhood experiences of sexual trauma and abuse. In addition, it is likely that memories of physical abuse experiences can also be encoded in this fashion.

It is beyond the scope of this report to attempt a comprehensive account of the psychological processes involved in these phenomena. Theories of conversion and somatization (Cloninger 1986; Ford 1983; Krohn 1978; Lazare 1981; Rangell 1959), the psychobiology of dissociation (Hilgard 1977; Putnam 1985, 1986), family systems (Avery 1982; Kreichman 1987; Krugman 1986), trauma and affects (Krystal 1978; van der Kolk 1986), and the impact of severe trauma on specific psychosexual and cognitive developmental phases (Eth and Pynoos 1985; Fish-Murray 1986; Goodwin 1982; Rothstein 1986; Terr 1983) all must be taken into account to understand the process more fully.

In addition, many patients with somatoform disorders will have a configuration of psychological difficulties also frequently described in victims of childhood sexual abuse. These include low self-esteem, negative self-identity, depression, suicide attempts, substance abuse, marital conflicts, and sexual problems (Bagley and Ramsay 1986; Browne and Finkelhor 1986; Gelinas 1983; Goodwin 1982; Herman 1981; Jehu and Gazan 1983; Meiselman 1978; Steele and Alexander 1981). Some of these patients may also meet criteria for posttraumatic stress disorder or a dissociative disorder. Specific treatment interventions related to the psychological consequences of child abuse are often helpful (Coons 1986; Goodwin 1982; Herman 1981). In addition, at least two studies suggest that child abuse victims may overuse medical services because of somatoform symptoms (Haber and Sitley 1987; Walker et al. 1988). Thus identification of these patients may permit more appropriate interventions to help them and to reduce the burden they place on the medical system.

Systematic research is also needed to study the association of child abuse and somatization. This can be done from the perspective of investigating abuse histories in patients meeting criteria for somatoform disorders as well as looking at the prevalence of somatoform disorders in abuse victims. Specifically, it would appear useful to devise controlled, prospective studies of incest in patients with pseudoseizures, both with and without concurrent true epilepsy. Physical abuse should also be considered as a variable, especially in male pseudoseizure patients, since childhood sexual abuse is thought to be much less common in males (Finkelhor 1984). In creating such studies, careful attention must be paid to defining specific study populations to minimize heterogeneity of the sample.

The evidence also seems compelling that an antecedent history of childhood sexual abuse should be studied as one of the important environmental factors related to the development of Briquet's syndrome/somatization disorder. Child abuse may be an etiologic factor in development of this disorder or, at least, the cause of a substantial unrecognized comorbidity in at least 25% to 50% of these patients. Another issue to be resolved is the relationship of somatization disorder with significant amnesia to the dissociative and posttraumatic stress disorders. Some of these patients may more parsimoniously receive a primary diagnosis of a dissociative disorder or chronic childhood-onset posttraumatic stress disorder with the somatization viewed as secondary to traumatization (Frederick 1986; Kreichman 1987; Krystal 1978). Other patients may be better conceptualized as having more than one disorder.

Multigenerational child abuse also should be considered as a variable in the reported familial association of Briquet's syndrome/somatization disorder, antisocial personality disorder, and attention-deficit disorder. Clearly all future studies seeking to separate genetic from environmental factors in the familial transmission of these conditions should control for histories of child abuse and trauma in the subjects.

The etiologic significance of childhood abuse, mistreatment, and trauma in the development of somatoform disorders was described by both Briquet and Freud. For different reasons, the importance of this observation has been relatively neglected by their followers. We should now begin to pursue more fully their insights concerning psychological trauma and somatization.

REFERENCES

Adams-Tucker C: Proximate effects of sexual abuse in childhood: a report on 28 children. Am J Psychiatry 139:1252–1256, 1982

American Psychiatric Association: Diagnostic and Statistical Manual of Mental Disorders, 3rd Edition. Washington, DC, American Psychiatric Association, 1980

American Psychiatric Association: Diagnostic and Statistical Manual of Mental

Disorders, 3rd Edition, Revised. Washington, DC, American Psychiatric Association, 1987

Anthony EJ: Hysteria in childhood, in Hysteria. Edited by Roy A. Chichester, New York, John Wiley, 1982, pp 145–164

Arkonac O, Guze SB: A family study of hysteria. N Engl J Med 268; 239–242, 1963

Avery NC: Family secrets. Psychoanal Rev 69:471–486, 1982

Bagley C, Ramsay R: Sexual abuse in childhood: psychosocial outcomes and implications for social work practice. Social Work in Human Sexuality 4:33–48, 1986

Barsky AJ, Klerman GL: Overview: hypochondriasis, bodily complaints, and somatic styles. Am J Psychiatry 140:273–283, 1983

Bliss EL: Multiple Personality, Allied Disorders and Hypnosis. New York, Oxford University Press, 1986

Bohman M, Cloninger CR, Sigvardsson S, et al: An adoption study of somatoform disorders, III: cross-fostering analysis and genetic relationship to alcoholism and criminality. Arch Gen Psychiatry 41:872–878, 1984

Breuer J, Freud S: Studies in hysteria (1893–1895), in The Standard Edition of the Complete Psychological Works of Sigmund Freud, Vol 2. Translated and edited by Strachey J. London, Hogarth Press, 1958

Briquet P: Traite de l'Hysterie. Paris, J Bailliere, 1859

Browne A, Finkelhor D: Impact of child sexual abuse: a review of the research. Psychol Bull 99:66–77, 1986

Bryer JB, Nelson BA, Miller JG, et al: Childhood sexual and physical abuse as factors in adult psychiatric illness. Am J Psychiatry 144:1426–1430, 1987

Cantwell DP: Psychiatric illnesses in the families of hyperactive children. Arch Gen Psychiatry 27:414–417, 1972

Cassem NH: Functional somatic symptoms and somatoform disorders, in Massachusetts General Hospital Handbook of General Hospital Psychiatry, 2nd Edition. Edited by Hackett T, Cassem NH. Littleton, MA, PSG Publishers, 1987, pp 126–153

Chodoff P: Hysteria and women. Am J Psychiatry 139:543–551, 1982

Chodoff P, Lyons H: Hysteria, the hysterical personality and "hysterical" conversion. Am J Psychiatry 114:734–740, 1958

Cleghorn RA: Hysteria: multiple manifestations of semantic confusion. Canadian Psychiatric Association Journal 14:539–551, 1969

Cloninger CR: Somatoform and dissociative disorders, in The Medical Basis of Psychiatry. Edited by Winokur G, Clayton P. Philadelphia, PA, WB Saunders, 1986, pp 123–151

Cloninger CR, Guze SB: Female criminals: their personal, familial, and social backgrounds: the relation of these to the diagnosis of sociopathy and hysteria. Arch Gen Psychiatry 23:554–558, 1970a

Cloninger CR, Guze SB: Psychiatric illness and female criminality: the role of sociopathy and hysteria in the antisocial woman. Am J Psychiatry 127:79–87, 1970b

Cloninger CR, Reich T, Guze SB: The multifactorial model of disease transmission, III: familial relationship between sociopathy and hysteria (Briquet's syndrome). Br J Psychiatry 127:23–32, 1975

Cloninger CR, Sigvardsson S, von Knorring AL, et al: An adoption study of somatoform disorders, II: identification of two discrete somatoform disorders. Arch Gen Psychiatry 41:863–871, 1984

Cloninger CR, Martin RL, Guze SB, et al: A prospective follow-up and family study of somatization in men and women. Am J Psychiatry 143:873–878, 1986

Coons PM: Treatment progress in 20 patients with multiple personality disorder. J Nerv Ment Dis 174:715–721, 1986

Coryell W: A blind family history study of Briquet's syndrome. Arch Gen Psychiatry 37:1266–1269, 1980

Davies RK: Incest: some neuropsychiatric findings. Int J Psychiatry Med 9:117–121, 1979

Derogatis LR: SCL-90-R Administration, Scoring, and Procedures Manual, II. Towson, MD, Clinical Psychometric Research, 1983

DeSouza C, Othmer E: Somatization and Briquet's syndrome: an assessment of their diagnostic concordance. Arch Gen Psychiatry 41:334–336, 1984

Dixon KN, Arnold LE, Calestro K: Father-son incest: underreported psychiatric problem? Am J Psychiatry 135:835–838, 1978

Donaldson MA, Gardner R: Diagnosis and treatment of traumatic stress among women after childhood incest, in Trauma and Its Wake. Edited by Figley CR. New York, Brunner/Mazel, 1985, pp 356–377

Draijer N: Long-term psychosomatic consequences of child sexual abuse, in The Free Woman: Women's Health in the 1990's. Edited by vanHall EV, Everaerd W. Cornforth (UK), The Parthenon Publishing Group, 1989, pp 696–709

Dubowitz V, Hersov V: Management of children with non-organic (hysterical) disorders of motor function. Dev Med Child Neurol 18:358–368, 1976

Ellenberger HF: The Discovery of the Unconscious. New York, Basic Books, 1970

Erikson E: Reality and actuality: an address. J Am Psychoanal Assoc 10:451–474, 1962

Eth S, Pynoos RS: Post-Traumatic Stress Disorder in Children. Washington, DC, American Psychiatric Association, 1985

Ey H: History and analysis of the concept, in Hysteria. Edited by Roy A. New York, John Wiley, 1982, pp 3–20

Farley J, Woodruff RA, Guze SB: The prevalence of hysteria and conversion symptoms. Br J Psychiatry 114:1121–1125, 1968

Feighner JP, Robins E, Guze SB, et al: Diagnostic criteria for use in psychiatric research. Arch Gen Psychiatry 26:57–63, 1972

Ferenczi S: Confusion of tongues between adults and the child (1933), in Final Contributions to the Problems and Methods of Psychoanalysis. New York, Basic Books, 1955, pp 155–167

Finkelhor D: Child Sexual Abuse: New Research and Theory. New York, Free Press, 1984

Finkelhor D: The sexual abuse of children: current research reviewed. Psychiatric Annals 17:233–241, 1987

Fish-Murray CC, Koby EV, van der Kolk BA: Evolving ideas: the effect of abuse on children's thought, in Psychological Trauma. Edited by van der Kolk BA. Washington, DC, American Psychiatric Press, 1986, pp 89–110

Ford CV: The Somatizing Disorders: Illness as a Way of Life. New York, Amsterdam, Elsevier Biomedical, 1983

Ford CV: The somatizing disorders. Psychosomatics 27:327–337, 1986

Ford CV, Folks DG: Conversion disorders: an overview. Psychosomatics 26:371–383, 1985

Frederick CJ: Post-traumatic stress disorder and child molestation, in Sexual Exploitation of Patients by Health Professionals. Edited by Burgess AW, Hartman CR. New York, Praeger, 1986, pp 133–142

Freud A: A psychoanalyst's view of sexual abuse by parents, in Sexually Abused Children and Their Families. Edited by Mrazek PB, Kempe CH. Oxford, Pergamon, 1981, pp 33–34

Freud S: On the psychical mechanism of hysterical phenomena: lecture (1893), in The Standard Edition of the Complete Psychological Works of Sigmund Freud, Vol 3. Translated and edited by Strachey J. London, Hogarth Press, 1958, pp 25–39

Freud S: The aetiology of hysteria (1896a), in The Standard Edition of the Complete Psychological Works of Sigmund Freud, Vol 3. Translated and edited by Strachey J. London, Hogarth Press, 1958, pp 187–221

Freud S: Further remarks on the neuropsychoses of defense (1896b), in The Standard Edition of the Complete Psychological Works of Sigmund Freud, Vol 3. Translated and edited by Strachey J. London, Hogarth Press, 1958, pp 157–185

Freud S: Heredity and the etiology of the neuroses (1896c), in The Standard Edition of the Complete Psychological Works of Sigmund Freud, Vol 3. Translated and edited by Strachey J. London, Hogarth Press, 1958, pp 141–156

Freud S: Fragment of an analysis of a case of hysteria (1905a), in The Standard Edition of the Complete Psychological Works of Sigmund Freud, Vol 7. Translated and edited by Strachey J. London, Hogarth Press, 1958, pp 3–122

Freud S: Three essays on the theory of sexuality (1905b), in The Standard Edition of the Complete Psychological Works of Sigmund Freud, Vol 7. Translated and edited by Strachey J. London, Hogarth Press, 1958, pp 125–243

Freud S: On the history of the psychoanalytic movement (1914), in The Standard Edition of the Complete Psychological Works of Sigmund Freud, Vol 14. Translated and edited by Strachey J. London, Hogarth Press, 1958, pp 3–66

Freud S: Introductory lectures on psychoanalysis, Part III: general theory of neurosis (1917), in The Standard Edition of the Complete Psychological Works of Sigmund Freud, Vol 16. Translated and edited by Strachey J. London, Hogarth Press, 1958, pp 358–377

Freud S: From the history of an infantile neurosis (1918), in The Standard Edition of the Complete Psychological Works of Sigmund Freud, Vol 17. Translated and edited by Strachey J. London, Hogarth Press, 1958, pp 3–122

Freud S: An autobiographical study (1925), in The Standard Edition of the Complete Psychological Works of Sigmund Freud, Vol 20. Translated and edited by Strachey J. London, Hogarth Press, 1958, pp 3–74

Freud S: Female sexuality (1931), in The Standard Edition of the Complete Psychological Works of Sigmund Freud, Vol 21. Translated and edited by Strachey J. London, Hogarth Press, 1958, pp 221–243

Freud S: New introductory lectures on psychoanalysis (1933), in The Standard Edition of the Complete Psychological Works of Sigmund Freud, Vol 22. Translated and edited by Strachey J. London, Hogarth Press, 1958, pp 1–182

Freud S: The Origins of Psychoanalysis: Letters to Wilhelm Fliess, Drafts and Notes: 1887–1902. Edited by Bonaparte M, Freud A, Kris A. New York, Basic Books, 1954

Furst SS: Psychic Trauma. New York, Basic Books, 1967

Galdston R: The domestic dimensions of violence. Psychoanal Study Child 36:391–414, 1981

Garcia EE: Freud's seduction theory. Psychoanal Study Child 42:443–469, 1987

Garrick T, Ostrov E, Offer D: Physical symptoms and self-image in a group of normal adolescents. Psychosomatics 29:73–80, 1988

Gelinas D: The persisting negative effects of incest. Psychiatry 46:312–332, 1983

Gomes-Schwartz G, Horowitz JM, Sauzier M: Severity of emotional distress among sexually abused preschool, school-age, and adolescent children. Hosp Community Psychiatry 36:503–508, 1985

Goodwin DW, Guze SB: Psychiatric Diagnosis, 2nd Edition. New York, Oxford University Press, 1979

Goodwin J: Sexual Abuse: Incest Victims and Their Families. Boston, MA, Wright/PSG, 1982

Goodwin J: Credibility problems in multiple personality disorder patients and abused children, in Childhood Antecedents of Multiple Personality. Edited by Kluft RP. Washington, DC, American Psychiatric Press, 1985, pp 1–19

Goodwin J, Geil C: Why physicians should report child abuse: the example of sexual abuse, in Sexual Abuse: Incest Victims and Their Families. Edited by Goodwin J. Boston, Wright/PSG, 1982, pp 155–168

Goodwin J, Simms M, Bergman R: Hysterical seizures: a sequel to incest. Am J Orthopsychiatry 49:698–703, 1979

Goodwin J, McCarthy T, DiVasto P: Prior incest in mothers of abused children. Child Abuse Negl 5:87–95, 1981

Goodyer IM: Epileptic and pseudoepileptic seizures in childhood and adolescence. J Am Acad Child Psychiatry 24:3–9, 1985

Greenacre P: The influence of infantile trauma on genetic patterns, in Psychic Trauma. Edited by Furst SS. New York, Basic Books, 1967, pp 108–153

Gross M: Incestuous rape: a cause for hysterical seizures in four adolescent girls. Am J Orthopsychiatry 49:704–708, 1979

Gross RJ, Doerr H, Caldirola D, et al: Borderline syndrome and incest in chronic pelvic pain patients. Int J Psychiatry Med 10:79–96, 1980–1981

Groth NA: Sexual trauma in the life histories of rapists and child molesters. Victimology 4:10–16, 1979

Guze SB: Conversion symptoms in criminals. Am J Psychiatry 121:580–583, 1964

Guze SB: The diagnosis of hysteria: what are we trying to do? Am J Psychiatry 124:491–498, 1967

Guze SB, Wolfgram ED, McKinney JE, et al: Psychiatric illness in the families of convicted criminals: a study of 519 first-degree relatives. Diseases of the Nervous System 28:651–659, 1967

Guze SB, Woodruff RA, Clayton PJ: Hysteria and antisocial behavior: further evidence of an association. Am J Psychiatry 127:957–960, 1971

Guze SB, Woodruff RA, Clayton PJ: Sex, age, and the diagnosis of hysteria (Briquet's syndrome). Am J Psychiatry 129:745–748, 1972

Haber JD, Sitley KN: The identification of abuse in a chronic care setting. Paper presented at the conference on Mental Disorders in General Health Care Settings: A Research Conference, Seattle, WA, June 1987

Hardwick PJ, Fitzpatrick C: Fear, folie and phantom pregnancy: pseudocyesis in a fifteen year old girl. Br J Psychiatry 139:558–560, 1981

Harrop-Griffiths J, Katon W, Walker E: Chronic pelvic pain: the relationship to psychiatric diagnosis and childhood sexual abuse. Paper presented at the conference on Mental Disorders in General Health Care Settings: A Research Conference, Seattle, WA, June 1987

Heffron WM, Martin CA, Welsh RJ, et al: Hyperactivity and child abuse. Can J Psychiatry 32:384–386, 1987

Herman JL: Father-Daughter Incest. Cambridge, MA, Harvard University Press, 1981

Herman J, Schatzow E: Recovery and verification of memories of childhood sexual trauma. Psychoanalytic Psychology 4:1–14, 1987

Herzog DB, Jellinek MS: Child psychiatric consultation, in Massachusetts General Hospital Handbook of General Hospital Psychiatry, 2nd Edition. Edited by Hackett TP, Cassem NH. Littleton, MA, PSG Publishers, 1987, pp 477–495

Hilgard ER: Divided Consciousness: Multiple Controls in Human Thought and Action. New York, John Wiley, 1977

Hosch IA: Munchausen by proxy. American Journal of Maternal Child Nursing 12:48–52, 1987

James J, Meyerding J: Early sexual experience and prostitution. Am J Psychiatry 134:1381–1385, 1977

Jehu D, Gazan M: Psychosocial adjustment of women who were sexually victimized in childhood or adolescence. Canadian Journal of Community Mental Health 2:71–82, 1983

Jones E: The Life and Work of Sigmund Freud, Vol 1. New York, Basic Books, 1953

Jones FD, Hales RE: Military combat psychiatry: a historical review. Psychiatric Annals 17:525–528, 1987

Jones JG, Butler HL, Hamilton B, et al: Munchausen syndrome by proxy. Child Abuse Negl 10:33–40, 1986

Kaminsky MJ, Slavney PR: Methodology and personality in Briquet's syndrome: a reappraisal. Am J Psychiatry 133:85–88, 1976

Kardiner A: The Traumatic Neuroses of War. New York, Paul B. Hoeber, 1941

Katon W, Egan K, Miller D: Chronic pain: lifetime psychiatric diagnosis and family history. Am J Psychiatry 142:1156–1160, 1985

Kaufman I, Peck AL, Tagiuri CK: The family constellation and overt incestuous relations between father and daughter. Am J Orthopsychiatry 24:266–279, 1954

Kellner R: Functional somatic symptoms and hypochondriasis: a survey of empirical studies. Arch Gen Psychiatry 42:821–833, 1985

Kenyon FE: Hypochondriacal states. Br J Psychiatry 129:1–14, 1976

Kernberg O: Borderline Conditions and Pathological Narcissism. New York, Jason Aronson, 1975

King EJ: Analysis of somatic dysfunction in adult survivors of father-daughter incest. Unpublished doctoral dissertation, Hofstra University, New York, 1986

Kluft RP (ed): Childhood Antecedents of Multiple Personality. Washington, DC, American Psychiatric Press, 1985

Kluft RP: Unsuspected multiple personality disorder: an uncommon source of protracted resistance, interruption, and failure in psychoanalysis. Hillside Clin Psychiatry 9:100–115, 1987a

Kluft RP: Update on multiple personality disorder. Hosp Community Psychiatry 38:363–373, 1987b

Kreichman AM: Siblings with somatoform disorders in childhood and adolescence. J Am Acad Child Adolesc Psychiatry 26:226–231, 1987

Kretschmer E: Hysteria, Reflex, and Instinct. New York, Philosophical Library, 1960

Krieger MJ, Rosenfeld AA, Gordon A, et al: Problems in the psychotherapy of children with histories of incest. Am J Psychother 34:81–88, 1980

Krohn A: Hysteria: the elusive neurosis. Psychol Issues Monograph 45/46, 1978

Kroll P, Chamberlain KR, Halpern J: The diagnosis of Briquet's syndrome in a male population. J Nerv Ment Dis 167:171–174, 1979

Krugman S: Trauma in the family: perspectives on the intergenerational transmission of violence, in Psychological Trauma. Edited by van der Kolk B. Washington, DC, American Psychiatric Press, 1986, pp 127–151

Krystal H: Trauma and affects. Psychoanal Study Child 38:81–117, 1978

Kubie LS: Manual of emergency treatment for acute war neuroses. War Medicine 4:582–598, 1943

LaBarbera JD, Dozier JED: Hysterical seizures: the role of sexual exploitation. Psychosomatics 21:897–903, 1980

Lazare A: The hysterical character in psychoanalytic theory: evolution and confusion. Arch Gen Psychiatry 25:131–137, 1971

Lazare A: Conversion symptoms. N Engl J Med 305:745–748, 1981

Leigh H (ed): Psychiatry in the Practice of Medicine. Menlo Park, CA, Addison-Wesley, 1983

Lewis M, Sarrel PM: Some psychological aspects of seduction, incest, and rape in childhood. J Am Acad Child Adolesc Psychiatry 8:606–619, 1969

Lewis WC, Berman M: Studies of conversion hysteria. Arch Gen Psychiatry 13:275–282, 1965

Libow JA, Schreier HA: Three forms of factitious illness in children: when is it Munchausen syndrome by proxy? Am J Orthopsychiatry 56:602–611, 1986

Lilienfeld SO, Valkenburg CV, Larntz K, et al: The relationship of histrionic personality disorder to antisocial personality disorder and somatization disorder. Am J Psychiatry 143:718–722, 1986

Liske E, Forster FM: Pseudoseizures: a problem in the diagnosis and management of epileptic patients. Neurology 14:41–49, 1964

Livingston R, Martin-Cannici C: Multiple somatic complaints and possible somatization disorder in prepubertal children. J Am Acad Child Adolesc Psychiatry 24:603–607, 1985

Loewenstein RJ: Anna O: Transference and countertransference acting out. Paper presented at the Annual Meeting of the American Psychiatric Association, San Francisco, CA, May 1989

Loewenstein RJ, Putnam FW, Duffy C, et al: Males with multiple personality disorder. Proceedings of the 3rd International Conference on Multiple Personality/Dissociative States (abstract), Chicago, 1986

Mai FM, Merskey H: Briquet's treatise on hysteria: a synopsis and commentary. Arch Gen Psychiatry 37:1401–1405, 1980

Mai FM, Merskey H: Briquet's concept of hysteria: an historical perspective. Can J Psychiatry 26:57–63, 1981

Marmer S: Psychoanalysis of multiple personality disorder. Int J Psychoanal 61:439–451, 1980

Martin RL, Cloninger RC, Guze SB: The evaluation of diagnostic concordance in follow-up studies, II: a blind, prospective follow-up of female criminals. J Psychiatr Res 15:107–125, 1979

Masson JM: The Assault on Truth. New York, Farrar, Strauss, & Giroux, 1983

Meadow R: Munchausen by proxy: the hinterland of child abuse. Lancet 2:343–345, 1977

Meadow R: Fictitious epilepsy. Lancet 2:25–28, 1984

Mears R, Horvath T: "Acute" and "chronic" hysteria. Br J Psychiatry 121:653–657, 1972

Meiselman KC: Incest: A Psychological Study of Causes and Effects with Treatment Recommendations. San Francisco, CA, Jossey-Bass, 1978

Merskey H: The Analysis of Hysteria. London, Bailliere Tindall, 1979

Miller LC: Louisville Behavior Checklist. Los Angeles, CA, Western Psychological Services, 1981

Millon T: Millon Clinical Multiaxial Inventory, 3rd Edition. Minneapolis, MN, Interpretive Scoring Systems, 1983

Mogielnicki RP, Mogielnicki NP, Chandler JE, et al: Impending child abuse: psychosomatic symptoms in adults as a clue. JAMA 237:1109–1111, 1977

Monson RA, Smith GR: Somatization disorder in primary care. N Engl J Med 308:1464–1465, 1983

Morrant JCA: In defense of Sigmund Freud against Masson's charge of cowardice. Can J Psychiatry 30:395–399, 1985

Morrison J: Childhood sexual histories in women with somatization disorder. Am J Psychiatry 146:239–241, 1989

Mrazek PB, Kempe CH: Sexually Abused Children and Their Families. Oxford, Pergamon, 1981

Mrazek PB, Mrazek DA: The effects of child sexual abuse: methodological considerations, in Sexually Abused Children and Their Families. Edited by Mrazek PB, Kempe CH. Oxford, Pergamon, 1981, pp 235–246

Orenstein DM, Wasserman AL: Munchausen syndrome by proxy simulating cystic fibrosis. Pediatrics 78:621–624, 1986

Othmer E, DeSouza C: A screening test for somatization disorder (hysteria). Am J Psychiatry 142:1146–1149, 1985

Oxman TE, Rosenberg SD, Schnurr PP, et al: Linguistic dimensions of affect and thought in somatization disorder. Am J Psychiatry 142:1150–1155, 1985

Perley MJ, Guze SB: Hysteria—the stability and usefulness of clinical criteria. N Engl J Med 266:421–426, 1962

Peters JJ: Children who are victims of sexual assault and the psychology of offenders. Am J Psychother 30:398–421, 1976

Prince M: The Dissociation of a Personality: A Biographical Study in Abnormal Psychology. New York, Longmans Green Co, 1905

Procter J: Hysteria in childhood. Am J Orthopsychiatry 28:394–407, 1958

Purtell JJ, Robins E, Cohen ME: Observations on clinical aspects of hysteria: quantitative study of 50 hysteria patients and 156 control subjects. JAMA 146:902–909, 1951

Putnam FW: Dissociation as a response to extreme trauma, in Childhood Antecedents of Multiple Personality. Edited by Kluft RP. Washington, DC, American Psychiatric Press, 1985, pp 65–97

Putnam FW: The scientific investigation of multiple personality disorder, in Split Minds, Split Brains: Historical and Current Perspectives. Edited by Quen JM. New York, New York University Press, 1986, pp 109–125

Putnam FW, Guroff JJ, Silberman EK, et al: The clinical phenomenology of multiple personality disorder: 100 recent cases. J Clin Psychiatry 47:285–293, 1986

Rangell L: The nature of conversion. J Am Psychoanal Assoc 7:632–662, 1959

Richtsmeier AJ, Waters DB: Somatic symptoms as family myth. Am J Dis Child 139:855–857, 1984

Robins E, Purtell JJ, Cohen ME: "Hysteria" in men: a controlled study of 38 patients so diagnosed and 194 control subjects. N Engl J Med 246:667–685, 1952

Robins LN: Deviant Children Grow Up. Baltimore, Williams & Wilkins, 1966

Robins LN, Helzer JE, Croughan J, et al: National Institute of Mental Health Diagnostic Interview Schedule. Arch Gen Psychiatry 38:381–389, 1981

Rothstein A (ed): The Reconstruction of Trauma: Its Significance in Clinical Work. New York, International Universities Press, 1986

Roy A: Psychiatric concepts: definitions and diagnosis of hysterical seizures, in Pseudoseizures. Edited by Riley TL, Roy A. Baltimore, MD, Williams & Wilkins, 1982b, pp 135–147

Roybal L, Goodwin J: The incest pregnancy, in Sexual Abuse: Incest Victims and Their Families. Edited by Goodwin J. Boston, MA, Wright/PSG, 1982, pp 125–138

Russell DEH: The incidence and prevalence of intrafamilial and extrafamilial sexual abuse of female children. Child Abuse Negl 7:133–146, 1983

Russell DEH: The Secret Trauma: Incest in the Lives of Girls and Women. New York, Basic Books, 1986

Schilder P: The concept of hysteria. Am J Psychiatry 95:1389–1413, 1939

Shengold LL: Child abuse and deprivation: soul murder. J Am Psychoanal Assoc 27:533–561, 1979

Sigvardsson S, von Knorring AL, Bohman M, et al: An adoption study of somatoform disorders, I: the relationship of somatization to psychiatric disability. Arch Gen Psychiatry 41:853–859, 1984

Silbert MH, Pines AM: Sexual child abuse as an antecedent to prostitution. Child Abuse Negl 5:407–411, 1981

Slater E: Diagnosis of "hysteria." Br Med J 1:1395–1399, 1965

Slater E: What is hysteria?, in Hysteria. Edited by Roy A. New York, John Wiley, 1982, pp 37–40

Slater ETO, Glithero E: A follow-up of patients diagnosed as suffering from "hysteria." J Psychosom Res 9:9–13, 1961

Slipp S: Interpersonal factors in hysteria: Freud's seduction theory and the case of Dora. J Am Acad Psychoanal 5:359–376, 1977

Smith GR, Monson RA, Ray DC: Psychiatric consultation in somatization disorder: a randomized controlled study. N Engl J Med 314:1407–1413, 1986

Spiegel D: Multiple personality disorder as a post-traumatic stress disorder. Psychiatr Clin North Am 7:101–110, 1984

Spitzer RL, Endicott J, Robins E: Research Diagnostic Criteria: rationale and reliability. Arch Gen Psychiatry 35:773–782, 1978

Standage KF: The etiology of hysterical seizures. Canadian Psychiatric Association Journal 20:67–73, 1975

Steele BF, Alexander H: Long-term effects of sexual abuse in childhood, in Sexually Abused Children and Their Families. Edited by Mrazek PB, Kempe CH. Oxford, Pergamon, 1981

Stefansson JG, Missina JA, Meyerowitz S: Hysterical neurosis, conversion type: clinical and epidemiological considerations. Acta Psychiatr Scand 53:119–138, 1976

Terr L: Chowchilla revisited: the effects of psychic trauma four years after a school-bus kidnapping. Am J Psychiatry 140:1543–1550, 1983

Van der Kolk B: Psychological Trauma. Washington, DC, American Psychiatric Press, 1986

Veith I: Hysteria: The History of a Disease. Chicago, IL, University of Chicago Press, 1965

Veith I: Four thousand years of hysteria, in Hysterical Personality. Edited by Horowitz MJ. New York, Jason Aronson, 1977

Volkmar FR, Poll J, Lewis M: Conversion reactions in childhood and adolescence. J Am Acad Child Adolesc Psychiatry 23:424–430, 1984

Wahler HJ: The Physical Symptoms Inventory: measuring levels of somatic complaining behavior. J Clin Psychology 24:207–211, 1968

Walker E, Katon W, Harrop-Griffiths J, et al: Relationship of chronic pelvic pain to psychiatric diagnoses and childhood sexual abuse. Am J Psychiatry 145:75–80, 1988

Warner R: The diagnosis of antisocial and hysterical personality disorders: an example of sex bias. J Nerv Ment Dis 166:839–845, 1978

Weeks RB: The sexually exploited child: South Med J 69:848–850, 1976

Woerner PL, Guze SB: A family and marital study of hysteria. Br J Psychiatry 114:161–168, 1968

Woodruff RA, Clayton PJ, Guze SB: Hysteria: studies of diagnosis, outcome, and prevalence. JAMA 215:425–428, 1971

Zeigler FJ, Imboden JB, Meyer E: Contemporary conversion reactions: a clinical study. Am J Psychiatry 116:901–910, 1960

Zoccolillo M, Cloninger CR: Parental breakdown associated with somatisation disorder (hysteria). Br J Psychiatry 147:443–446, 1985

APPENDIX.   DSM-III-R Somatoform Disorders

1. Diagnostic criteria for body dysmorphic disorder
   A. Preoccupation with some imagined defect in appearance in a normal-appearing person. If a slight physical anomaly is present, the person's concern is grossly excessive.
   B. The belief in the defect is not of delusional intensity, as in delusional disorder, somatic type (i.e., the person can acknowledge the possibility that he or she may be exaggerating the extent of the defect or that there may be no defect at all).
   C. Occurrence not exclusively during the course of anorexia nervosa or transexualism.
2. Diagnostic criteria for conversion disorder
   A. A loss of, or alteration in, physical functioning suggesting a physical disorder.
   B. Psychological factors are judged to be etiologically related to the symptom because of a temporal relationship between a psychosocial stressor that is apparently related to a psychological conflict or need and initiation or exacerbation of the symptom.
   C. The person is not conscious of intentionally producing the symptoms.
   D. The symptom is not a culturally sanctioned response pattern and cannot, after appropriate investigation, be explained by a known physical disorder.
   E. The symptom is not limited to pain or to a disturbance in sexual function.
   Specify: single episode or recurrent.
3. Diagnostic criteria for hypochondriasis
   A. Preoccupation with the fear of having, or the belief that one has, a serious disease, based on the person's interpretation of physical signs or sensations as evidence of physical illness.
   B. Appropriate physical evaluation does not support the diagnosis of any physical disorder that can account for the physical signs or sensations or the person's unwarranted interpretation of them, **and** the symptoms in A are not just symptoms of panic attacks.
   C. The fear of having, or belief that one has, a disease persists despite medical reassurance.
   D. Duration of the disturbance is at least six months.
   E. The belief in A is not of delusional intensity, as in delusional disorder, somatic type (i.e., the person can acknowledge the possibility that his or her fear of having, or belief that he or she has, a serious disease is unfounded).

---

4. Diagnostic criteria for somatization disorder
   A. A history of many physical complaints or a belief that one is sickly, beginning before the age of 30 and persisting for several years.
   B. At least 13 symptoms from the list below. To count a symptom as significant, the following criteria must be met:
      (1) no organic pathology or pathophysiologic mechanism (e.g., a physical disorder or the effects of injury, medication, drugs, or alcohol) to account for the symptom or, when there is related organic pathology, the complaint or resulting social or occupational impairment is grossly in excess of what would be expected from the physical findings
      (2) has not occurred only during a panic attack
      (3) has caused the person to take medicine (other than over-the-counter pain medication), see a doctor, or alter life-style

Symptom list:

Gastrointestinal symptoms:
   (1) **vomiting (other than during pregnancy)**
   (2) abdominal pain (other than when menstruating)
   (3) nausea (other than motion sickness)
   (4) bloating (gassy)
   (5) diarrhea
   (6) intolerance of (gets sick from) several different foods

Pain symptoms:
   (7) **pain in extremities**
   (8) back pain
   (9) joint pain
   (10) pain during urination
   (11) other pain (excluding headaches)

Cardiopulmonary symptoms:
   (12) **shortness of breath when not exerting oneself**
   (13) palpitations
   (14) chest pain
   (15) dizziness

Conversion or pseudoneurologic symptoms:
   (16) **amnesia**
   (17) **difficulty swallowing**
   (18) loss of voice
   (19) deafness
   (20) double vision
   (21) blurred vision

(22) blindness
(23) fainting or loss of consciousness
(24) seizure or convulsion
(25) trouble walking
(26) paralysis or muscle weakness
(27) urinary retention or difficulty urinating

Sexual symptoms for the major part of the person's life after opportunities for sexual activity:
(28) **burning sensation in sexual organs or rectum (other than during intercourse)**
(29) sexual indifference
(30) pain during intercourse
(31) impotence

Female reproductive symptoms judged by the person to occur more frequently or severely than in most women:
(32) **painful menstruation**
(33) irregular menstrual periods
(34) excessive menstrual bleeding
(35) vomiting throughout pregnancy

Note: The seven items in boldface may be used to screen for the disorder. The presence of two or more of these items suggests a high likelihood of the disorder.

5. Diagnostic criteria for somatoform pain disorder
   A. Preoccupation with pain for at least six months.
   B. Either (1) or (2):
      (1) appropriate evaluation uncovers no organic pathology or pathophysiologic mechanism (e.g., a physical disorder or the effects of injury) to account for the pain
      (2) when there is related organic pathology, the complaint of pain or resulting social or occupational impairment is grossly in excess of what would be expected from the physical findings

6. Diagnostic criteria for undifferentiated somatoform disorder
   A. One or more physical complaints, e.g., fatigue, loss of appetite, gastrointestinal or urinary complaints.
   B. Either (1) or (2):
      (1) appropriate evaluation uncovers no organic pathology or pathophysiologic mechanism (e.g., a physical disorder or the effects of injury, medication, drugs, or alcohol) to account for the physical complaints
      (2) when there is related organic pathology, the physical complaints or resulting social or occupational impairment is grossly in excess of what would be expected from the physical findings

C. Duration of the disturbance is at least six months.

D. Occurrence not exclusively during the course of another somatoform disorder, a sexual dysfunction, a mood disorder, an anxiety disorder, a sleep disorder, or a psychotic disorder.

CHAPTER 6

Disturbances of "Self" in Victims of Childhood Sexual Abuse

Frank W. Putnam, M.D.

In this chapter, I will discuss a conceptual model for understanding the array of symptoms and pathologic behaviors manifested by victims of childhood sexual abuse. While working with adults who were victims of childhood sexual abuse, I have repeatedly observed disturbances in what I would characterize as the person's self-representations. It is my premise that many of the symptoms and behaviors manifested by adult victims of childhood sexual abuse can be understood as expressions of disturbances in one or more of these representations of self; treatment must address these issues to be effective.

I will begin by briefly discussing self-representations and their developmental course in the individual. I will document the range of disturbances of self-representations in victims of childhood sexual abuse and explore a possible underlying psychobiologic mechanism for these disturbances. Finally, I will examine the implications of this model for treatment and research.

REPRESENTATIONS OF SELF

Anyone who surveys the literature on the "self" quickly discovers that there are many terms (e.g., self-concept, self-image, self-object, body image, ego, identity) that are used by various authorities to denote an individual's psychological representations of self. These terms reflect differences in the many theoretical orientations that have been brought to bear on our understanding of self. The degree to which these different

113

constructs can be equated is debatable. Rather than attempt to sort out a confusing literature and to detail similarities and reconcile differences in the terminology and ideology of various authorities, I have chosen for heuristic purposes to lump all of these constructs into the general category of self-representations. This will permit readers to substitute their own understanding of these terms based on their own theoretical and experiential perspective. In instances where I cite an author's data, I will use his or her terminology to convey the context of the investigator's work.

While there is no single, well-accepted definition of *self*, Stern (1985) observed that the self and its boundaries are at the heart of our understanding of human nature.

> While no one can agree on exactly what the self is, as adults we still have a very real sense of self that permeates daily social experience. It arises in many forms. There is the sense of a self that is a single, distinct, integrated body; there is the agent of actions, the experiencer of feelings, the maker of intentions, the architect of plans, the communicator and sharer of personal knowledge. Most often these senses of self reside out of awareness, like breathing, but they can be brought to and held in consciousness. We instinctively process our experiences in such a way that they appear to belong to some kind of unique subjective organization that we commonly call the sense of self. (pp. 5–6)

Development of Representations of Self

Virtually all developmental descriptions of the origin of self representations (e.g., self-concept, self-image, body image) agree that these representations begin in the first year of life and are initially based on the infant's sensorimotor experiences (Stern 1985). Most authors see the infant as gradually developing a sense of "me/not me." From about age 7 months on, infants play games that serve to delineate the baby's own body image from the mother's (Mahler et al. 1975). By the age of 1 year, children demonstrate clear evidence of self-recognition, such as responding differentially to themselves in a mirror (McCandles and Trotter 1977). By age 3 years they can recognize sexual differences and have developed a gender identity. This process corresponds with the development of libidinal object constancy and presumably also reflects the development of a constancy in the child's sense of self-object (Mahler et al. 1975).

Wylie (1961) demonstrated that individual differences in self-esteem are evident by kindergarten. As children grow older, they report their self-representations in an increasingly abstract and individualized manner (Eder et al. 1987). Sheikh and Beglis (1973) found that second graders described themselves concretely (e.g., "I am a boy; I live on Main Street"). At about fourth grade, children frequently include remarks such as, "I get good grades in spelling; I have a lot of friends" that indicate a growing sense of their own individuality. By sixth grade, many children include remarks about their future and their relationships with the opposite sex; girls talk about physical appearances (Papalia and Olds 1975).

Virtually all authorities on adolescence see the individual's primary developmental task during this period as the establishment of adult identities, including sexual identity (as opposed to gender identity). Adolescence, derived from the Latin meaning "to grow into maturity," is a period that is marked by profound physiologic and psychological changes, beginning with pubescence and ending in the early 20s. Major physical changes such as the development of secondary sex characteristics and the typical adolescent growth spurt must be integrated into the repertoire of body images, while cognitive changes such as the development of Piagetian formal operations bring new levels of self-awareness.

Adolescence, the fifth of Erikson's (1950) eight ages of man, is dominated by a developmental crisis involving identity versus role confusion (see also Papalia and Olds 1975). Erikson, who delved into the mystery of adolescence as much as anyone, emphasized that the adolescent search for identity is not a "maturational malaise" but a healthy process resulting in a strengthened adult ego. During this period, the individual may exhibit profound swings in his or her sense of self, including at times temporary surrender of individual identity to processes such as hero worship and overidentification with a group or significant individual.

While many textbooks and theorists abruptly end their inquiry into the development of self-representation with the onset of adulthood, others are showing that self-representations continue to undergo profound revisions through an individual's life (Horowitz 1979; Stern 1985). The ability of adults to continue to alter their self-representations is, of course, a fundamental capacity on which psychotherapy operates and one of the abilities that must be systematically enlisted by therapists working with individuals who have serious disturbances in self-representation.

Factors Influencing Self-Representations

Most authorities point to socialization as the principal factor that shapes all forms of self-representation (Ausubel 1954; Craig 1979; Epstein 1973; Honess and Yardley 1987; McCandles and Trotter 1977; Rae 1982; van der Welde 1985). While self-representations are internal psychological experiences, they are primarily derived from one's perceptions of other's perceptions and from expectations of one's self (Dinkmeyer 1965; Papalia and Olds 1975). Self-representations are largely social products arising out of experiences with other people—primarily parents, siblings, relatives, peers, teachers, and the general community (Dinkmeyer 1965; Honess and Yardley 1987).

Trust and security appear to be major prerequisites for the establishment of healthy self-representations in infants and toddlers (Dinkmeyer

1965; Schaffer 1971; Spitz 1965; Stone and Church 1979). Coopersmith's (1967) widely cited studies on self-esteem in preadolescents indicated that self-concepts are based on a child's self-perceived degree of success in four areas. These areas are: 1) significance (the way the child feels love and approval by the important people in his or her life), 2) competence (in performing tasks that he or she feels are important), 3) virtue (his or her attainment of moral and ethical standards defined by significant others), and 4) power (the extent to which the child can influence his or her own life and the lives of others) (Papalia and Olds 1975).

In addition to the global factors enumerated by Coopersmith (1967), a number of psychological mechanisms play an important role in incorporation and refinement of self-representations. Identification, defined by Freud (1949) as "the endeavor to mould a person's own ego after the fashion of one that has been taken as a model" (p. 63), is a particularly powerful mechanism in forming self-concepts. Kagan (1965) postulated that there are two major goals that drive all forms of identification: 1) a feeling of power or mastery over the environment and 2) the attainment of love and affection. Attainment of these goals leads to a decrease in anxiety over helplessness and loneliness.

Anna Freud (1937) and others (Kagan 1965) observed the operation of behaviors that are similar to an aggressive or threatening model. She termed this process, "identification with the aggressor." The motivation for this imitation of behavior is presumed to be anxiety over anticipated aggression or domination by the threatening model (Kagan 1965). The collective experiences of therapists working with victims of childhood sexual abuse, as well as the statistics on child abuse committed by adults abused as children (Kaufman and Zigler 1986) and studies of aggression in abused children and adolescents (Burgess et al. 1987; Friedrich et al. 1986), all provide ample evidence of such an identification with the aggressor occurring in abused children. Seghorn et al. (1987), for example, found extremely high rates of sexual and physical abuse in the childhood histories of incarcerated rapists and child molesters.

A second important mechanism in the development of self-representations is the effects of expectancies. There is a wealth of evidence to show that the expectancies of others have a tremendous influence on how an individual behaves (Jones 1986). The experiment of Rosenthal and Jacobson (1968) in which teachers were led to expect that certain first-through sixth-grade students were going to "bloom" academically, in fact, resulted in these randomly chosen children doing significantly better than peers who were not labeled in this fashion. Although this study was controversial and often criticized on methodological grounds, subsequent studies have confirmed their finding that teachers operating under an incorrect expectancy behave in such a way as to bring about confirmation of that expectancy in their students (Jones 1986).

A specific expectancies process, the self-fulfilling prophecy, is particularly malignant when it becomes a downward cycle of increasingly negative expectations held by an individual about him- or herself and socially reinforced by significant others. No one who has worked with abused, neglected, or deprived children or adolescents can fail to be impressed by the relentlessness of this process as it undercuts self-esteem and produces an increasingly deteriorating sense of self resulting in evermore negative self-presentations.

Self-Esteem

Volumes have been devoted to the subject of self-esteem. The scope of this chapter, however, limits me to a few brief comments. Self-esteem in children seems to be strongly influenced by early family dynamics, particularly the rewarding of good behaviors rather than the punishment of bad (Coopersmith 1967). Dynamically, self-esteem reflects the degree to which idealized self-expectations correspond to more reality-based self-representations (Higgins 1987; McCallon 1967). A large discrepancy between the real and idealized selves is generally associated with a low sense of self-esteem. Again, the interactive effects of expectancy and the self-fulfilling prophecy can lead to a spiraling reinforcement of high or low self-esteem.

DISTURBANCES OF SELF IN ABUSED CHILDREN

While there are repeated clinical observations of disturbances of sense of self in child and adult victims of childhood abuse, there is surprisingly little systematic research on the effects of sexual and/or physical abuse on self-representations. Almost nothing is known about the impact of abuse on children of different ages (Augoustinos 1987). The limited data in the literature suggest that there is a trend toward sexual abuse at earlier ages being more traumatic (Browne and Finkelhor 1986), but the Tufts New England Medical Center (1984) study, which specifically addressed this question, concluded that the age at which abuse begins is less important than the number of stages of development through which abuse persists. A number of instruments and scales are available to assess disturbances in self-representations in children, and hopefully some of these will be incorporated into future prospective studies.

Clinical Evidence of Disturbed Self-Representations

There are a number of reports indicating major disturbances in self-esteem and self-concepts in abused children. Martin and Beezley (1977) found that "very few [abused] children thought well of themselves" (p. 374).

Half of their sample showed "obvious low self-esteem" and often appeared unresponsive to praise. Kinard (1980, 1982) found that abused children differed significantly from nonabused children on certain items of the Piers-Harris Children's Self-Concept Scale (Piers and Harris 1969). More severe abuse was associated with a greater likelihood of having a negative self-image (Kinard 1982). She interpreted her data as suggesting that "their sense of identity is not well formed" (p. 694) and speculated that the persistence of this lack of identity into adulthood may explain the role-reversal phenomenon (Green 1982), in which battering parents abuse children for attributes they dislike in themselves.

Green (1978a), likewise, noted a high frequency of self-deprecation in his study of 20 abused children. Green (1982) hypothesized that:

> The preverbal infant who is repeatedly assaulted acquires an unpleasurable awareness of "self," consisting of painful sensation and painful affects linked to primary objects. This painful self-awareness becomes transformed into a de-valued self-concept with the development of cognition and language. These children ultimately regard themselves with the same displeasure and contempt that their parents directed towards them. The young children who were re-peatedly punished, beaten, and threatened with abandonment assume that it was a consequence of their own behavior, regardless of their actual innocence. (p. 255).

Humphrey et al. (1978) reported also observing the tendency of abused children to incorporate negative parental attitudes and to believe that they deserve to be abused.

Disturbances in sexual identity have been repeatedly reported by cli-nicians working with sexually abused children. Precocious sexualized be-haviors and eroticization are the most commonly reported sign of sexual abuse in children (Friedrich et al. 1986; Putnam, unpublished observa-tions). Burgess and Holmstrom (1975) found that repeated sexual abuse during latency appeared to disrupt normal development of the concept of sexuality. Kaufman et al. (1954) found evidence of confusion in sexual identification in the Rorschach responses of daughters of father-daughter incest. These disturbances in sexuality and sexual identity often result in secondary traumatization for these children by complicating their treat-ment and placement (Krieger et al. 1980; Yates 1982). In adulthood the same process results in serious disturbances of marital relationships, dys-functional sexuality, and prostitution (Gelinas 1983).

Disturbances in body image, while rarely systematically documented, are obvious to clinicians and often expressed destructively by self-muti-lation or expressed symbolically by conversion reactions. Hjorth and Har-way (1981) found significant differences between physically abused adolescents' and normal adolescents' drawings of human figures; there is good reason to suspect that similar differences would be manifest by sexually abused children. Green (1978b) found a much higher rate of self-destructive behavior (40.6%) in his physically abused children than in control children (6.7%). He postulated that disturbances in self-esteem resulted in the development of self-destructive behaviors. It is likely that the same dynamic drives the self-destructive behavior of sexually abused children. A similar percentage (57.7%) of self-injurious behaviors was found in incest victims by de Young (1982), with a typical age of onset between 9.7 and 12.4 years.

Conversion disorders, a manifestation of bodily-image disturbance, are strongly associated with histories of sexual trauma in children and adolescents (Kriechman, 1987; Volkmar et al. 1984). In addition, the disturbances of identity that accompany dissociative reactions, primarily depersonalization, elicited by traumatic experiences (Putnam 1985) are thought to play a significant role in triggering some self-destructive behaviors in sexually abused children (de Young 1982).

Factors Contributing to Poor Self-Concepts in Abused Children

A number of interactive factors probably make a significant contribution to the development of negative self-representations in abused children. A rapidly growing number of studies suggest that severely abused children are at risk for delays in cognitive and locomotor development (Ammerman et al. 1986; Coons 1986). Although the data are more impressive for physical abuse, several authors have documented learning and attentional problems in sexually abused children (Adams-Tucker 1982; Kaufman et al. 1954). Poor peer relationships (Green 1978a; Humphrey et al. 1978; Martin and Beezley 1977), social withdrawal and isolation (Adams-Tucker 1982; Coons 1986; Green 1978a; Martin and Beezley 1977), depression (Blumberg 1981; Coons 1986; Kaufman et al. 1954), and maladaptive behaviors such as aggression (George and Main 1979; Hoffman-Plotkin and Twentyman 1984; Kinard 1980, 1982; Reidy 1977) and oppositional behavior (Adams-Tucker 1982; Martin and Beezley 1977) are all likely to produce negative responses in peers and significant others leading to the downward spiral of self-esteem, self-representations, and self-presentations discussed in the preceding section.

Data on the relationship of abuser to victim (Browne and Finkelhor 1986; Bryer et al. 1987; Williams and Fuller 1987) indicate that most sexually abused children are victimized by close relatives, who would normally serve as objects for identification and introjection. The processes of internalization of the important aspects of significant others (e.g., identification and introjection) are most powerfully operative during middle childhood and adolescence (Zinner and Shapiro 1972) and would be expected to contribute to serious behavioral disturbances in abused children.

DISTURBANCES OF SELF IN ADULT VICTIMS OF CHILDHOOD SEXUAL ABUSE

A number of symptoms commonly reported in adults who were victims of incest or other childhood sexual abuse can be understood as manifestations of continued major disturbances in the victim's sense of self. Perhaps the single most commonly reported adult outcome of childhood sexual abuse is a serious disturbance in the individual's sense of self-esteem (Browne and Finkelhor 1986; Coons 1986). Studies by Bagley and Ramsay (1985), Courtois (1979), Herman (1981), and Williams and Fuller (1987) all document the much higher frequency of a negative "self-image" in abuse victims compared to nonabused controls.

Self-destructive behavior expresses a profound disturbance in the sense of self. Suicidal ideation and behavior, self-mutilation, and other forms of self-destructive behavior are common in adult victims of childhood sexual abuse. Briere's (1984) extensive survey of "walk-ins" to a community health center documented a much higher incidence of suicide attempts in sexual abuse victims than in nonabused clients. Other clinical researchers (Bagley and Ramsay 1985; Herman 1981; Sedney and Brooks 1984) have found similar results.

Disturbances in sexual identity and sexual functioning are universally noted in sex abuse victims (Browne and Finkelhor 1986; Coons 1986). Meiselman (1978) found 87% of her sexually abused sample had serious sexual dysfunction compared to 20% of nonabused control subjects from the same clinical setting. Similar results, although of a lesser magnitude, have been reported by Herman (1981), Langmade (1985), and Briere (1984). Promiscuity (Courtois 1979; de Young 1982; Herman 1981) has been reported as an outcome of childhood sexual abuse, although data from Fromuth's (1983) study indicate that sexual abuse victims may not have significantly more sexual partners than nonabused controls. Brown and Finkelhor (1986) interpreted this finding as suggesting "that the 'promiscuity' of sexual abuse victims may be more a function of their negative self-attributions, already well documented in the empirical literature, than their actual sexual behavior" (p. 71). Some clinical researchers (Burgess et al. 1987; Goodwin and DiVasto 1982; Gundlach 1977; Johnson and Shrier 1987) suggested that sexual orientation may be altered by childhood sexual abuse; others (e.g., Browne and Finkelhor 1986) have found no association.

Goodwin et al. (1981) found evidence of a disturbance in parental identity in incest victims compared to a nonabused control group. They found that 24% of mothers in abusing families had a history of incest compared to 3% of their controls. The phenomenon of revictimization in adulthood (e.g., rape, wife beating) is frequently reported in adults with a childhood history of abuse (Briere 1984; Browne and Finkelhor 1986; Carmen et al.

1984; Coons and Milstein 1984; Fromuth 1983; Gelinas 1983; Hilberman 1980; Hilberman and Munson 1978; Putnam et al. 1986). Some investigators have postulated that revictimization is due to the imprinting of a "victim identity" in early childhood. Dissociative symptoms and disorders are common in victims of childhood sex abuse (Coons 1986; Gelinas 1983; Putnam et al. 1986). These symptoms produce disturbances in identity (Putnam 1985) and are thought to play an important role in the dynamics of self-destructive behavior (Burgess et al. 1987; de Young 1982; Pao 1969; Raine 1982).

A POSSIBLE PSYCHOBIOLOGIC MECHANISM

One of the major contributions that may accrue from the study of the effects of childhood trauma is the cross-linkage of dynamic, developmental, and biologic models of psychopathology. Perhaps nowhere else is the complementarity of these different domains of knowledge more apparent than in understanding the effects of child abuse. As illustrated above, sexual abuse during childhood produces a range of psychological and biologic effects that span the course of development and lead to major psychopathology during adult life (Beck and van der Kolk 1987; Bryer et al. 1987; Burgess et al. 1987; Carmen et al. 1984; Gelinas 1983; Herman 1986a). Any theory that attempts to grapple with these effects must cut across these different spheres of knowledge in understanding the mechanisms through which this trauma impacts on its victims.

The altered states of consciousness model, perhaps more correctly termed the *alternative states* (Zinberg 1977) or the *discrete states of consciousness* model (Tart 1977), permits the specification of behavioral states in a manner that can be operationalized in both dynamic and biologic terms. This concept dates to the early 19th century and has been repeatedly invoked in one form or another by a variety of clinicians and theoreticians over the past century to explain major shifts in mental processes. The terms, *state of consciousness* or *mental state*, are freely used in today's clinical literature and connote one of the major assumptions underlying our daily clinical formulations of behavior. While the widespread and often causal use of these terms have sometimes resulted in a trivialization of the concept, the states of consciousness model provides a powerful investigational paradigm for understanding the symptoms and mechanisms of disturbances in sense of self observed in victims of childhood trauma (Putnam 1988).

Definition and Principles of an Altered States of Consciousness Model

Emde et al. (1976) observed that *state* is a "low-level" concept that has found favor with researchers in behavior and physiology because it is

easily operationalized. Most formal and informal definitions of state emphasize that a state is a recurrent interactive organization of consciousness
that organizes or structures perception, cognition, and behavior. Hutt
et al. (1969) referred to a state as a constellation of certain patterns of
physiologic variables and/or patterns of behaviors that seem to repeat
themselves and that appear to be relatively stable. Emde et al. (1976),
applying *state* in a developmental context, observed: "We have found it
useful to think of the concept of state as referring to a group of variables
at a given point in development which determine readiness to act on the
one hand, and readiness to react on the other" (p. 29). Horowitz (1979)
observed that:

> States are commonly recognized during a clinical interview because of changes
> in facial expression, intonation and inflection in speech, focus and content of
> verbal reports, degree of self reflective awareness, general arousal, shifts in
> degree and nature of empathy, and other communicative qualities. (p. 31)

Horowitz et al. (1980) observed that "certain self-images and role relationship models predominate in each state: we infer that these are or-
ganizing principles which are partly responsible for the repetition of a
given state over time" (p. 1159).

Discrete states of consciousness, with their state-specific alterations in
sense of self, can be triggered by external stimuli such as abreactions or
phobic attacks, or activated by specific trains of thought such as the
depressive states observed by Seligman (1975) and Beck (1976). Discrete
states of consciousness are exchanged or switched (Horowitz 1979; Putnam
1988), and traumatically induced altered states of consciousness are particularly susceptible to activation by environmental stimuli (Gelinas 1983;
Putnam 1988; Solomon et al. 1987). There is growing evidence to indicate
that discrete states of consciousness are associated with unique state-
dependent psychobiologies (Lydic 1987) and that switches in states of
consciousness are accompanied by changes in neurotransmitter levels and
other biologic markers (Bunney and Murphy 1974; Putnam 1986; Wolff
et al. 1985). Powerful state-dependent memory and state-dependent
learning phenomena have been documented to accompany discrete state
changes in psychiatric disorders such as bipolar illness (Weingartner et al.
1977) and multiple personality disorder (Ludwig et al. 1972; Nissen et al.
1988; Silberman et al. 1985).

While there are a number of pathologic states of consciousness in addition to dissociative states (e.g., catatonic states, anxiety states), Ludwig
(1983) pointed out that all altered states of consciousness, dissociative
states included, share a set of common characteristics in varying degrees.
These are:

> a) alterations in thinking, whereby archaic modes of thought predominate;
> b) disturbed time sense; c) a sense of loss of control; d) changes in emotional

expression; e) body image changes; f) perceptual distortions; g) change in meaning or significance; h) feelings of rejuvenation; and i) hypersuggestibility. (p. 94)

There is overwhelming evidence documenting the activation of dissociative states of a response to psychological, physical, and sexual trauma (Putnam 1985). Most authorities on dissociation have emphasized that it often represents an initially adaptive process to significant trauma (Braun and Sachs 1985; Ludwig 1983; Putnam 1985). Ludwig (1983) enumerated a number of adaptive functions served by dissociation:

1) the automatization of certain behaviors, 2) the efficiency and economy of effort, 3) the resolution of irreconcilable conflicts, 4) escape from the constraints of reality, 5) the isolation of catastrophic experiences, 6) the cathartic discharge of certain feelings, and 7) the enhancement of herd sense (e.g. the submersion of the individual ego for the group identity, greater suggestibility, etc). (p. 93)

The dissociative disorders exist at one end of a spectrum of dissociative phenomena ranging from simple microdissociative experiences, which Hilgard (1977) termed "the dissociation of everyday life," to extreme forms such as multiple personality (Bernstein and Putnam 1986). Dissociation is judged pathologic only when it produces a major disturbance in identity and memory (Bernstein and Putnam 1986; Putnam 1985). In its pathologic forms, such as psychogenic amnesia, fugue states, chronic depersonalization, and multiple personality disorder, pathologic dissociation can be understood as a sustained entry into an altered state (or states) of consciousness with attendant alterations in the individual's sense of self.

DISTURBANCES OF SELF IN A DISCRETE STATES OF CONSCIOUSNESS MODEL

Fragmentation or Loss of Sense of Self

A traumatically induced, altered states of consciousness model provides insight into the fragmentation of sense of self commonly described in incest victims (Burgess et al. 1987; Rieker and Carmen 1986). Psychiatric disorders frequently diagnosed in incest survivors include 1) borderline personality disorder, with its identity diffusion and disturbance of core sense of self; 2) multiple personality disorder, with its alternation of radically different identities; and 3) eating disorders, with their distortions of body image. The breaks in continuity of self, continuity of behavior, and continuity of memory resulting from dissociative state amnesic gaps contribute to a fragmentation of the incest victim's sense of self. The loss of significant childhood and adolescent memories commonly encountered in incest victims (Herman 1986b) deprives the individual of autobiographical memory, which is a central element in one's sense of self (Eder et al.

1987; Stern 1985). Rubin (1985) noted that "autobiographical memory is the source of our sense of self: the feeling that we are the same person with the same personality over time" (p. 42).

Concerns About Control

Impulsivity and concerns about control or loss of control of self and/or others, so commonly noted during therapy with incest victims, must stem, in part, from the victims' repeated experiences of loss of self-control accompanying environmentally triggered altered states of consciousness, such as flashbacks, abreactions, panic attacks, and regressive states. The extreme sense of vulnerability that many incest victims feel toward environmental triggers of dysphoric states also contributes to social withdrawal and isolation as well as the development of phobic avoidance and anxiety responses. The high rates of substance abuse seen in incest victims may represent attempts at stabilizing one's state or preventing entry into dysphoric states.

Identity Disturbances

A variety of identity disturbances are often present in incest victims. These include issues of sexual identity, often resulting in sexual dysfunction (Browne and Finkelhor 1986), and identity as a victim, often leading to pathologic relationships and revictimization in adulthood. Extreme forms of identity disturbance occur with multiple personality disorder and gender identity disorders (Coons and Milstein 1986). Early childhood identification processes, such as identification with the aggressor, may result in state-dependent pathologic introjects that can be activated by internal and external triggers, resulting in behaviors that subsequently cause guilt and lower self-esteem.

Body-Image Disturbances

Incest victims exhibit an array of body-image disturbances, ranging from feeling ugly or unclean (Williams and Fuller 1987) to profound disturbances in their sense of gender identity and age identity. Many of these disturbances are probably secondary to the major shifts in body image that occur with abreactions and other altered states of consciousness. Regression, often observed in sex abuse victims in crisis, can be understood as the reinstitution of stored body images from earlier stages of life (Horowitz 1966). Symptoms such as self-mutilation, which may occur in dissociative states (de Young 1982) or represent an attempt to stave off the numbing dysphoria of depersonalization, are another expression of body-image dysfunction in incest victims. Out-of-body experiences reported by some incest victims may produce a sense of detachment and alienation from one's physical self. Somatic symptoms and conversion reactions, relatively common in incest victims, may express yet another state-dependent form of body-image disturbance.

Low Self-Esteem

As discussed above, self-esteem is determined in part by the degree of discrepancy between idealized self-images and reality-based self-images. Investigators and clinicians have universally observed that incest victims suffer from low self-esteem (Browne and Finkelhor 1986; Coons 1986). This low self-esteem may be secondarily produced, in part, by the many disturbances in self-image discussed above. Lacking a solid, consistent, continuous sense of self to compare against often overidealized self-images, incest victims are doubly vulnerable to disturbances in their self-esteem. Their vulnerability to environmentally triggered flashbacks, interpersonal difficulties, and identity confusion further leads to feelings of helplessness and lack of control over sense of self or behavior.

IMPLICATIONS FOR TREATMENT AND RESEARCH

Treatment

The recognition that childhood sexual abuse often produces serious disturbances in a variety of forms of self-representation has significant implications for the diagnosis and treatment of these patients. Clinicians should systematically look for a history of childhood sexual abuse in any patient who shows a significant disturbance in one or more representations of self (e.g., conversion reactions, self-mutilation, pervasive poor self-esteem, fragmentation of self, loss of autobiographical memory, multiple or pathologic alter identities). Specific techniques or tests that probe self-image or body image (e.g., drawing or video modeling) may be useful in uncovering and documenting disturbances in self and may serve as possible screening instruments in populations known to be at risk for sexual abuse.

Treatment should address the specific disturbances of self found in victims of childhood sexual abuse. In many instances, adjunctive treatment modalities (e.g., art therapy, movement therapy) may be more effective with certain disturbances of self (e.g., body-image distortions) than conventional psychotherapy. The reconstitution of self through the recovery and chronologic sequencing of missing autobiographical memories can play an important role in the therapeutic process. This reconstruction process is often accompanied by abreactions that activate latent self-images and liberate dissociated affects. The bringing of dissociated material into consciousness leads to greater self-awareness and decreased vulnerability to environmental triggers. The state-dependency of traumatic memories and affects in sex abuse victims makes this material and associated self-concepts relatively impervious to standard psychotherapy. In many instances, hypnosis is a useful adjunctive technique for breaching amnesic barriers and retrieving dissociative state-dependent material for psychotherapeutic processing.

Therapists must help the patient recognize and rework pathologic identifications and introjects (e.g., victim identities and identification with the aggressor pathologies). In cases such as multiple personality disorder, where the patient has developed multiple identities to compartmentalize traumatic memories and affects, the therapist must help the patient process and integrate these dissociated identities into a more unified sense of self. The discrete states of consciousness model is useful in helping the therapist understand and work with the state-dependency of memories, behaviors, and biologic sensitivities frequently noted in these individuals (Putnam 1984).

Research

The discrete states of consciousness paradigm provides a unique perspective that permits the integration of well-accepted psychoanalytic concepts such as ego states and object relations with modern neurobiology and developmental psychology. The application of this model to the investigation of disturbances of self found in victims of childhood sexual trauma may provide the isomorph necessary to link these previously disparate domains of knowledge into a more unified understanding of mind and body.

SUMMARY

In this chapter I have briefly reviewed the literature on the development of self-representation, noting the important role of early socialization experiences and identifying mechanisms and processes particularly vulnerable to pathologic disruption in abused children. The existence of an array of disturbances of self-representations manifested by children, adolescents, and adults who were sexually victimized in childhood is documented. A possible explanatory psychobiologic paradigm, the discrete states of consciousness model, is briefly presented and some implications for treatment and research are discussed.

REFERENCES

Adams-Tucker C: Proximate effects of sexual abuse in childhood: a report on 28 children. Am J Psychiatry 139:1252–1256, 1982

Ammerman RT, Cassisi JE, Hersen M, et al: Consequences of physical abuse and neglect in children. Clinical Psychology Review 6:291–310, 1986

Augoustinos M: Developmental effects of child abuse: recent findings. Child Abuse Negl 11:15–27, 1987

Ausabel D: Theory and Problems of Adolescent Development. New York, Grune & Stratton, 1954

Bagley C, Ramsay R: Disrupted childhood and vulnerability to sexual assault: long-term sequels with implications for counselling. Paper presented at the Conference on Counselling the Sexual Abuse Survivor, Winnipeg, Canada, February 1985

Beck AT: Cognitive Therapy and Emotional Disorders. New York, International Universities Press, 1976

Beck JC, van der Kolk B: Reports of childhood incest and current behavior of chronically hospitalized psychotic women. Am J Psychiatry 144:1474–1476, 1987

Bernstein EM, Putnam FW: Development, reliability, and validity of a dissociation scale. J Nerv Ment Dis 174:727–735, 1986

Blumberg ML: Depression in abused and neglected children. Am J Psychother 35:342–355, 1981

Braun BG, Sachs RG: The development of multiple personality disorder: predisposing, precipitating, and perpetuating factors, in Childhood Antecedents of Multiple Personality. Edited by Kluft RP. Washington, DC, American Psychiatric Press, 1985, pp 37–64

Briere J: The effects of childhood sexual abuse on later psychological functioning: defining a "post-sexual-abuse syndrome." Paper presented at the Third National Conference on Sexual Victimization of Children, Washington, DC, April 1989

Browne A, Finkelhor D: Impact of child sexual abuse: a review of the literature. Psychol Bull 99:66–77, 1986

Bryer JB, Nelson BA, Miller JB, et al: Childhood sexual and physical abuse as factors in adult psychiatric illness. Am J Psychiatry 144:1426–1430, 1987

Bunney WE, Murphy DL: Switch process in psychiatric illness, in Factors in Depression. Edited by Kline NS. New York, Raven, 1974, pp 139–158

Burgess AW, Hartman CR, McCormack A: Abused to abuser: antecedents of socially deviant behaviors. Am J Psychiatry 144:1431–1436, 1987

Burgess AW, Holmstrom LL: Sexual trauma in children and adolescents. Nurs Clin North Am 10:551–557, 1975

Carmen E, Rieker PP, Mills T: Victims of violence and psychiatric illness. Am J Psychiatry 141:378–383, 1984

Coons PM: Psychiatric problems associated with child abuse: a review, in Psychiatric Sequelae of Child Abuse. Edited by Jacobsen JJ. Springfield, IL, Charles C Thomas, 1986, pp 169–200

Coons PM, Milstein V: Rape and post-traumatic stress in multiple personality. Psychol Rep 55:839–845, 1984

Coons PM, Milstein V: Psychosexual disturbances in multiple personality: characteristics, etiology and treatment. J Clin Psychiatry 47:106–110, 1986

Coopersmith S: The Antecedents of Self-Esteem. San Francisco, CA, WH Freeman, 1967

Courtois C: The incest experience and its aftermath. Victimology 4:337–347, 1979

Craig GJ: Child Development. Englewood Cliffs, NJ, Prentice-Hall, 1979

de Young M: Self-injurious behavior in incest victims: a research note. Child Welfare 61:577–584, 1982

Dinkmeyer DC: Child Development: The Emerging Self. Englewood Cliffs, NJ, Prentice-Hall, 1965

Eder RA, Gerlach SG, Perlmutter M: In search of children's selves: development of the specific and general components of the self-concept. Child Dev 58:1044–1050, 1987

Emde RN, Gaensbauer TJ, Harmon RJ: Emotional expression in infancy: a biobehavioral study. Psychol Issues 10: Monograph 37, 1976

Epstein S: The self-concept revisited. Am Psychol 28:404–416, 1973

Erikson EH: Childhood and Society. New York, WW Norton, 1950

Freud A: The Ego and Mechanisms of Defense. London, Hogarth Press, 1937

Freud S: Group Psychology and the Analysis of the Ego. London, Hogarth Press, 1949

Friedrich WN, Urquiza AJ, Beilke RL: Behavior problems in sexually abused young children. J Pediatr Psychol 11:47–57, 1986

Fromuth ME: The long term psychological impact of childhood sexual abuse. Unpublished doctoral dissertation, Auburn University, Auburn, AL, 1983

Gelinas DJ: The persisting negative effects of incest. Psychiatry 46:312–332, 1983

George C, Main M: Social interactions of young abused children: approach, avoidance and aggression. Child Dev 50:306–318, 1979

Goodwin J, DiVasto P: Female homosexuality: a sequel to mother-daughter incest, in Sexual Abuse: Incest Victims and Their Families. Edited by Goodwin J. Boston, MA, Wright-PSG, 1982, pp 117–124

Goodwin J, McCarth T, DiVasto P: Prior incest in mothers of abused children. Child Abuse Negl 5:87–96, 1981

Green AH: Psychopathology of abused children. Journal of the American Academy of Child Psychiatry 17:356–371, 1978a

Green AH: Self-destructive behavior in battered children. Am J Psychiatry 135:579–582, 1978b

Green AH: Child abuse, in Psychopathology in Childhood. Edited by Lachenmeyer J, Gibbs M. New York, Gardner Press, 1982, pp 244–267

Grunlach RH: Sexual molestation and rape reported by homosexual and heterosexual women. J Homosex 2:367–384, 1977

Herman JL: Father-Daughter Incest. Cambridge, MA, Harvard University Press, 1981

Herman JF: Histories of violence in an outpatient population. Am J Orthopsychiatry 65:137–141, 1986a

Herman JL: Recovery and verification of memories of childhood sexual trauma. Paper presented at the Annual Meeting of the American Psychiatric Association, May 1986b

Higgins ET: Self-discrepancy: a theory relating self and affect. Psychol Rev 94:319–339, 1987

Hilberman E: Overview: the "wife-beater's wife" reconsidered. Am J Psychiatry 137:1336–1347, 1980

Hilberman E, Munson K: Sixty battered women. Victimology 2:460–470, 1978

Hilgard ER: Divided Consciousness: Multiple Controls in Human Thought and Action. New York, John Wiley, 1977

Hjorth CW, Harway M: The body image of physically abused and normal adolescents. J Clin Psychol 37:863–866, 1981

Hoffman-Plotkin D, Twentyman CT: A multimodal assessment of behavioral and cognitive deficits in abused and neglected preschoolers. Child Dev 55:794–802, 1984

Honess T, Yardley K: Self and social structure: an introductory review, in Self and Identity: Psychosocial Perspectives. Edited by Yardley K, Honess T. New York, John Wiley, 1987, pp 67–96

Horowitz MJ: Body image. Arch Gen Psychiatry 14:456–460, 1966

Horowitz MJ: States of Mind: Analysis of Change in Psychotherapy. New York, Plenum, 1979

Horowitz MJ, Wilner N, Marmar C, et al: Pathological grief and the activation of latent self-images. Am J Psychiatry 137:1157–1162, 1980

Humphrey FJ, Ackerman L, Strickler E: Child abuse: psychological antecedents and sequelae. Pennsylvania Medicine 8:10–12, 1978

Hutt SJ, Lenard HG, Prechtl HFR: Psychophysiological studies in newborn infants, in Advances in Child Development. Edited by Lipsitt LP, Reese HW. New York, Academic, 1969, pp 103–124

Johnson RL, Shrier D: Past sexual victimization by females of male patients in an adolescent medicine clinic population. Am J Psychiatry 144:650–652, 1987

Jones EE: Interpreting interpersonal behavior: the effects of expectancies. Science 234:41–46, 1986

Kagan J: The concept of identification, in Readings in Child Development and Personality. Edited by Mussen PH, Conger JJ, Kagan J. New York, Harper & Row, 1965, pp 315–326

Kaufman I, Peck AL, Tagiuri CK: The family constellation and overt incestuous relations between father and daughter. Am J Orthopsychiatry 24:266–275, 1954

Kaufman J, Zigler E: Do abused children become abusive parents? Am J Orthopsychiatry 57:186–192, 1986

Kinard EM: Emotional development in physically abused children. Am J Orthopsychiatry 50:686–696, 1980

Kinard EM: Emotional development in physically abused children. Am J Orthopsychiatry 52:82–91, 1982

Kriechman AM: Siblings with somatoform disorders in childhood and adolescents. J Am Acad Child Adolesc Psychiatry 26:226–231, 1987

Krieger MJ, Rosenfeld AA, Gordon A, et al: Problems in the psychotherapy of children with histories of incest. Am J Psychother 34:81–88, 1980

Langmade CJ: The impact of pre- and postpubertal onset of incest experiences in adult women as measured by sex anxiety, sex guilt, sexual satisfaction and sexual behavior. Dissertation Abstracts International 44:917B, 1985 (University Microfilms No 3592)

Ludwig AM: The psychobiological functions of dissociation. Am J Clin Hypn 26:93–99, 1983

Ludwig AM, Brandsma J, Wilbur C, et al: The objective study of a multiple personality: or, are four heads better than one? Arch Gen Psychiatry 26:298–310, 1972

Lydic R: State-dependent aspects of regulatory physiology. J Federation of American Societies of Experimental Biology 1:6–15, 1987

Mahler MS, Pine F, Bergman A: The Psychological Birth of the Human Infant. New York, Basic Books, 1975

Martin HP, Beezley P: Behavioral observations of abused children. Dev Med Child Neurol 19:373–387, 1977

McCallon EL: Self-ideal discrepancy and the correlates sex and academic achievement. Journal of Experimental Education 35:45–49, 1967

McCandles BR, Trotter RJ: Behavior and Development. New York, Holt, Rinehart & Winston, 1977

Meiselman K: Incest. San Francisco, CA, Jossey-Bass, 1978

Nissen MJ, Ross JL, Willingham DB, et al: Memory and awareness in a patient with multiple personality disorder. Brain & Cognition 8:117–134, 1988

Pao P: The syndrome of delicate self-cutting. Br J Med Psychol 42:195–207, 1969

Papalia DE, Olds SW: A Child's World: Infancy Through Adolescence. New York, McGraw-Hill, 1975

Piers E, Harris D: The Piers-Harris Children's Self-Concept Scale. Nashville, TN, Counselor Recordings and Tests, 1969

Putnam FW: The psychophysiological investigation of multiple personality disorder: a review. Psychiatr Clin North Am 7:32–40, 1984

Putnam FW: Dissociation as a response to extreme trauma, in Childhood Antecedents of Multiple Personality. Edited by Kluft RP. Washington, DC, American Psychiatric Press, 1985, pp 65–97

Putnam FW: The scientific investigation of multiple personality disorder, in Split Minds, Split Brains. Edited by Quen JM. New York, New York University Press, 1986, pp 109–126

Putnam FW: The switch process in multiple personality and other state-change disorders. Dissociation 1:24–32, 1988

Putnam FW, Guroff JJ, Silberman EK, et al: The clinical phenomenology of multiple personality disorder: review of 100 recent cases. J Clin Psychiatry 47:285–293, 1986

Rae WA: Body images of children and adolescents during physical illness and hospitalization. Psychiatric Annals 12:1065–1073, 1982

Raine WJB: Self-mutilation. J Adolesc 5:1–13, 1982

Reidy TJ: The aggressive characteristics of abused and neglected children. J Clin Psychol 33:1140–1145, 1977

Rieker PP, Carmen E: The victim-to-patient process: the disconfirmation and transformation of abuse. Am J Orthopsychiatry 56:360–370, 1986

Rosenthal R, Jacobson L: Pygmalion in the Classroom. New York, Winston, 1968

Rubin DC: The subtle deceiver: recalling our past. Psychology Today 19:39–46, 1985

Schaffer HR: The Origins of Human Social Relations. New York, Academic, 1971

Sedney MA, Brooks B: Factors associated with a history of childhood sexual experience in a nonclinical female population. Journal of the American Academy of Child Psychiatry 23:215–218, 1984

Seghorn TK, Prentky RA, Boucher MS: Childhood sexual abuse in the lives of sexually aggressive offenders. J Am Acad Child Adolesc Psychiatry 26:262–267, 1987

Seligman MEP: Helplessness: On Depression, Development and Death. San Francisco, CA, WH Freeman, 1975

Sheikh AA, Beglis JF: Development of self-concept in Negro and White children. Paper presented at the biennial meeting of the Society for Research in Child Development, Philadelphia, PA, March 29–April 1, 1973

Silberman EK, Putnam FW, Weingartner H, et al: Dissociative states in multiple personality disorders: a quantitative study. Psychiatry Res 15:253–260, 1985

Solomon Z, Garb R, Bleich A, et al: Reactivation of combat-related posttraumatic stress disorder. Am J Psychiatry 144:51–55, 1987

Spitz R: The First Year of Life. New York, International Universities Press, 1965

Stern DN: The Interpersonal World of the Infant. New York, Basic Books, 1985

Stone LG, Church J: Childhood and Adolescence. New York, Random House, 1979

Tart C: Putting the pieces together: a conceptual framework for understanding discrete states of consciousness, in Alternative States of Consciousness. Edited by Zinberg N. New York, Free Press, 1977, pp 158–219

Tufts New England Medical Center, Division of Child Psychiatry: Sexually exploited children: service and research report. Final report for the Office of Juvenile Justice and Delinquency Prevention. Washington, DC, U.S. Department of Justice, 1984

van der Velde CD: Body images of one's self and of others: developmental and clinical significance. Am J Psychiatry 142:527–537, 1985

Volkmar FR, Poll J, Lewis M: Conversion reactions in childhood and adolescence. J Am Acad Child Adolesc Psychiatry 23:424–430, 1984

Weingartner H, Miller HA, Murphy DL: Mood-state dependent retrieval of verbal associations. J Abnorm Psychol 86:276–283, 1977

Williams WV, Fuller W: Adult victims of childhood sexual abuse in a clinical population. Paper presented at the annual meeting of the American Orthopsychiatry Association, Washington, DC, March 1987

Wolff EA, Putnam FW, Post RM: Motor activity and affective illness. Arch Gen Psychiatry 42:288–294, 1985

Wylie RC: The Self Concept. Lincoln, NE, University of Nebraska Press, 1961

Yates A: Children eroticized by incest. Am J Psychiatry 139:482–484, 1982

Zinberg NE: The study of consciousness states: problems and progress, in Alternative Stress of Consciousness. Edited by Zinberg N. New York, Free Press, 1977, pp 1–36

Zinner J, Shapiro R: Projective identification as a mode of perception and behavior in families of adolescents. Int J Psychoanal 53:523–530, 1972

CHAPTER 7

Secrets of Adolescence: Incest and Developmental Fixations

Rosalyn Schultz, Ph.D.

> But that I am forbid
> To tell the secrets of my prison house,
> I could a tale unfold
> —Shakespeare, Hamlet Act I

Following a brief overview of normal adolescence and the evolution of both secrets and self-representation, I will describe several developmental inhibitors associated with secrecy that interfere with the capacity to negotiate the developmental challenges of adolescence and thus prevent the female victim of prolonged and habitual incest from consolidating a cohesive self-representation. The defensive structure and treatment implications also are addressed.

The ego psychological and object relations perspective of the following discussion emphasizes the incest victim's unsuccessful negotiation of the primary developmental task of adolescence (Deutsch 1944): relinquishing the emotional ties of the past and creating new ones. The path of inquiry revolves primarily around the vicissitudes of attempting to keep secrets of incest during adolescence and the consequences for adult functioning. Some repetitions are unavoidable, since I discuss variations on the themes as they relate to the incest victim's fears of disclosure, loss of maternal protection, pseudomaturity, collusion with the family conspiracy, and avoidance of her peer group. I have selected father-daughter incest because this dyad has the most traumatic consequences for the victim (Russell 1986), comprises the majority of studied incestuous relationships (Alter-

Reid et al. 1986; Pelletier and Handy 1986), and is the constellation representing the majority of my clinical experience with victims of incest.

Adults who were victims of incest as children or adolescents may suffer any of a wide spectrum of emotional distress and mental disorders. Despite the variety of their clinical presentations, they share in common a crippled self-representation (Eisnitz 1984–1985; Ulman and Brothers 1988). In connection with and as a consequence of this, they fail to develop crucial aspects of ego functioning and have a distorted self-perception that affects all aspects of their adult sense of identity (Brooks 1985; Giovacchini 1984; Herman 1981; Herman and Hirschman 1981; Meiselman 1978; Putnam, Chapter 6, this volume; Rosenthal and Doherty 1985; Sgroi 1989; Sheugold 1989; Steele 1986b; Ulman and Brothers 1988).

One young woman said:

> I flunked "Living 101." I can hold a job, but my personal life is a mess . . . just a string of fucked up relationships with men. Why do I only find men who treat me like a worthless old piece of furniture? Why do I keep looking for love when I can't stand being touched? I know I'm supposed to like sex; I feel like a freak. What does it matter, anyhow . . . I can't look in the mirror because I can't stand what I see. I feel ugly . . . I'm always trying to please so I have to keep feelings locked away.

Although adult incest survivors may manifest any of a multitude of clinical syndromes, they do not often present with classic and well-defined disorders. Underlying a myriad of defensive and adaptive mechanisms, they are generally confused as to who they are and their purpose in life. Consequently, they perceive themselves as helpless and vulnerable, worthless and inadequate. They have a crippled view of themselves because their individual existence was denied during childhood or adolescence. They were treated as objects to be exploited and violated. As described by Reich (1960), such trauma "can seriously interfere not only with the formation of defenses, but also with the integration and general development of the ego" (p. 220).

Giovacchini (1984, 1986) noted that difficulties with adaptation and self-esteem are related to defects in early nurturance and soothing received by the child, defects that affect the ego's executive system and the identity sense, hence the self-representation. In this chapter, a broad concept of the self-representation as the central powerhouse is employed, similar to that formulated by Eisnitz (1969) as "the mental representation of the self and its cathexis" (p. 19). This includes such concepts as body ego (from which the self-representation evolves), self-image, sense of identity, and conscious and unconscious attitudes and emotions connected with the self. The self-representation and its maintenance are mainly ego functions, but involve id and superego elements as well.

The consolidation of the self-representation, normally accomplished by the end of adolescence and accompanied by the completion of phase-specific developmental tasks (Blos 1962, 1968), is not successfully negotiated by the incest victim (O'Brien 1987). As with other adults who have developmental deficits, they are unable to develop a firm sense of autonomy and identity. Instead, the adaptive and defensive mechanisms adopted to protect against a heightened state of helpless vulnerability persist into adulthood, affecting all areas of functioning.

Many troubled adolescents use secrecy as a protective vehicle in their struggles to support their faltering self-esteem and identity (Coppolillo et al. 1981; Ekstein and Caruth 1972; Hoyt 1978). A pathologic defense, this secrecy differs from the healthy maintaining of one's personal privacy.

For adolescent victims of incest, the need for secrecy is heightened even more and affects both their self-perception and their perception of others. Because of ongoing external threats and internal fears of prohibition and danger (Summit 1983), they attempt to protect themselves against abandonment and psychic dissolution and to preserve the cohesion of the pathologic family pattern (Avery 1982–1983; Russell 1986). By working to keep the incestuous activity hidden, they are unable to establish their own personal privacy in the service of self-cohesion (Kluft, personal communication, 1988), safety from intrusion (Bettelheim 1979), and enhanced separation and individuation (Blanck 1966; Gross 1951).

OVERVIEW OF NORMAL ADOLESCENCE

Freud (1905) regarded the detachment from dependency on the parents as one of the most significant and painful psychical achievements. However, the developmental tasks that lead the adolescent into adulthood, including character formation, proceed optimally only if the adolescent can maintain continuity with the family and with the past (Blos 1968). Parental ties are loosened, earlier conflicts and trauma are reactivated and resolved, and a sexual identity solidified. At the same time, external sources of identity and self-esteem are gradually replaced by internal sources, and new object ties are established. Faced with such difficult tasks, the adolescent's ego resorts to numerous defense mechanisms, including denial, isolation, disavowal, splitting, and dissociation to combat the experience of helplessness. Deutsch (1944) described a "clash" between progressive and regressive forces, which Blos (1979) considered a prerequisite for progressive development.

Adolescence can be described as a time when the personality melts, heats into a molten volcano, then ultimately hardens into its characterological core (Spiegel 1951). If the ego remains rigid or fixated in response to its new demands, an impoverishment of the emotional life (Freud 1937) will profoundly affect the development of object relationships and adult functioning.

SECRETS

Overview

The Latin origin of the word *secret* is *sécernere*, meaning to set apart, to secrete, to separate out. Freud (see Tausk 1933) noted that the child's first successful lie, its first secret, emerges with the initial capacity for separation and individuation, and this marks the end of the infant's assumption that all thoughts are received from others (i.e., the infant begins to experience a private identity unknown to its parents). As elaborated by Ekstein and Caruth (1972): "all lying, all secreting, derives . . . from the capacity to put apart, to separate me from thee, mine from thine, self from object" (p. 201).

This developmental milestone is reached during the anal phase (Tausk 1933). "The child learns that . . . he can hold back, that he can keep something to himself" (Hoyt 1978, p. 232). In his seminal paper, "The Secret," Gross (1951) described the anal origins of the secret and emphasized that:

> it is the content of the secret which occupies the limelights, and appears as a possession which must not be given up. When the anal regime begins to disintegrate, the secret gradually loses the character of a possession, and is manifested in a conflict between the urge to retain and the urge to surrender (p. 44).

With the approach of the genital stage, secrecy is placed in the service of the oedipal conflict, and there is an increase in exhibitionism (Gross 1951). Gross considered that the secret first becomes meaningful during the oedipal period. With subsequent maturation, the secret becomes a potential gift to be used to initiate intimacy (Ekstein and Caruth 1972; Gross 1951; Hoyt 1978).

Because the word *secret* is derived from the same root as *secretions* and because of the secretive nature of the intimate bodily processes, secrecy is often unconsciously associated with the private secretions (excremental and genital) of the body (Gross 1951). In this way, the content of secrets are closely linked in the mind with issues of control and power (Ekstein and Caruth 1972; Gross 1951; Jacobs 1980); conflicts between expulsion and retention (Gross 1951; Margolis 1974; Meares 1976; Sulzberger 1953); and shame associated with exposure of one's body, its function in elimination, and sexuality (Bettelheim 1979; Greenson 1967; Hoyt 1978; Meares 1976). Greenson (1967) related the contents of the secret to shameful and loathsome secretions or the opposite, that is, very valuable products to be hoarded. In addition, he considered secrecy and the confession of secrets to be related to exhibitionism, scoptophilia, and teasing.

Secrecy Versus Privacy

Both the maintaining and revealing of secrets are ubiquitous in the human condition; several authors have noted its necessity for identity formation (Blanck 1966; Coppolillo et al. 1981; Ekstein and Caruth 1972; Gross 1951; Margolis 1966; Meares 1976). However, secrecy can also be a pathologic defense connoting prohibition and the need to conceal, inhibiting the capacity for genital primacy by reinforcing isolation (Hoyt 1978) rather than promoting identity and individuation.

In contrast to the pathologic need to keep secrets, which is defensive, the healthy ability to maintain privacy (i.e., a sense of separateness without fear or anxiety) enhances the development of the individual. This is first observed during the anal phase when children discover that they can exercise personal choice either to withhold or divulge private information (Caruth 1985; Margolis 1966). The adolescent's heightened need for secrets may be a brief repetition of the earlier anal phase (Tarachow 1966). During the phallic phase, masturbation may also serve the purpose of reinforcing separation from the primary object by providing a sense of personal privacy (Blanck 1966). The ability to preserve privacy thus contributes to developing self-determination and autonomy (Erikson 1959; Piaget 1962) and a sense of individualism and ego identity (Bettelheim 1979). In healthy adolescents, privacy promotes progressive development of autonomous functioning.

Jacobs (1980) described a situation in which a child is driven to secrecy because the mother attempts to obstruct the child's normative need for privacy and separateness. The mother's invasiveness affects both the child's ability to separate from her as well as the child's capacity to retain his or her own clear and separate boundaries.

Similarly, the adolescent who is unable to contain private information (i.e., divulges all thoughts and feelings to the mother, his or her "best friend") is also demonstrating pathologic attachment needs. This may indicate the wish to return to what Ekstein and Caruth (1972) referred to as "the secretless state of infantile fusion and communion" (p. 206).

During adolescence, closed bedroom doors, private phone calls to peers, and hidden diaries are common expressions of a heightened need for privacy. During this transitional phase between childhood and adulthood, maintaining such "privileged information" is a healthy vehicle that assists the adolescent in containing regressive swings; promoting separation from the family and intimacy with new objects; and developing a separate, distinct identity and integrated self-representation.

In contrast, for victims of incest, as with other conflicted adolescents who have difficulty with the reopening of earlier developmental problems, secrets are utilized to stabilize their diminished self-esteem and insecure identity, to calm their abandonment anxieties, to deny their isolation, and to defend against regressions. Like a magnet, the secret attracts many things and is a factor in psychic functioning. The incest victim's secrets are indications of pathologic circumstances during adolescence and contribute to developmental fixations.

SELF-REPRESENTATION

The self-representation, a theoretical and abstract construct, has never been agreed on in the literature. Sandler (1987) noted it does not exactly correspond to the Freudian concept of ego, described by Rapaport (1957–1958) as the person, the self, and consciousness. However, it is generally agreed that the self-representation is an ego structure encompassing all levels of the personality and forming its core (Eisnitz 1969, 1981; Giovacchini 1986; Greenson 1954; Hartmann 1951; Sandler 1987).

Hartmann (1951) distinguished between the ego (a substructure of the personality), the self (the subjective sense of being or the person), and the self-representation (the unconscious, preconscious, and conscious images of the body and body states in the ego system). This conceptual framework led Jacobson (1954) to describe the ego as including both object representations and self-representations. The self-representation forms an integral part of a representational world, described by Sandler (1987) as a stage set within a theater (the ego) with characters (object and self-representations) on stage representing various object and self-images. This metaphor helps to clarify the concept that both self-representations and object representations exist within the same mind (Spiegel 1959).

Eisnitz (1969) described the self-representation as a barometer by which to gauge psychic structure. Variations constantly occur in the self-representation under the influence of instinctual drives; the impact of external environment; and as a result of one's activities, thoughts, and fantasies, thus providing a construct in which to view clinical phenomena (Sandler 1987).

The self-representation is an ego subsystem that incorporates various aspects of one's sense of identity (Giovacchini 1986), including both conscious and unconscious elements of self-perception. The self-representation defines the feelings that will be integrated into a person's identity, which must be harmonized with the rest of the ego to be securely balanced (Giovacchini 1984). Without a synthesis of internal and external perceptions, the identity sense fragments. The ego then fails to achieve integration. A well-functioning self-representation is also necessary for the recognition of one's body and self-boundaries (Sandler 1987).

The healthy adolescent's struggle for freedom and independent individuality gradually solidifies and leads to the development of a "*Weltanschauung*," described by Anna Freud (1937) as the way we "view the world." Newly formulated opinions, ideas, and ideals reflect not only

instinctual and emotional freedom but also freedom of thought and action
(Jacobson 1961). Subsequently, adolescent vacillations of self-esteem and
identity subside and "an autonomous, grown-up, and sexually mature
person [emerges who is able to] create and accept a corresponding consistent and durable self-representation" (Jacobson 1961, p. 179).

Incest victims may have either fragile and vulnerable or stable self-
representations dominated by feelings of inadequacy. Their self-esteem
is diminished (Brooks 1985; Eisnitz 1981, 1984–1985; Finkelhor 1985;
Gelinas 1983; Shapiro 1987; Steele 1986b; Ulman and Brothers 1988) and
they feel ineffective. They can face neither inner nor outer reality. Closely
related to this impairment in self-perception and lowered self-esteem is
the incest victim's impaired sense of identity (Steele 1986b). As is true
for many individuals with character disorders, the incest victim attempts
to stabilize and complete the self-representation by clinging to objects
(Eisnitz 1969, 1981; Meissner 1984; Reich 1953, 1960) to gain a sense of
identity or to enhance a faltering identity (Erikson 1959).

According to Eisnitz (1984–1985), even the healthiest incest victims
are unable to develop an effective internalized system to sustain self-
esteem and maintain a stable self-representation. The self-representation
lacks continuity from the past to the future and so does not allow the
disengagement from parental ties or the formation of a secure and cohesive
sense of identity.

DEVELOPMENTAL INHIBITORS

In the following discussion on inhibitors of adolescent development related to keeping the secrets of incest, I focus on pathologic consequences
for the negotiation of crucial tasks related to consolidating a healthy self-
representation.

Realistic Fears of Disclosure

The incest victim's anxiety regarding blame, punishment, abandonment,
or family disruption is reinforced by the realistic fears of the dangers
surrounding disclosure. As described by Ferenczi (1949): "The children
feel physically and morally helpless, their personalities are not sufficiently
consolidated in order to be able to protest . . . for the overpowering force
and authority of the adult can rob them of their senses" (p. 228). Consequently, the majority of incest victims do not disclose their secret during
childhood or adolescence (Goodwin 1982; Herman 1981; Russell 1986;
Sgroi 1989; Summit 1983).

In a retrospective study by Schultz et al. (1987) that included 148 incest
victims having either multiple personality disorder or posttraumatic stress
disorder, the mean age at which patients made the disclosure of their

incest experiences was 24 years. The majority first disclosed the incest during treatment, to the therapist participating in the questionnaire survey. Of those patients who reported disclosing the incest before age 18 (34% multiple personality disorder, 45% posttraumatic stress disorder), the mean age was 11.5 years. The study also reported that many were not believed (75% multiple personality disorder, 34% posttraumatic stress disorder) by the source first informed (mother, school personnel, or mental health resource), and a significant percentage of both groups were either punished or removed from their home after disclosure.

Such findings underscore the realistic fears incest victims have that the recipient of their secret will betray this trust. The following is a 12-year-old girl's experience following her disclosure of paternal incest. It illustrates many rational reasons for incest victims to suppress the information. The letter appeared in Abigail Van Buren's (1987) newspaper column and is entitled "Promises, Promises—A Child's View of Incest."

> I asked for your help and you told me you would if I told you the things my dad did to me. It was really hard for me to say all those things, but you told me to trust you—then you made me repeat them to 14 different strangers.
>
> I asked you for privacy and you sent two policemen to my school in front of everyone, to go downtown for a talk in their black and white car—like I was the one being busted.
>
> I asked you to believe me, and you said that you did, then you connected me to a lie detector, and took me to court where lawyers put me on trial like I was a liar. I can't help it if I can't remember times or dates or explain why I couldn't tell my mom. Your questions got me confused—my confusion got you suspicious.
>
> I asked you for help and you gave me a doctor with cold metal gadgets and cold hands . . . just like my father, who said it wouldn't hurt, just like my father, who said not to cry. He said I look fine—good news for you. You said, bad news for my case.
>
> I asked you for confidentiality and you let the newspaper get my story. What does it matter that they left out my name when they put in my father's and our home address? Even my best friend's mother won't let her talk to me anymore.
>
> I asked for protection and you gave a social worker who patted my head and called me Honey (mostly because she could never remember my name). She sent me to live with strangers in another place, with a different school.
>
> Do you know what it's like to live where there's a lock on the refrigerator, where you have to ask permission to use the shampoo, and where you can't use the phone to call your friends? You get used to hearing, "Hi, I'm your new social worker, this is your new foster sister, dorm mother, group home." You tiptoe around like a perpetual guest and don't even get to see your own puppy grow up.
>
> Do you know what it's like to have more social workers than friends?
>
> Do you know what it feels like to be the one that everyone blames for all the trouble? Even when they were speaking to me, all they talked about was

lawyers, shrinks, fees, and whether or not they'll lose the mortgage. Do you know what it's like when your sisters hate you, and your brother calls you a liar? It's my word against theirs. I'm 12 years old and he's the manager of a bank. You say you believe me—who cares, if nobody else does.

I asked you for help and you forced my mom to choose between us—she chose him, of course. She was scared and had a lot to lose. I had a lot to lose too—the difference was you never told me how much.

I asked you to put an end to the abuse—you put an end to my whole family. You took away my nights of hell and gave me days of hell instead. You've exchanged my private nightmare for a very public one.

Cindy, age 12*

Loss of Maternal Protection and Attachment Needs

Although many incest victims have stated that the incestuous activity was the most damaging event in their lives (Lindberg and Dystad 1985a), the serious breaches in the maternal protection, analogous to what Winnicott (1960) referred to as a "holding environment," have been described by many investigators (Brooks 1983; Eisnitz 1984–1985; Gartner and Gartner 1988; Giovacchini 1964; Lustig et al. 1966) as the most harmful trauma for the incest victim. In the absence of a "holding environment," the adolescent may protect herself against increased attachment needs by keeping the incest secret.

Trauma was defined by the ancient Greeks (Rappaport 1968) to mean: a wound, a hurt, a damage, and, in an implied sense, a heavy blow or defeat. In contemporary times, *trauma* has been described as the flooding of the psyche by stimuli in excess of its ability to cope (Steele 1986a). Protection against an excess quantity of stimulation (Steele 1986a) as well as against an excess intensity of stimulation are of paramount importance. Freud (1920) described the protection against excessive stimulation as a "protective shield" (*Reizchutz*) and described as traumatic any excitation powerful enough to break through the protective shield. The deficits and failures in this protection determine the amount of psychic damage that may occur.

In contrast to the healthy child's development of a relative immunity to trauma by gradual and age-appropriate exposure to tolerable amounts of stimulation (Edgcumbe and Gavshon 1985), incest victims are generally deprived of this crucial experience, an essential for normal development, long before overt incestuous activity commences. Incest is a symptom of family dysfunction (Lustig et al. 1966; Summit and Kryso 1978) that often includes serious disturbances in the mother-daughter relationship. Such

*Taken from the "Dear Abby" column by Abigail Van Buren, © 1987. Universal Press Syndicate. Reprinted with permission. All rights reserved.

disturbances are likely to be manifested throughout childhood (Brooks 1983; Eisnitz 1984–1985; Gartner and Gartner 1988; Justice and Justice 1979; MacVicar 1979; Rosenthal and Doherty 1985; Soll 1984–1985; Steele 1986b). Although the psychodynamics of the mother-child relationship vary, the defective mothering results in the child experiencing the impact of a traumatic environment without having acquired the relative immunity from trauma noted above. This increased vulnerability may prove a factor from the beginning of life, so that distortions of ego development and defects occur both in preobject and later phases (Gartner and Gartner 1988; Giovacchini 1987), leading to fixations in development. Because protection from internal and external dangers is not available from the mother (primary caretaker), the incest victim is exposed to injurious over-stimulation; the "dosage" of trauma experienced is age- or phase-inappropriate and too great, relative to the strength of the ego (Edgcumbe and Gavshon 1985). The ego is unable successfully to bind the ensuing anxiety (Reich 1960). The victim of incest experiences what has been described by Khan (1964) as a cumulative trauma that "builds up silently and invisibly throughout childhood right up to adolescence, and leaves its mark on all crucial phases of psychosexual development" (p. 273).

Such trauma interferes with the development of self-soothing and the ability to absorb heightened overstimulation. This may result in a wide range of symptoms, defined by Giovacchini (1987) as "the behavioral and subjective manifestations of defense mechanisms" (p. 200). Such symptoms during adolescence are well documented, ranging from action discharge behaviors such as promiscuity (Deisher et al. 1982; Finkelhor 1985; Goodwin 1989; Lindberg and Dystad 1985), substance abuse (Goodwin 1989; Herman 1981; Lindberg and Dystad 1985b; Shapiro and Dominiak 1990; Silbert and Pines 1981), delinquency (Steele 1986b), seizures (Goodwin et al. 1979), pregnancy (Goodwin 1982; Herman and Hirschman 1981; Russell 1986), running away (Carper 1979; Finkelhor 1985; Goodwin 1989; Herman 1981; Herman and Hirschman 1981; McCormack et al. 1986), self-mutilation (Brooks 1985; Goodwin 1982; Richards 1988; Shapiro 1987), and suicide gestures (Finkelhor 1985; Goodwin 1981; Herman 1981; Herman and Hirschman 1981; Lindberg and Dystad 1985b), to withdrawal behaviors and depression (Brooks 1985; Lindberg and Dystad 1985b; MacVicar 1979). Whatever the reactions to this defect in self-regulation, all have the common denominator of vulnerability. The adolescent attempts to fend off the fear of being overwhelmed through symptom formation (Krystal 1978), described by McDougall (1982–1983) as an attempt to self-cure the traumatic state.

Secrecy may also assist the adolescent incest victim to deal with fears of internal dissolution. A patient of Meares (1976) feared that if she told her secrets, she would have nothing left inside and would be invisible.

You're invisible now
You've no secrets left to conceal. (Bob Dylan 1965)

Secrecy structures the heightened stimulus, that is, binds anxiety, and defends against feelings of helplessness, inadequacy, and disintegration.

Another patient, an adult incest survivor, is described by Blitzsten et al. (1950) as reacting with panic and extreme rage when her analyst asked her to reveal the contents of her dream, hence to look at her secret. "The violence of her objection was so great that she even sometimes jumped up from the couch and huddled in a corner" (p. 14). The authors described her specific reaction as unlike the anal characteristic of withholding for fear of devaluation, but rather as expressing an intolerable fear that she would destroy a part of herself (internal dissolution or disintegration) if the dream (secret) were to be revealed. "By being looked at and discussed, the dream might come alive and destroy her" (p. 14).

Realistic fears of family dissolution if the incest secret is disclosed may also increase attachment needs and reinforce the adolescent's self-demand for secrecy. In addition, the cumulative impact of overstimulation perceived as assaultive (Giovacchini 1984) and the experience of maternal abandonment from childhood through adolescence may increase dependency needs and markedly affect the self-representation. Absence of the internalized equivalent of the "protective shield" (self-soothing) throughout childhood increases oral-dependent drives and attachment needs. In a psychological sense, the adolescent incest victim continues to need soothing and nurturing from the mother.

Gordon (1955) suggested that adult incest survivors may reenact the incestuous behavior with other men "primarily as revenge against her rejecting mother and as a defense against her masochistic dependence on her" (p. 292). Kaufman et al. (1954) supported this hypothesis: they reported significant oral deprivation and oral sadism on the Rorschachs (Rorschach 1954) of female adolescent victims of incest. These findings were substantiated on the victims' Thematic Apperception Test (Murray 1943) perceptions of the mother figures as cruel, unjust, and depriving.

According to psychoanalytic theory, dependency is associated with the oral drive and early pregenital impulses (Abraham 1916; Giovacchini 1987). Several authors have suggested that incest is an elaboration of the girl's oral attachment to the mother, concealing pregenital wishes to be loved and protected by her (Blos 1979; Brooks 1983; Gordon 1955; Marmor 1953). During adolescence, the incest victim may hold on to the secret of incest to remain attached to the mother and not disrupt the family unity, however pathologic. The fact that the formula "If you obey, you will be protected" captures the adolescent's longing for omnipotent protection and comfort helps to explain the psychological effectiveness of authority (Fenichel 1945).

Such heightened attachment needs may continue into incest victims' adulthood and perpetuate the need to keep secrets, profoundly affecting the ability to protect their own children. In their attempts to master the trauma, many repeat it by selecting husbands who collude with them in reenacting it, this time making their daughter the victim (Gelinas 1983; Meiselman 1978). They reverse roles with their own mothers, turning passive into active and thus identifying with the aggressor. This is an example of the repetition compulsion, first described by Freud (1914) as repeating rather than remembering.

This is illustrated in the experience of Mrs. W. She did not reveal her own incestuous experience with her father from ages 5 to 12 until she had entered treatment with me at age 41. During the course of treatment, she began to "wonder" if her 8-year-old daughter was involved in a sexual relationship with her husband. Her monetary and psychological dependence on her husband, reflecting her own feelings of helplessness and inadequacy to function autonomously, made it very difficult for her to acknowledge clues to the incestuous relationship between her daughter and her husband. She wanted to keep the secret to preserve her marriage and to protect herself from the fear of internal dissolution.

Mrs. W's mother did not reveal her own childhood incest experience with her father until she was on her deathbed at the age of 86.

Pseudomaturity

Reversal of roles with the mother may begin long before adulthood and is a sign of pathology in the parent and contributor to pathology in the child or adolescent (Bowlby 1973, 1980, 1982). As described in the study by Kaufman et al. (1954), mothers of incest victims displaced their hostility toward their own mothers onto this chosen daughter, forcing her to become their helper and advisor. "They relinquished their responsibilities as parents so that they, in effect, became daughters again, and the daughter a mother . . .they deserted the fathers, who then became involved in the incestuous relationship with the daughters" (pp. 270–271). Consequently, victims of incest serve as selfobjects for the sexually abusive father and nonparticipating mother (Ulman and Brothers 1988).

One reason that the adolescent incest victim may accept the mother's demands to become the caretaker is that the facade of maturity may assist her in keeping her dependency needs secret. Often central to the incestuous dynamics in the family (Pelletier and Handy 1986), such role reversal, or parentification (Gelinas 1983), promotes pseudomature behavior (Kaufman et al. 1954). However, as stated by Lustig et al. (1966), "this involves an unconscious contract exchanging compliance in one area for autonomy in other, perhaps more critical, areas" (p. 36). Pseudomaturity in the area of sexual activity and caretaking is a thin veneer covering heightened anxiety due to insufficient soothing and protection from the maternal object.

Still, role reversal gives the adolescent female a sense of competency in her search for self-esteem and is often accompanied by an "illusion of self-sufficiency" (Modell 1975) that may reinforce her need to hold the secret of incest. For example, this spurious maturity is evident during the adolescence of multiple personality disorder incest victims. The development of additional alternate personalities, some of which may appear to be quite precocious and mature, gives such patients an illusion of separateness and independence that covers strong dependency needs.

Survivors of incest may continue to keep their dependent orientation secret as adults by constructing defenses to protect against crippling feelings of inadequacy and deprivation. Their overcompensatory maneuvers include a false self that has the appearance of total autonomy. As described by Giovacchini (1987), such an ego orientation "is a defensive superstructure defending against a fundamental core dependency" (p. 286). Compulsive caregiving and compulsive self-sufficiency describe a type of independence (Bowlby 1973, 1982) that covers deficiency in self-reliance by catering to the needs of others and/or denying the existence of any needs of one's own. Reversal of roles with the mother may also be an attempt to contain the dysfunctional family since the mother is generally not available to fulfill her maternal and marital commitments (Gartner and Gartner 1988; Herman 1981; Swanson and Biaggio 1985).

The "secret within a secret" includes another aspect of reversal of roles with the mother. Some adolescents involved in a paternal sexual relation find comfort in the sexual experience. Rosenfeld et al. (1977) noted that incestuous relationships are frequently attempts by the daughters to obtain caring and warmth from their fathers, who are often the only source of affection in their environment (Kaufman et al. 1954; Swanson and Biaggio 1985). Father may be perceived as the protector, mother as the castrator (Gordon 1955).

In addition, although the majority of incest terminates at puberty (Gelinas 1983), some adolescents do not want to give it up because of the genital pleasure. As one patient revealed to me: "When I was a little girl, Daddy's penis hurt me, but when I got older it stopped hurting and felt good." Although Ferenczi (1949) stated that the victim of incest has no desire for sexual relations, Abraham (1907) was the first to refute this hypothesis by emphasizing that a child could unconsciously desire it. However, as discussed earlier, the desire for father may be a veneer covering a deeper oral disturbance of the relation to the mother (Gordon 1955; Marmor 1953; Reich 1932). Strivings for the paternal phallus may represent pregenital strivings for the mother's breast (Gordon 1955). In either case, the secret pleasures of the penis generally remain deeply buried and are filled with shame.

Even for the normal adolescent, the struggles with developmental tasks may be associated with shame and a sense of inadequacy (Severino et al. 1987), but the experience of shame is heightened for the incest victim because it is linked with an inner sense of badness and a loss of an idealized self-image (Sandler 1987; Severino et al. 1987). Fenichel (1945) noted: "Shame as motive for defense is mainly directed against exhibitionism and scoptophilia" (p. 139). It is an attempt to hide and to refuse to look because of a constant fear of being criticized, ostracized, or punished (Fenichel 1945). The function of shame, therefore, is similar to the function of keeping secrets: to hide a defective sense of self (Severino et al. 1987).

Adults who are incest survivors have failed to develop a capacity to tolerate shame because of their inability to acknowledge their defective self-images. They may perceive themselves as "damaged goods" (O'Brien 1987), and shame may be the consequence of an internalized defective body image (Severino et al. 1987). Diminished self-esteem (feelings of powerlessness) and inferiority may be compensated by narcissistic object choices (Eisnitz 1969, 1984–1985; Reich 1953, 1960). Reich (1953, 1960) described two predominant patterns: first is a dependent and compliant attachment to one man, who becomes the admired and indispensable idealized object; second is a series of brief, dependent infatuations. Such narcissistic object choices may enhance the fragile self-representation by bolstering or replacing damaged parts (Eisnitz 1969, 1981).

Family Collusion and Conspiracy of Silence

The incest victim's secrecy reinforces illusions, as the adolescent struggles to deny reality both to the external world and to her internal structure. By keeping the incest secret, the adolescent attempts to provide for the other family members what remains unavailable to her: a protection against dissolution. She loyally maintains the secret of incest to guard against punishment and family breakup (Herman 1981; Lister 1982; Russell 1986; Summit 1983) while she herself is denied the opportunity to hold together an adequate self-representation. By bearing the secret, she controls anxiety and preserves her dependency on her mother; thus she cannot develop autonomy (Avery 1982–1983). In addition, to break the conspiracy of silence might be felt as an act of betrayal of the supposedly trusting relationship with her father, for she may feel that she caused the sexual activity and is responsible for it (Finkelhor 1985; Shapiro 1987). Other incest victims believe that they were selected because they were "bad" (Summit and Kryso 1978) and thus deserve to be treated as objects. Forward and Buck (1978) described the profound self-loathing of adult incest survivors that contributes to their belief that they do not deserve emotional, physical, or material satisfaction.

Internalization of the unwritten law of secrecy (the French root for *loyalty* is *loi*, law) also gives the adolescent a sense of direction and meaning (Lutz 1984). Such loyalty may temporarily "fix" (neutralize) her damaged self-representation by preserving the early object ties, warding off terror of loss and separation. In addition, a desire to "cure" the parent (Lister 1982) may also assist the adolescent in retaining the secret.

Consequently, a gratifying sense of power over the parents and control over one's self by holding the secret may provide an illusory self-esteem. However, the self-representation is not genuinely enhanced, for the secret is split off, its reality denied, and the possibility of detachment from the incestuous object diminished.

Because of deficiencies in the self-evaluating functions (Reich 1960), the adolescent incest victim is unable to react and behave in a fashion determined by her own inner needs, and follows the edicts of the external world (Lustig et al. 1966). Such compliance perpetuates her self-perception of being a "pawn" (or a "hole" rather than being "whole"); reinforces her profound experience of inadequacy, worthlessness, and dependency; and further contributes to her defective self-representation. Compliance with external edicts also serves to diminish vulnerability by decreasing fear of losing love or being subjected to hostility. However, feelings of safety by adapting to others comes at the expense of autonomy, a stable self-representation, the modulation of affects, self-esteem, self-respect, and dignity.

When such patients enter treatment, they frequently experience a heightened pathologic need to comply with what they believe that the therapist's expectations will be of them. Unable to initiate interaction, they may wait for the therapist's direction and respond with attempts to conform to what they assume to be expected. If the therapist colludes with this "false self" described by Winnicott (1960), the "true self" remains hidden away, inhabiting the inner core of the personality (Meissner 1982–1983). However,

> Even in the most extreme case of compliance and the establishment of a false personality, hidden away somewhere there exists a secret life that is satisfactory because of its being creative and original to that human being. Its unsatisfactoriness must be measured in terms of its being hidden, its lack of enrichment through experience. (Winnicott 1971, p. 68)

Avoidance of Peer Group

The peer group plays a pivotal role in the assimilation of new objects outside the nuclear family and in establishing an autonomous identity (van der Kolk 1987). Sullivan (1940) suggested that the peer group confirms self-worth, permitting separation from the parents. Erikson (1956)

stated that the adolescent's ability to develop intimacy with peers is related to the ensuing adult capacities for closeness and intimacy.

Because the adolescent incest victim perceives the entire external world
as dangerous and overwhelming, she does not have the autonomy to move
toward new objects, and determinedly avoids significant peer relationships. In O'Brien's (1987) study of 60 female adolescent incest victims,
none of them reported having had adequate and sustained relationships
with their peers; the family remained the main socializing force. Maintaining the secret surrounding the incest contributes to the adolescent's
avoidance of relationships outside the family.

The incest victim withdraws from peers as a defense against her fear
of disclosure of the secret, and she projects her self-perception of worthlessness and blame onto the external world. On the other hand, the secret
may help her to maintain boundaries, assisting in differentiating between
inside and outside (Winnicott 1986); to experience self-esteem ("I've got
something no one else has"); and to establish a feeling of separateness,
described by Fairbairn (1952) as feeling "different from other people"
(p. 22).

Secrecy may also reflect an ego defect. The adolescent may be unable
to form new introjects if they are perceived as threatening and abandoning, or proscribed and punishable. Schafer (1968) defined an introject as
an inner existence that one feels and by which one is influenced.

Just as the maternal introject is always instrumental in the formation
of the self-representation (Giovacchini 1984), perhaps the peer group, as
well as the therapist, can be understood as "transitional introjects" that
aid in the tasks of loosening dependent family ties, proceeding toward
autonomous functioning and developing a cohesive self-representation.
Thus the secret "protects" the incest victim from what are perceived as
traumatic involvements outside the family.

Alice is a 36-year-old former incest victim. When she was a child and
adolescent, her mother constantly told her such "truths" as that she wished
that Alice had never been born because she (Alice) was a "worthless piece
of shit." Alice utilized dissociation and splitting mechanisms to defend
against intolerable affects and projected them into the external world,
from which she withdrew. During treatment with me, Alice's maternal
destructive introjects were projected in the transference. Consequently,
she experienced my interpretations as hurtful accusations and painful
"truths" that disrupted her psychic equilibrium. My efforts to impart
understanding were perceived as traumatic depreciations, similar to the
chronic ruptures in maternal protection that she had experienced throughout childhood and adolescence. She perceived my words as threatening
ruptures, penetrating the protective walls of denial and disavowal that
had been constructed in her attempt to maintain some sense of boundaries, separateness, and self-esteem. Because of her distorted perception,

treatment was an arduous task. She perceived the "holding environment" that I was attempting to provide as dangerous and the "food" that I offered by way of my interpretations as noxious.

Incest victims are filled with disruptive introjects that contribute to a distorted relationship with the external world, as illustrated in the clinical vignette above. Beginning with destructive maternal caretaking, negative percepts have been split off rather than assimilated into the ego. Consequently, the incest victim may be unable to bring new percepts inside because they are perceived as destructive, as well as intrusive and overwhelming.

Maintaining the secret prevents the victimized adolescent from adequately exploring the interpersonal world outside of her family. Consequently, the age-appropriate broadening of interests and pursuit of new objects with which to identify to replace preoedipal ties generally are not feasible. Without having other love objects to turn to, the adolescent cannot complete development (Blum 1987; Pelletier and Handy 1986) for she is unable to affirm her self-worth and loosen infantile dependencies.

SECRECY AND THE DEFENSIVE STRUCTURE

During normal adolescence, defensive adaptations are increased in attempts to cope with increased instinctual turmoils and bodily changes. Incest victims fear object loss and thus experience additional threats to the integrity of the self-representation. Therefore they cling to the object, leading to a fixation of emotional development. This makes the task of coping with the external world more difficult, and the more intolerable the reality, the greater the tension and the more inaccessible the internal situation (Lorenzer 1968).

Rather than using repression, which can be considered a "blanket" in as much as it acts as a cover to render perceptions unconscious, incest victims use disavowal and denial in attempts to repudiate reality, or "blank it," from consciousness.

The truth is not denied entirely, however, for this would sever all contact with reality. Instead, the adolescent victim may distort reality by thinking, "If the world doesn't know about it then it doesn't exist." The defensive maneuvers of splitting and dissociation are utilized also to keep contradictory and intolerable affects split off from consciousness of inner reality.

Secrecy is also a way of splitting off the traumatic experience and an attempt to blank out or deny reality. As stated by Avery (1982–1983), the family secret is "split off but it is not discarded. It forms an unconscious template on which covert family relationships are organized" (p. 481). Consequently, secrecy is an adaptive defense in the victim's attempt to protect both the family and the self from dissolution.

However, such splitting further fragments the already fragile ego, leading to further impairment of the sense of identity. The possibility of developing an expanded and altered sense of self is diminished. Erikson (1968) stated that reality and truth are essential in formation of identity during adolescence. Brooks (1985) stated that the unavailability of "truth seeking" to the incest victim, whose secret is split off, leads to premature closure of identity development.

Splitting off the secret of incest also profoundly affects the ego functions of memory and perception (Jacobs 1980). The family collusion implicitly communicates to the incest victim that conscious awareness of what is seen and experienced must be deleted or distorted. As described by Blum (1987): "The enforced silence may be a fantasy elaboration of the parent's actual attitudes, but it may also become internalized along with impairment of curiosity and alterations in the sense of reality" (p. 618).

Adults who are chronically preoccupied with secrets and secrecy may have a personality organization that includes a secretive mode of relating to the world, described by Coppolillo et al. (1981) as an ego distortion. Gitelson (1958) called these ego distortions highly organized clinical phenomena whose etiology is not readily apparent, each case representing a particular adaptation to a particular internal and external environment, which was impressed on the entirety of personality development. For many adult survivors, a secretive mode of relating is embedded as a persistent character trait, becomimg more important for their psychic economy than the content of the secret itself. Gross (1951) described the secret as capable of regenerating itself: "The secret, once surrendered, is lost only insofar as its content is concerned. The vessel which contained it endures, ready to be filled with new content" (p. 38).

TREATMENT IMPLICATIONS

The harboring of secrets by adult incest survivors serves multidetermined defensive and adaptive functions, but I limit my discussion in this section to those encompassing the issues of autonomy and sense of identity.

During the course of treatment, adult incest survivors, like others who have a secretive mode of relating to the world, reenact through the transference situation all or many of the original uses and meanings of secrets and secrecy. Gross (1951) suggested that a full transference develops only after patients are finally able to reveal one of their secrets to the therapist.

The fundamental rule in psychoanalytic treatment, the *sine qua non*, is free association, which requires that the patient must not keep secrets (Greenson 1967; Hoyt 1978). The patient is directed not to withhold conscious secrets so that unconscious secrets can be uncovered (Ekstein and Caruth 1972). The necessity to follow this fundamental rule (*die Grundregel*) was first emphasized by Freud (1913) when he noted that harboring conscious secrets, which he considered an intentional overt resistance, would permit memories, thoughts, and impulses to remain hidden behind this shelter and thus elude examination. Secrets can deliberately be kept in many ways, including the declared withholding of information (explicit secrets), the passive refusal to submit to the basic rule of keeping no secrets (silence), and the attempt to conceal the presence of secrets (lies). Freud (1913) compared a patient consciously withholding material from the therapist to a village allowing one spot to be a haven from the police. Eventually, all the riffraff of the village would congregate there and thus escape detection. However, as pointed out by Hoyt (1978): "Rules are generally established to control behavior that would otherwise occur. . . . The fundamental rule is no exception: the keeping and telling of secrets occurs frequently and plays an important role in the course of psychotherapy" (p. 231).

The therapist must be cautious that the fundamental rule of treatment, the *sine qua non*, does not become the therapist's "sin" *qua non*. The therapist must not commit the sin of becoming a superego figure (police officer) with rules against secrets (riffraff).

Both Greenson (1967) and Gross (1951) considered the secret to be a form of resistance, that is, directed against a drive, but it is generally understood that the unconscious motive for keeping the secret, rather than its hidden content, needs to be analyzed first (Greenson 1967). Greenson argued that "it is an error to use coercion, threats, or pleadings to get the patient to tell his secret" (p. 231). The term *resistance* is frequently misused by those therapists who assume that all patients are able to respond otherwise. However, not all patients are able to free associate. It is imperative for the therapist working with incest survivors to recognize that what appears to be resistance may be inherent incapacity due to structural defects and characterological maldevelopment (Giovacchini 1986).

In addition, we must understand that the healthy keeping of secrets is adaptive and does not require countercathectic energy. According to Blanck (1966), they "should, therefore, be left intact or even reinforced . . . to help the patient understand his defensive structure" (p. 8). For example, a defense that operates as a resistance in analysis may also serve the function of primary autonomy (Hartmann 1951), and a secret may have the adaptive function of maintaining a core identity (Caruth 1985).

Incest survivors may keep secrets to prevent leaking, or secreting, their sense of identity in a way similar to that of the autistic child who stuffed the holes in his body to prevent his leaking out through them (Tustin 1981). In essence, the patient must be allowed the freedom to keep secrets until the impaired ego is capable of genuine choice. As noted by Blanck (1966): "Not until the ability to say 'no' is well established can one also say 'yes' without loss of autonomy" (p. 11).

Consequently, keeping secrets may serve both pathologic and healthy functions simultaneously. A major goal of treatment is to recognize these functions and assist such patients in holding and containing the split off and dissociated affects surrounding the rupture in maternal protection. Just as going to sleep may help infants adapt to intense distress (McDougall 1982–1983), secrecy may assist the incest victim to "put to sleep" intolerable affects that are forbidden expression.

To illustrate, an adult incest survivor, Miss L, began treatment by saying that she wanted to "put the past behind her." I soon learned that during her adolescence her father would get into bed with her during the night and penetrate her genitally as he lay behind her. She remained "sleeping" during these sexual experiences and they were never directly acknowledged. This attempt to "blank" affects, perceptions, and underlying regressive wishes reinforced her experience of being dead, ineffective, and worthless.

Throughout treatment, Miss L attempted to protect herself in a similar fashion by avoiding content and ignoring my interpretations. The patient gave me a Christmas gift. Rather than collude with her pathology by blindly opening the box and accepting the gift, over the next several sessions, I attempted to determine the unconscious meaning of her gesture. After her initial feeling of being rejected because I did not open the box immediately, she was able to let me know that the contents symbolized what she hoped to become in treatment. I understood that the gift represented her secret "true" self, the healthy core of her identity that she kept deeply hidden, so I returned the box to her unopened. I informed her that I would participate in holding her destructive and distorted forces but would not intentionally take away her healthy characteristics, as represented by the gift.

Was the attempted gift giving a sign of health or pathology? It may be considered healthy for she was attempting to reveal to me her secret "true" self. However, it may also be considered pathologic, for she was reenacting her childhood incestuous experience in numerous ways. First, she frequently used the phrase "it doesn't matter," recalling her avoidance behavior by remaining asleep as well as her self-perception as an object without substance and worth. If I had taken her gift, I would have acted as her father, robbing her of her self-esteem and her hidden self-perception that she does "matter." Second, by accepting her gift, I would have colluded with her oral-dependent strivings and wish to merge with me as a maternal object via giving up her sense of identity. Finally, she was very reluctant to reveal the contents of the box and explore the meaning. Again, was this resistance or healthy adaptation? On the one hand, her decision to say "no," not revealing the content of the box, might promote autonomy and self-esteem—both healthy functions of maintaining the secret. In addition, she may have unconsciously felt that I was not receptive to her "true" self and wanted to protect me from her "dangerous thoughts." On the other hand, her reluctance to reveal the contents of the box may also be understood as a pathologic attempt, similar to her childhood attempt, to keep content out of the relationship and remain disconnected from me as well as from her own thoughts, feelings, and actions.

As therapists working with such patients, we must recognize both the healthy and pathologic functions of secrets; we must accept but not collude with such patients' needs to avoid, distort, blank, or dissociate fundamental truths and affects, nor can we participate in what Langs (1982) referred to as "lie or lie-barrier therapy." Painful truths may be perceived as dangerous, and it is vital that we understand how the persistent pathologic needs for secrecy contribute to the distorted perception of the self as only a reflection of the external world. Lack of self-observation and inner deadness are reflected in a poorly defined identity sense and a defective self-representation.

Without treatment, the structural defects, developmental fixations, blurred ego boundaries, and overcompensatory defenses and adaptations persist. As adults, incest survivors manifest a multitude of possible aberrant behavior patterns and handicapping symptoms. However, at the core of their psychopathology, a defective self-representation remains, around which develops a multitude of clinical presentations.

Consequently, although secrecy ensures incest victims against further loss (Avery 1982–1983; Lister 1982), it contributes to their remaining in the mire of adolescence, bound to infantile objects and unable to become more independent of the external world. Adult incest survivors remain in a state of what Blos (1968) called a "prolonged adolescence" because of inability to negotiate developmental tasks. Rather than developing a continuity of experience, such patients sustain a series of developmental fixations.

Speaking metaphorically, these individuals live in houses having rooms that are locked, rooms that are empty, and rooms filled only with furnishings identical to those of their parents. Our task as therapists is to help such patients to open the locked rooms, to tolerate what emerges, and to develop their own sense of "taste" and autonomy.

SUMMARY

Incest victims' intense need for secrecy during adolescence profoundly affects consolidation of personality development at the end of this transitional phase. Intended to protect the self and the family from dissolution, secrecy inhibits disengagement from pathologic objects and their internalized representations, thus contributing to fixations and leading to an inability to form an integrated self-representation and to function autonomously as adults.

REFERENCES

Abraham K: The experiencing of sexual traumas as a form of sexual activity (1907), in The Selected Papers on Psychoanalysis. Translated by Bryan D, Strachey A. New York, Basic Books, 1960, pp 47–63

Abraham K: The first pregenital stage of the libido (1916), in The Selected Papers on Psychoanalysis. Translated by Bryan D, Strachey A. New York, Basic Books, 1960, pp 248–279

Alter-Reid K, Gibbs MS, Lachenmeyer JR, et al: Sexual abuse of children: a review of the empirical findings. Clinical Psychology Review 6:249–266, 1986

Avery NC: Family secrets. Psychoanal Rev 69:471–486, 1982–1983

Bettelheim B: Some comments on privacy, in Surviving and Other Essays. New York, Knopf, 1979, pp 399–411

Blanck G: Some technical implications of ego psychology. Int J Pychoanal 47:6–13, 1966

Blitzsten NL, Eissler RS, Eissler KR: Emergence of hidden ego tendencies during dream analysis. Int J Psychoanal 31:12–17, 1950

Blos P: On Adolescence: A Psychoanalytic Interpretation. New York, Free Press, 1962

Blos P: Character formation in adolescence. Psychoanal Study Child 23:245–263, 1968

Blos P: Modifications in the classical psychoanalytic model of adolescence. Adolesc Psychiatry 7:6–25, 1979

Blum H: The role of identification in the resolution of trauma: the Anna Freud Memorial Lecture. Psychoanal Q 56:609–627, 1987

Bowlby J: Attachment and Loss, Vol 2: Separation. New York, Basic Books, 1973

Bowlby J: Attachment and Loss, Vol 3: Sadness and Depression. New York, Basic Books, 1980

Bowlby J: Attachment and Loss, Vol 1: Attachment, 2nd Edition. New York, Basic Books, 1982

Brooks B: Preoedipal issues in a postincest daughter. Am J Psychother 37:129–136, 1983

Brooks B: Sexually abused children and adolescent identity development. Am J Psychother 39:401–410, 1985

Carper JM: Emergencies in adolescents: runaways and father-daughter incest. Pediatr Clin North Am 26:883–894, 1979

Caruth EG: Secret bearer or secret barer? Contemporary Psychoanalysis 21:548–562, 1985

Coppolillo HP, Horton PC, Haller L: Secrets and the secretive mode. Journal of the American Academy of Child Psychiatry 20:71–83, 1981

Deisher R, Robinson G, Boyer D: The adolescent female and male prostitute. Pediatr Ann 11:819–825, 1982

Deutsch H: The Psychology of Women, Vol 1. New York, Grune & Stratton, 1944

Dylan B: "Like A Rolling Stone." M Witmark, 1965

Edgcumbe R, Gavshon A: Clinical comparisons of traumatic events and reactions. Bulletin of the Anna Freud Centre 8:3–21, 1985

Eisnitz AJ: Narcissistic object choice, self representation. Int J Psychoanal 50:15–25, 1969

Eisnitz AJ: The perspective of the self-representation: some clinical implications. J Am Psychoanal Assoc 29:309–336, 1981

Eisnitz AJ: Father-daughter incest. International Journal of Psychoanalysis and Psychotherapy 10:495–503, 1984–1985

Ekstein R, Caruth E: Keeping secrets, in Tactics and Techniques in Psychoanalytic Therapy. Edited by Giovacchini PL. New York, Science House, 1972, pp 200–215

Erikson EH: The problem of ego identity. J Am Psychoanal Assoc 4:56–121, 1956

Erikson EH: Identity and the Life Cycle. New York, International Universities Press, 1959

Erikson EH: Identity, Youth and Crisis. New York, WW Norton, 1968

Fairbairn WR: An Object Relations Theory of the Personality. New York, Basic Books, 1952

Fenichel O: The Psychoanalytic Theory of Neurosis. New York, WW Norton, 1945

Ferenczi S: Confusion of tongues between the adult and the child. Int J Psychoanal 30:225–230, 1949

Finkelhor D: The traumatic impact of child sexual abuse: a conceptualization. Am J Orthopsychiatry 55:530–541, 1985

Forward S, Buck C: Betrayal of Innocence: Incest and Its Devastation. Los Angeles, CA, Tarcher, 1978

Freud A: The Ego and the Mechanisms of Defense (1937), Revised Edition. New York, International Universities Press, 1966

Freud S: Three essays on sexuality (1905), in The Standard Edition of the Complete Psychological Works of Sigmund Freud, Vol 7. Translated and edited by Strachey J. London, Hogarth Press, 1953

Freud S: On beginning treatment (1913), in The Standard Edition of the Complete Psychological Works of Sigmund Freud, Vol 12. Translated and edited by Strachey J. London, Hogarth Press, 1958

Freud S: Remembering, repeating and working through (1914), in The Standard Edition of the Complete Psychological Works of Sigmund Freud, Vol 12. Translated and edited by Strachey J. London, Hogarth Press, 1958

Freud S: Beyond the pleasure principle (1920), in The Standard Edition of the Complete Psychological Works of Sigmund Freud, Vol 18. Translated and edited by Strachey J. London, Hogarth Press, 1955

Gartner A, Gartner J: Borderline pathology in post-incest female adolescents: diagnostic and theoretical considerations. Bull Menninger Clin 52:101–113, 1988

Gelinas D: The persisting negative effects of incest. Psychiatry 46:312–331, 1983

Giovacchini PL: The submerged ego. Journal of the American Academy of Child Psychiatry 3:430–442, 1964

Giovacchini PL: Character Disorders and Adaptive Mechanisms. Northvale, NJ, Jason Aronson, 1984

Giovacchini PL: Developmental Disorders: The Transitional Space in Mental Breakdown and Creative Integration. Northvale, NJ, Jason Aronson, 1986

Giovacchini PL: A Narrative Textbook of Psychoanalysis. Northvale, NJ, Jason Aronson, 1987

Gitelson M: On ego distortion. Int J Psychoanal 39:245–257, 1958

Goodwin J: Suicidal attempts in sexual abuse victims and their mothers. Child Abuse Negl 5:217–221, 1981

Goodwin J: Sexual Abuse: Incest Victims and Their Families, 2nd Edition. Chicago, IL, Year Book, 1989

Goodwin J, Simms M, Bergman R: Hysterical seizures: a sequel to incest. Am J Orthopsychiatry 49:698–703, 1979

Gordon L: Incest as revenge against the preoedipal mother. Psychoanal Review 42:284–292, 1955

Greenson RR: The struggle against identification. J Am Psychoanal Assoc 2:200–217, 1954

Greenson RR: The Technique and Practice of Psychoanalysis. New York, International Universities Press, 1967

Gross A: The secret. Bull Menninger Clin 15:37–44, 1951

Hartmann H: Technical implications of ego psychology (1951), in Essays on Ego Psychology. New York, International Universities Press, 1964, pp 142–154

Herman JL: Father-Daughter Incest. Cambridge, MA, Harvard University Press, 1981

Herman JL, Hirschman L: Families at risk for father-daughter incest. Am J Psychiatry 138:967–970, 1981

Hoyt MF: Secrets in psychotherapy: theoretical and practical considerations. International Review of Psychoanalysis 5:231–241, 1978

Jacobs JJ: Secrets, alliances, and family fictions: some psychoanalytic observations. J Am Psychoanal Assoc 28:21–42, 1980

Jacobson E: The self and the object world: vicissitudes of their infantile cathexes and their influences on ideational and affective development. Psychoanal Study Child 9:75–127, 1954

Jacobson E: Adolescent moods and the remodeling of psychic structures in adolescence. Psychoanal Study Child 16:164–183, 1961

Justice B, Justice R: The Broken Taboo. New York, Human Sciences Press, 1979

Kaufman I, Peck AL, Tagiuri CK: The family constellation and overt incestuous relations between father and daughter. Am J Orthopsychiatry 24:266–279, 1954

Khan MR: Ego distortion, cumulative trauma, and the role of reconstruction in the analytic situation. Int J Psychoanal 45:272–279, 1964

Krystal H: Trauma and affects. Psychoanal Study Child 33:81–116, 1978

Langs R: The Psychotherapeutic Conspiracy. Northvale, NJ, Jason Aronson, 1982

Lindberg FH, Dystad LJ: Post-traumatic stress disorders in women who experienced childhood incest. Child Abuse Negl 9:329–334, 1985a

Lindberg FH, Dystad LJ: Survival responses to incest: adolescents in crisis. Child Abuse Negl 9:521–526, 1985b

Lister ED: Forced silence: a neglected dimension of trauma. Am J Psychiatry 139:872–876, 1982

Lorenzer A: Some observations on the latency of symptoms in patients suffering from persecution sequelae. Int J Psychoanal 49:316–318, 1968

Lustig N, Dresser JW, Spellman SW, et al: Incest: a family group survival pattern. Arch Gen Psychiatry 14:31–40, 1966

Lutz SE: Contextual family therapy with the victims of incest. J Adolesc 7:319–327, 1984

MacVicar K: Psychotherapeutic issues in the treatment of sexually abused girls. Journal of the American Academy of Child Psychiatry 18:342–353, 1979

Margolis GJ: Secrecy and identity. Int J Psychoanal 47:517–522, 1966

Margolis GJ: The psychology of keeping secrets. Int J Psychoanal 1:291–296, 1974

Marmor J: Orality in the hysterical personality. J Am Psychoanal Assoc 1:656–671, 1953

McCormack A, Janus MD, Burgess AW: Runaway youths and sexual victimization: gender differences in an adolescent runaway population. Child Abuse Negl 10:387–395, 1986

McDougall J: Alexithymia, psychosomatosis, and psychosis. International Journal of Psychoanalysis and Psychotherapy 9:379–388, 1982–1983

Meares R: The secret. Psychiatry 39:258–265, 1976

Meiselman K: Incest: A Psychological Study of Causes and Effects With Treatment Recommendations. San Francisco, CA, Jossey-Bass, 1978

Meissner WW: Notes on the potential differentiations of borderline conditions. International Journal of Psychoanalysis and Psychotherapy 9:3–49, 1982–1983

Meissner WW: The Borderline Spectrum: Differential Diagnosis and Developmental Issues. Northvale, NJ, Jason Aronson, 1984

Modell AH: A narcissistic defence against affects and the illusion of self-sufficiency. Int J Psychoanal 56:275–282, 1975

Murray HA: Thematic Apperception Test. Cambridge, MA, Harvard University Press, 1943

O'Brien JD: The effects of incest on female adolescent development. J Am Acad Psychoanal 15:83–92, 1987

Pelletier G, Handy LC: Family dysfunction and the psychological impact of child sexual abuse. Can J Psychiatry 31:407–412, 1986

Piaget J: Play, Dreams and Imitation in Childhood. New York, WW Norton, 1962

Rapaport D: A historical survey of psychoanalytic ego psychology. Bulletin of the Philadelphia Association of Psychoanalysis 7/8:105–120, 1957–1958

Rappaport EA: Beyond traumatic neurosis. Int J Psychoanal 49:719–731, 1968

Reich A: Analysis of a case of brother-sister incest (1932), in Annie Reich: Psychoanalytic Contributions. New York, International Universities Press, 1973, pp 1–22

Reich A: Narcissistic object choice in women. J Am Psychoanal Assoc 1:22–42, 1953

Reich A: Pathologic forms of self-esteem regulation. Psychoanal Study Child 15:215–232, 1960

Richards AD: Self-mutilation and father-daughter incest: a psychoanalytic case report, in Fantasy, Myth, and Reality: Essays in Honor of Jacob A. Arlow, M.D. Edited by Blum HP, Kramer V, Richards AK, et al. Madison, CT, International Universities Press, 1990, pp 465–478

Rorschach H: Rorschach. New York, Grune & Stratton, 1954

Rosenfeld AA, Nadelson CC, Krieger M, et al: Incest and sexual abuse of children. Journal of the American Academy of Child Psychiatry 16:327–339, 1977

Rosenthal PA, Doherty MB: Psychodynamics of delinquent girls' rage and violence directed toward mother. Adolesc Psychiatry 12:281–289, 1985

Russell DE: The Secret Trauma: Incest in the Lives of Girls and Women. New York, Basic Books, 1986

Sandler J: From Safety to Superego. New York, Guilford, 1987

Schafer R: Aspects of Internalization. New York, International Universities Press, 1968

Schultz R, Braun BG, Kluft RP: The relationship between post-traumatic stress disorder and multiple personality disorder, in Dissociative Disorders 1987: Proceedings of the Fourth International Conference on Multiple Personality/ Dissociative States. Edited by Braun BG. Chicago, IL, Rush University, 1987, p 14

Severino SK, McNutt ER, Feder SL: Shame and the development of autonomy. J Am Acad Psychoanal 15:93–106, 1987

Sgroi SM: Handbook of Clinical Intervention in Child Sexual Abuse. Lexington, MA, DC Heath, 1989

Shapiro S: Self-mutilation and self-blame in incest victims. Am J Psychother 41:46–54, 1987

Shapiro S, Dominiak G: Common psychological defenses seen in the treatment of sexually abused adolescents. Am J Psychother 44:68–74, 1990

Sheugold L: Soul Murder: The Aftereffects of Childhood Abuse and Deprivation. New Haven, CT, Yale University Press, 1989

Silbert MH, Pines AM: Sexual child abuse as an antecedent to prostitution. Child Abuse Negl 5:407–411, 1981

Soll MH: The transferable penis and the self-representation. International Journal of Psychoanalysis and Psychotherapy 10:473–493, 1984–1985

Spiegel LA: A review of contributions to a psychoanalytic theory of adolescence. Psychoanal Study Child 6:375–393, 1951

Spiegel LA: The self, the sense of self, and perception. Psychoanal Study Child 14:81–109, 1959

Steele BF: Child abuse, in The Reconstruction of Trauma: Its Significance in Clinical Work (Monograph 2). Edited by Rothstein A. New York, International Universities Press, 1986a, pp 59–72

Steele BF: Notes on the lasting effects of early child abuse throughout the life cycle. Child Abuse Negl 10:283–291, 1986b

Sullivan HS: Conceptions of Modern Psychiatry. New York, WW Norton, 1940

Sulzberger CF: Why it is hard to keep secrets. Psychoanalysis 2:37–44, 1953

Summit R: The child sexual abuse accommodation syndrome. Child Abuse Negl 7:177–193, 1983

Summit R, Kryso J: Sexual abuse of children: a clinical spectrum. Am J Orthopsychiatry 48:237–251, 1978

Swanson L, Biaggio MK: Therapeutic perspectives on father-daughter incest. Am J Psychiatry 142:667–674, 1985

Tarachow S: Coprophagia and allied phenomena. J Am Psychoanal Assoc 14:685–700, 1966

Tausk V: On the origin of the "influencing machine" in schizophrenia. Psychoanal Q 2:519–556, 1933

Tustin F: Autistic States in Children. London, Routledge & Kegan Paul, 1981

Ulman RB, Brothers D: The Shattered Self: A Psychoanalytic Study of Trauma. Hillsdale, NJ, Analytic Press, 1988

Van Buren A: Promises, promises—a child's view of incest. Universal Press Syndicate, Kansas City, MO, September 24, 1987

van der Kolk BA: The role of the group in the origin and resolution of the trauma response, in Psychological Trauma. Edited by van der Kolk BA. Washington, DC, American Psychiatric Press, 1987, pp 153–171

Winnicott D: The Maturational Process and the Facilitating Environment. New York, International Universities Press, 1960

Winnicott D: Playing and Reality. New York, Basic Books, 1971

Winnicott D: Holding and Interpretation: Fragment of an Analysis. New York, Grove Press, 1986

CHAPTER 8

The Cognitive Sequelae of Incest

Catherine G. Fine, Ph.D.

"It changed my way of thinking.
I think all men are out there
for what they can get."
(From Russell 1986, p. 9)

This comment could be uttered by an angry spouse or an embittered lover; it could reflect unresolved oedipal issues in a neurotic patient; it could be a radical feminist's sociopolitical statement. In actuality, it was said by a victim of brother-sister incest.

The object of this chapter is to explore the cognitive domain of incest victims. It will attempt to capture their world and speculate about the processes that lead to its creation and maintenance. In the first section of the chapter, I will briefly review the cognitive, affective, and behavioral presentations of incest survivors. This will be followed by an inquiry into the defensive mechanisms mobilized by victims of abuse from a cognitive-developmental perspective and a review of their fairly standard and steadfastly rigid distorted beliefs. A cognitive-developmental approach will be employed to attempt to explain the process through which the false assumptions are established and reinforced. Implications for treatment will be considered in the last section.

INCEST: COGNITIVE, AFFECTIVE, AND BEHAVIORAL PHENOMENOLOGIES

Incest and its consequences are being increasingly addressed in the popular as well as scholarly literature. Clinicians and patients alike are lifting the shroud that long concealed this once secret trauma (Finkelhor 1984; Gelinas 1983; Herman 1981; Russell 1986). They address both the short-term and far-reaching negative effects that incest victims experience.

161

These negative consequences are the result of the betrayal of a significant relationship by an "alleged" caretaker (Gelinas 1983; Goodwin 1982; Russell 1986). The reported sequelae of incest are many; they can affect every area of an individual's life. Incest in childhood and adolescence impacts on how victims think and feel and on the way in which they behave.

The problems of incest victims pervade the cognitive, affective, and behavioral realms. Their phenotypal symptom complexes are fluid and disguised and may include characteristic that are commonly associated, with any number of other mental disorders (Gelinas 1983). They are often misattributed by the patient, and sometimes by the therapist, to ongoing daily problems in living or to problems based on fantasized seductions by the opposite-sex parent, rather than being recognized as rooted in historical trauma and forced sexuality with a parent or someone in a quasi-parental or other familial role. There is no single indicator or unitary clue pathognomonic of past or present incestuous involvement. The incest survivor's symptoms are diverse and will vary as a function of patients' ages, expectations of treatment, definition of their problems (and therefore the type of therapist with whom they have chosen to work), and so on.

The Behavioral Realm of the Incest Survivor

An exploration of different behavioral presentations of incest victims according to the ages at which patients are assessed suggests that children may enter the mental health system because of learning disabilities or attention-deficit disorder (Fish-Murray et al. 1987). Adolescents may be brought to therapy or court ordered to therapy because they are runaways, promiscuous, or involved in prostitution and/or polysubstance abuse (Gelinas 1983). Adult women may present for treatment with marital difficulties or sexual dysfunctions (Herman 1981). These behavioral manifestations may express or result from attempts to ward off unacceptable feelings or still more unacceptable impulses; they often appear to be actual behavioral reenactments of abuse scenes. Although these reenactments constitute a present-day reliving of past abuse, they unfortunately also recreate opportunities for revictimization.

The Affective Realm of the Incest Survivor

The affective presentation of incest victims is remarkably nonspecific. The identifying complaint that brings the patient to treatment is often vague and can be suggestive of any number of affective disorders. In the words of Tamara (a pseudonym):

> I'm not sure why I'm here . . . I'm just unhappy . . . I've been this way for years . . . nothing ever works out for me . . . I probably shouldn't be here. . . .

I'm sure I'm wasting my time, this won't work out either . . . other doctors have said it was genetic.

In some ways, her problem *was* genetic, but in the psychoanalytical rather than the traditional psychobiologic sense: her biologic father had forced sexual intercourse on her starting in elementary school.

Feelings of depression and anxiety are by far the more common emotions described by these victims, although panic attacks, multiple phobias, and hypomania are also reported. Acute emotional reactions are often triggered by situations (or people or places) that, through stimulus generalization, have become associated with their abuser(s) or the abuse(s). Any sensory modality can be mobilized to transmit the message: danger. For example, triggers to panic attacks can be men, men with certain characteristic features, a swimming pool, the smell of cigars, or even a time of year. Obviously, the more generalized the stimulus trigger, the more disabled the patient will be and the more likely she may be to seek treatment.

The Cognitive Realm of the Incest Survivor

Although these panic reactions to perceived danger may appear spontaneous and instantaneous to the outside observer, much of the information about the stimulus circumstance has already been processed repeatedly at a cognitive level and has become, for better or worse, overlearned. Hence, the incest victim's cognitive make-up can be understood as a defensive by-product of the physical and sexual abuse sustained by a young and developmentally maturing child who is trying to make sense of her frightening circumstances. The abuse victim has created ways of understanding herself and the world around her that allow her to gain some predictive edge over its many inconsistencies and seeming incongruities. Because the perceived reality of sexually abused children is different from that of other children (Fish-Murray et al. 1987), it is safe to assume that their understanding of people, of themselves, and of situations will also differ. In other words, incest victims think differently from nonvictims, and consequently their feelings and their behaviors will also differ.

Incest victims, like other survivors of traumatic stress, have had some of their fundamental beliefs about themselves and their world shattered (Janoff-Bulman 1985). Epstein (1973, 1979) postulated that these two belief systems form one's perception of reality. Incest victims may have endured and survived the trauma(s), but their reality is shattered. They construct or reconstruct a world based on distorted beliefs and misguided assumptions that will determine their causal attributions, set up their strategies for predicting outcomes, and dictate their life views. There are marked dissimilarities between the thinking of victims and nonvictims;

these differences will increase with the age of onset of the abuse, its total duration, the number of perpetrators, and the actual violence of the assaults. Incest beginning at a younger age, persisting over a longer period of time, and involving several individuals (Hartman et al. 1987) and marked by more violent altercations increases the likelihood of more deeply rooted alterations in thinking.

INCEST AND TRAUMA

Surveys on incest and child sexual abuse and its detrimental consequences (Finkelhor 1984; Russell 1986) are increasing in the contemporary scientific literature. Although they recognize that some survive incest with minimal consequences, they discredit with emphasis earlier reports that proposed that, in general, incest may not be traumatic (Henderson 1975; Weiner 1962). Rascovsky and Rascovsky (1950) suggested that tolerating incestuous involvement may be the lesser of two evils, the alternative being psychosis.

Enduring incest is not the alternative to psychosis, but dissociation may well be. Dissociation is a defense mechanism mobilized as the abuse is ongoing; it is an attempt to "escape from the present" (Spiegel et al. 1988) in which the child is physically trapped. The child's helplessness when being abused is internalized and transformed and becomes the background against which all additional psychological phenomena will evolve. If dissociation represents the severing of the association of one thing from another (Frischholz 1985), then dissociation in traumatic circumstances serves the purpose of removing from the individual's awareness parts of the event or the event in toto. Initially designed to decrease temporarily the anxiety of the overwhelming circumstances befalling the child, dissociation can become a more permanent and preferred strategy that leads incest victims to be amnestic for the actual abuse as well as other informational or affective nuclei proximally and/or semantically connected to the abuse.

The presence of dissociation and its concomitant phenomena after a trauma is not a new concept. Historically, Despine (Despine 1840; Fine 1988) and Janet (1889) documented cases of dissociation secondary to trauma more than 100 years ago. Their observations are congruent with those of contemporary investigators such as Kluft (1984), Putnam (1985), and Spiegel (1984). These authors anticipated the possibility of encountering dissociative symptoms, and perhaps even a dissociative disorder, when a trauma has been documented in a patient's life history.

A more extreme example of dissociative disorder is multiple personality disorder (MPD). Of patients with MPD, 97% have experienced physical and sexual abuse, 68% incestuously (Putnam et al. 1986). The illustrative examples for this chapter will be taken from an MPD subsample who were sexually molested by a close relative.

It is understood that all incest victims do not develop MPD and that all do not have such extreme disorders of identity and memory as are common in this disorder (Nemiah 1981). However, dissociative phenomena are common to the point of being characteristic of non-MPD incest victims as well (Gelinas 1983). MPD patients who demonstrate more encapsulated and discrete psychopathologic phenomena provide more explicit demonstrations of the effects of dissociation on cognition than incest victims with less well-defined dissociative symptoms.

If therapists know which cognitive styles may reflect dissociation in MPD, their index of suspicion will be raised to the less dramatic dissociative pathologies common throughout the incest-related syndromes. Understanding the cognitive world of the MPD victim will facilitate detection of incest in non-MPD victims and help to establish a working relationship between therapist and patient more rapidly. Therefore, in this chapter, MPD will be used as the paradigmatic model against which other perhaps less dramatic dissociative phenomena and cognitive distortions commonly found in incest victims can be compared.

In the context of the often distorted reality of the incest victim, the task of initiating and maintaining a therapeutic alliance is forwarded when the therapist is consistent and predictable. These attributes are more likely achieved when the therapist is grounded within a flexible explanatory model, such as Braun's (1988) model of dissociation, which includes a strong cognitive component.

BRAUN'S BASK MODEL OF DISSOCIATION

Braun's (1988) BASK model of dissociation has considerable descriptive and explanatory power despite (or perhaps because of) its parsimony. It states that people, when in nondissociated states, experience events almost simultaneously across four dimensions: they have Knowledge of the events, they can associate Behaviors to those events, they have Sensations (physical/physiologic and/or proprioceptive) during them, and feel Affects as well. In a dissociated state, any one or all of these interconnections can be severed and recombined.

Dissociated ego states, which are patterns of behavior and experiences bound by a common principle, yet separated from one another by differentially permeable boundaries (Kluft 1987; Watkins and Watkins 1982), are based on independent ostensibly "free-floating" parts, on incomplete combinations of these disassociated elements, or on groups of complete or incomplete event-parts escalating into increasingly complex structures.

Each of these dissociated ego states may carry with it a cognitive experience that shapes that part's affect. Uncovering this cognitive mode is very much like listening for Luborsky's (1984) "red thread" within a symptom-context approach in his work on patients' core conflictual relationships. Discovering the red thread of the patient's cognitive reality hopefully will protect the therapy from disruptions by the patient's resistances and the therapist's countertransferential withdrawal as both struggle against inner obstacles to face the patient's genuinely painful material.

In the treatment of abuse victims, it is essential to discover and confront both the cognitive distortions and their often overdetermined reactions rather than engaging in the pursuit of increasingly complex ruminations or distracting issues that foster spiraling confusion, derailing of the treatment, helplessness on the part of the patient, and a sense of impotence and exasperation on the part of the therapist. Therefore, in the next section of this chapter, I will examine the cognitive world of adults incestuously victimized as children and systematically review the cognitive distortions the therapist is likely to encounter as treatment proceeds.

THE COGNITIVE REALITIES OF CHILDHOOD VICTIMS OF ABUSE

Many MPD patients share the same distorted thinking present in their non-MPD depressive cohorts; indeed, depressive symptomatology is present in more than 80% of MPD patients (Putnam et al. 1986). Depressogenic thoughts (Beck et al. 1979) are also the unfortunate plight of incest victims. Although the distorted thinking in depressed patients Beck et al. speak of shares surface similarities with the thinking of incest survivors, the cognitive distortions of child sexual abuse victims are more established and have the quality of deep-rooted perceptual deficits. They respond fairly unsuccessfully to traditional cognitive maneuvers.

The distortions that form the bases of MPD patients' cognitive realities stem from faulty information processing of the varieties described by Beck et al. (1979). They lead to the following determinants of thought: 1) dichotomous thinking, 2) selective abstraction, 3) arbitrary inference, 4) overgeneralization, 5) catastrophizing, 6) time distortion, 7) distortions of self-perceptions, 8) excessive responsibility, 9) circular thinking, and 10) misassuming causality.

Case Example

The same MPD patient will be used to illustrate the 10 cognitive distortions for two purposes. First, it will allow the reader to become more familiar with, and thus more connected to, the life of this one patient. Second, it will help stress the fact that all these cognitive distortions can coexist and interplay with one another. As noted above, certain characteristics of MPD patients facilitate the demonstration of the issues under consideration.

Elayne H (a pseudonym) is nearly 30 years old now. Her MPD was diagnosed 3 years ago. Prior to that she spent 6 years of therapy under the diagnosis of schizophrenia and was treated with major tranquilizers. A few personalities who can pass for one another had attended the first 6 years of therapy while the others watched, commented, and occasionally interfered. Elayne H's descriptions of the voices she heard and the influences she felt playing on her were considered signs of schizophrenia. Suicide attempts, which in reality were attempted "inner murders" (one alter trying to kill another), occurred when the previous therapist would get too close to discovering her history of incest and abuse.

Dichotomous thinking.   Dichotomous thinking is a response set in which there is a tendency to classify experiences into one of two extreme categories. Depending on the personality or ego state being addressed, the thinking may be polarized from the positive extreme to the negative.

One of the driving forces and major distortions of the host personality of this patient is an attempt to maintain an idealized view of the father. He was always represented as a handsome, tall, brilliant professional man who trained at the best schools, competitively gained access to the better positions in his field, provided superbly for his family, financed the patient's excellent education, and was a pillar of the community. She (the host) met the new therapist during the evaluation for MPD and tried to convince the therapist that she came from a prominent and respectable family. It took 31 months from that initial interview (two sessions per week) before she acknowledged and reexperienced some of the abuse that had been forced on her by the father.

In the course of therapy, one angry alter of this same patient (at the therapist's request) stopped dealing drugs and prostituting herself. She had felt impelled "to make men pay." At the beginning of treatment, she had no idea why she felt angry all the time and, more importantly, why this rage was acted out specifically against men. She eventually came to understand that the abuse of which she originally had no knowledge—abuse at the hands of her father—was the driving force behind these behaviors. In the course of treatment, she became able to modulate her feelings about men and, prior to fusing with another alter 35 months after the onset of treatment, expressed the desire to become genuinely sexually involved with a man and experience orgasm.

> It's not like before . . . I knew there would always be men, the kind of men that would pay me . . . now I'm worried about finding a good man. . . . Do you know anybody?

Selective abstraction.   Selective abstraction represents a stimulus set in which certain elements or characteristics of an event are taken out of context. Some salient features do not seem to be integrated into the event's perception. As a consequence, the meaning of the whole event is derived from an incomplete/constricted data base, which often leads not only to ambiguous semantics, but also to some conclusions that are patently incorrect.

An angry alter in Elayne H would refuse to talk to "that weakling" passive alter because the latter had submitted to the abuse.

> I ain't seen no gun held to her head; I don't gotta speak to no pushovers.

As part of the exploration into her past, the angry alter saw the abuser hurting the passive one and the passive one just lying there. The angry alter felt that the abuser could have been stopped, overpowered, kicked, bitten, or something. The angry alter, when looking at the abuse scene, genuinely did not see the knife in the abuser's hand; nor did she see the background of lit candles around the bed, candles that would be used to cauterize the cuts the father would inflict to her vagina or around her nipples. Once the therapist understood one of the reasons for which the angry alter shunned the more passive one, both angry alter and therapist together could slowly reexamine the abuse scene and complete it.

Arbitrary inference. Arbitrary inference is a response set that involves drawing specific conclusions without the evidence in support of them. The overlap between this and the first two categories is self-evident.

As treatment progressed, it became increasingly clear to Elayne H's host personality that there were more facets to her father than she had initially recognized. Even though she was bright (her IQ was over 130 and she had almost completed a doctoral degree), she had selectively chosen to base her impressions of her father on selected aspects of her father's behaviors and accomplishments and infer general conclusions about all aspects of his personality based on the positive aspects consonant with her "father knows best" image of him. Redressing those long-held and distorted beliefs has been gruelingly painful for her, but necessary for her recovery.

Overgeneralization. Overgeneralization is a response set in which incorrect conclusions are drawn from a restricted sample or from nonexistent data. It is often the response set that corresponds to the stimulus set of selective abstraction and works hand in hand with dichotomous thinking.

> My father is bad—he is a man—I cannot trust him—therefore I can trust no man.

This syllogism is endorsed by many of Elayne H's alters. One of the personalities who held this belief chose to exclude 50% of the population from her interactional repertoire and has been involved in a long series of unsuccessful lesbian relationships.

Catastrophizing and decatastrophizing. Catastrophizing is a response set, which when first mobilized in the abused child was not a distortion but an acknowledgment of a reality. The child's circumstances were truly catastrophic. Unfortunately, the persistence of cognitions that tend to catastrophize events act as conditioned stimuli, which maintain conditioned emotional responses.

One of Elayne H's teenage personalities flees from any form of medication. She recalls her father forcing her to take large quantities of diazepam so that she would not fight him off as he raped her. This personality was recently in a restaurant with a date. A woman at a nearby table took out a pill box. A series of connected thoughts raced through this personality's mind: pillbox-pills-drowsy-rape. She panicked, screamed at the woman, and climbed out the window to escape. Fortunately for my patient, it was a ground-floor restaurant. On the other hand, the *la belle indifférence* stance that can prevail when some alters decatastrophize any event, regardless of its seriousness, can be equally destructive to the patient.

Another of Elayne H's personalities took a serious fall. The skin was broken; no treatment was sought. An infection ensued. The symptoms were ignored until they became so severe that the patient was admitted directly to an intensive care unit and administered intravenous antibiotics. A serious situation was decatastrophized because child personalities were frightened of hospitals (the abusing father had assaulted her in her hospital bed when she has been admitted for some procedures unrelated to her abuse). They absorbed the pain and throbbing of the infection; this allowed the adult alters to minimize the seriousness of the condition, with near-disastrous consequences.

Time distortion. Time distortion is a response set in which an individual thinks that she is in a different year/month/day/season and feels and acts accordingly.

One of Elayne H's personalities still struggling with the diagnosis of MPD and attempting to deny it came to a July appointment wearing a bulky sweater. She half-jokingly asked whether there had been worldwide hemispheric weather reversals that could account for summer weather in January. Needless to say, my explanation (i.e., the time loss and distortion often experienced in MPD) was less plausible to her than her own (i.e., surge of carbon dioxide in the atmosphere, rapid greenhouse effect since last appointment, and 90-degree weather in January).

Distortions of self-perceptions. Distortion of self-perceptions is a response set typical of abused individuals. MPD patients' personalities, through autohypnotically induced hallucinations, literally see themselves as different. They think differently and, as a consequence, feel and act differently. Maintaining their perceived physical distinctiveness is very important to many personalities.

It is understood that challenging an authoypnotically created image is fairly fruitless, and usually is as productive as challenging the delusions of a schizophrenic patient. Such efforts actually can be counterproductive. Some therapists spend more time disagreeing with their MPD patients over the personalities' perceived physical characteristics than getting to the business of therapy. More importantly, such interventions reinforce these patients' belief that they lack credibility and remind them of times when, as children, they were often called liars (Kluft 1985). For less exaggerated dissociative pathologies, the distortions can take the form of poor body image; feeling smaller, heavier, or less attractive than others.

In the course of a session with another therapist also involved in her care, that therapist tried to confront a child personality with the biologic fact of her adulthood. She challenged the child's distorted perception by putting a mirror to that personality's face. The child personality perceived this as an attempt at disqualifying her self-perceived reality. She thought that this therapist was trying to tell her that she did not exist. She refused to come back to treatment for 3 months.

Excessive responsibility or excessive irresponsibility.   Excessive responsibility is a response set that typically leads to excessive reactions to opportunities for self-flagellation, self-blame, and guilt. In MPD, cognitions associated with excessive responsibility tend to overwhelm the younger personalities, those who are cognitively-developmentally arrested, as well as the adult personalities.

Excessive irresponsibility is the converse of excessive responsibility. It often leads adolescent and/or angry adult alters to behave in ways in which they set themselves up for continued abuse through their negligence or ignorance.

One of Elayne H's child personalities maintained that she must have been a "bad girl" and deserved to be punished:

> Daddies don't do things "like this" to little girls, unless they are bad . . . real bad.

She is still unable to grasp that her father could be mentally ill. ("He doesn't look sick to me!") Her alternative explanation is that if she were not the one who was bad, then he must not have loved her. That is why he hurt her. She is taking excessive responsibility for the sustained abuse.

A turning point in the therapy with the angry adolescent alter mentioned above, who irresponsibly prostituted herself, came when she became concerned that she would switch into one of the child alters when "turning a trick" and could therefore be an abuser herself. Until that point she considered it "their problem."

Circular thinking.   Circular thinking is a response set where the premise for the conclusion becomes the conclusion, and the conclusion can become the premise, and so on. It is a fairly common cognitive style across personalities and is easily challenged in adult alters. However, the developmental level of a given personality puts a ceiling on the ability to analyze and dispel circular thinking. It may be more helpful to child personalities who are developmentally arrested to help them grow up first before attempting any change in circular thinking.

A previously mentioned example in the section on excessive responsibility is of a child personality who does not understand why the abuse is ongoing.

> I am bad, therefore I deserve to be hurt. I am hurt because I am bad.

Misassuming causality.   Misassuming causality is a response set that is often connected to taking of excessive responsibility as well as to responding to circular reasoning. It is a stance that maintains an alter in fixed styles of thinking, constricted affect, and predetermined behaviors. It involves difficulties in predicting events from precursor incidents as well as the drawing of unfortunate connections between unrelated events.

As Elayne H's host personality was coming to grips with a less glorified image of her father, she would revert at times to saying:

> He is a good man. You have told me I don't always know what I am doing; therefore maybe I did something that I don't remember and just got him a bit angry.

The cognitive distortions of non-MPD incest victims are more similar than dissimilar to the cognitive distortions described in victims of MPD. The essential difference lies in the intensity with which the faulty belief is held and its genuine resilience to interpretation and/or challenge. MPD patients represent the subgroup with the most clearly evident and most strongly entrenched distortions. In both MPD and non-MPD incest victims, the distortions pervade every arena and influence every decision in the survivor's life. Non-MPD incest victims present with milder cognitive idiosyncrasies than MPD incest survivors. Therefore, differentiating them from a more traditional depressive nonincestuously abused subgroup should be based on the fact that nonabused depressive patients will more likely restrict their distortions to certain specific arenas rather than to all aspects of their life, whereas with incestuously abused victims the distortions will tend to pervade their total experience of reality.

THE EVOLUTION OF COGNITIVE DISTORTIONS

In the preceding section, I described some of the cognitive distortions that therapists encounter in their clinical interaction with victims of incest.

These distortions resemble those commonly encountered by cognitive therapists in their work with nonsexually abused depressed patients. As stated earlier, the thinking of abuse victims, although sharing surface similarities with nonabuse patients, is intrinsically different. Rather than the deep-rooted distorted beliefs reinforced by learning typical of depressive patients, the thinking of abuse survivors can have a delusional quality reminiscent of an actual deficit in cognitive and/or perceptual realms. It is hypothesized that these deficits result from the interferences of dissociative phenomenology with the evolving perceptual and cognitive structures of the child's mind. In the section to follow, I will initially review normal cognitive development in children and then the effect of abuse on that same development. The consequences of dissociation on the evolving cognitive processes will be explored as well as the impact of dissociation on both cognitive schemes and cognitive schemas.

Perception and cognition traditionally work together to help an individual make sense of the world through the development of the symbolic function. According to Piaget (1969), this function is the essence of human intelligence. It is not present in the newborn, who has no images to facilitate the recall of details and who cannot imagine what lies in the future (Cowan 1978). The foundation on which the symbolic function is constructed is a perceptual one. Perception is the organization and interpretation of sensations, which are the raw changes in the central nervous system following stimulation of sensory receptors (Nash 1970). It serves as a precursor to symbolic meaning. It is determined by factors both intrinsic and external to the perceiver (body states, moods, motivations) (Allport 1955; Piaget 1969) and is thus multidetermined. Perception makes the external world accessible for both interpretation and eventual reworking by cognitive structures.

Cognitive Development in Normal Children

The evolution of perceptual-cognitive structures has been described by Piaget (1960a, 1960b, 1964, 1969, 1971), an interactionist, who postulated the existence of four developmentally interrelated and contiguous stages through which all normal children progress. These are the sensorimotor stage, the preoperational stage, the concrete operational stage, and the stage of formal operations.

Advancement from the sensorimotor stage to the formal operations stage is accomplished through adaptation and organization. The process of adaptation reflects the two choices any animal has to ensure survival: the animal can modify the environment to meet its needs (assimilation) or modify itself to mold to the environment (accommodation) (Cowan 1978). Organization represents a supraordinate process that involves the coordination of assimilative and accommodative functions (Piaget 1960b).

It is therefore understood that adaptation is the sum total of accommodative and assimilative processes.

A closer examination of accommodation reveals that its function is primarily representational: its purpose is to encode, store, and retrieve accurate images of specific events or objects. These representations are called schemas and are forever mutable and changing. Although schemas are not carbon copies of the external event or object, they do reflect its salient features and are thus figurative. After the initial accommodative process, the event or object is a symbol without a meaning. To become meaningful, assimilation must occur or else every event or object appears new and unintelligible (Cowan 1978).

Assimilation includes the event in a general conceptual structure, which Piaget (1960b) called an operative scheme. A scheme is an organized system of action, a structural unit that is repeatable and generalizable across situations (Cowan 1978). In summary, schemas are particular, accommodative, and figurative; whereas schemes are general, assimilative, and operative. Both are necessary for symbolic meaning to occur. Accommodation, assimilation, schemas, and schemes, are the processes and dynamic templates that are mobilized in the course of cognitive development.

The movement from one developmental stage to another requires four elements: maturation, social interaction, physical experience, and (most importantly) equilibration. Equilibration is a process of balanced assimilation and accommodation between the organism and the environment as well as the balancing of internal cognitive structures. Typically, a discrepancy in the environment will lead the organism to perceive a state of imbalance, which will require a shift in the schemas and perhaps in the schemes to reestablish an equilibrium (Piaget 1964). Once equilibrium is again achieved, the organism will perceive the environment in terms of this organization—the implication being that schemas and schemes orient the organism to the environment and help give it predictability (Neisser 1976).

Effect of Abuse on Cognitive Development

The age of onset of abuse, its intensity, and its duration will differentially affect the child's accommodative and assimilative functions. Fish-Murray et al. (1987) reported that abuse affects the organism's capacity to accommodate, rendering self-correction difficult. The cognitive structures are more fixed than variable and lack optimal flexibility. There is no doubt that an environment that is abusive will lead to cognitive schemas that reflect the abuse history of the organism, nor is there any doubt that cognitive inflexibility will impair the organism in its adjustment to a nonabusive environment. One could speculate from clinical observation that some schemas remain untouched by abuse whereas others may be shattered or lamed. This may explain the differential cognitive lacunae observed in abuse survivors.

Abuse may affect not only accommodation; it may also interfere with assimilation. It appears that there is no modulating the assimilative function; the outcome is all-or-none. One either assimilates or one does not. If assimilation does not occur, some of the cognitive schemas may remain fixed at a previous level of ontogenic development and never get generalized into schemes. The schemas may remain meaningless and non-integrated, or they may reflect a meaning acquired at a preceding developmental level and thus be incomplete and/or immature. Another possibility is saccadic or alternating assimilation, in which the assimilative function is turned on and off like a switch. When certain cognitive schemas are overwhelmed by either the amount or the nature of external information (and are therefore unable to incorporate essential environmental data), the assimilative function may temporarily shut off. This state of affairs may lead to nonassimilation of certain schemas or to faulty assimilation into inappropriate schemes, the by-products of which are the cognitive distortions discussed earlier.

Examples of differential assimilation of cognitive schemas, nonassimilation, or assimilation into faulty or inaccurate schemes are frequent in incestuously molested MPD patients. Although not de rigueur, it is common to encounter personalities within one MPD patient who have no knowledge, no memory, and no understanding or mastery over certain cognitive domains, whereas other personalities may excel in the identical arenas. The clinical evidence points to two ongoing phenomena to explain this confusion: cognitive regression and cognitive substitution or replication. Therefore, the dissociative strategies that will help the abused child survive one form of destruction (death) will prove harmful to her ability to create a safe and predictable reality as an adult.

Illustrative examples of selected cognitive schemas and schemes present among some of the personalities in the index MPD patient described previously may prove helpful. It should be understood that these examples reflect already established and therefore reworked schemas and schemes and consequently probably differ from the original, more microscopic encodings that are closer to the initial perceptual experience.

One of the child alters who remembered being hurt by the father had a schema that read: "Daddy hurt me." This same alter's scheme derived from the previous schema enlarged the sample of people to fear from father to all men and read: "Men hurt me." This scheme was reinforced in the child alter's mind when she would become co-conscious with the adolescent alter, who was a prostitute. Another child alter who had similar memories and started with a seemingly similar schema added an additional element to the schema: "Daddy loves me." For her, the scheme became:

"To be hurt means to be loved." An adolescent alter connected with this second child alter would always get involved with violent men who would physically abuse her. She often brags about "liking bruisers" and speaks of them as "real men, and great lovers," even subsequent to several hospitalizations for broken bones.

The preferred use of dissociation during and after abuse. It is understood that dissociative processes are mobilized in abuse victims to help them negotiate the impact of the overwhelming stress imposed by the violations to the self (Kluft 1984; Spiegel 1984). These dissociative episodes may initially correspond to microdissociative phenomena, which, when chained, eventually create a substrate fertile for the development of a true dissociative disorder (Braun and Sachs 1985). Young (1988) suggested that personalities in MPD are formed in this cumulative way rather than emerging spontaneously as complete entities. Whether rapidly or in a more progressive manner, parts of the mind can become segregated from the common flow of consciousness. These parts may keep some characteristics of the original stream of consciousness or add and delete idiosyncratic elements.

In Braun's (1988) previously described BASK model of dissociation, he suggested that an event can be dissociated into its four components: behavior, affect, sensation, and knowledge. A child's knowledge, however, is only developing; it is still in the formative stages during which the cognitive schemas and schemes are evolving. It is heuristically plausible that not only does abuse sever knowledge from the three other dimensions as described by Braun, but abuse may force the knowledge dimension to shatter into smaller units of information, into fragments of knowledge. Knowledge may be broken down into its schematic elements.

The actual consequences of a reduction of cognitive structures to their elemental parts by random dissociative intrusions may be different when it occurs in children than when it occurs in adolescents or adults. In adults, the major evolution of the cognitive schemas or schemes has already occurred. The cognitive structures of a child, on the other hand, are still in a period of exponential growth.

Piaget's (1971) epigenetic perspective is useful in considering the consequences of dissociation on children's thinking. Comparing the effects of dissociation on the knowledge dimension of an adult mind versus the mind of a child is not unlike considering the differential cytogenic effects of radiation or chemical agents on established cells versus germ cells. The cells that evolve consequent to the tampering of germ cells often lead to mutant strains of cells, which, if they survive, may be aberrations (DeRobertis et al. 1970). In the same way, cognitive aberrations in adolescence and adulthood can be the result of interference by dissociative phenomena in the development of the cognitive schemas of children and their regrouping into distorted cognitive schemes.

The consequences of dissociation for cognitive schemas and cognitive schemes. Heuristically, one might speculate that dissociation consequent to abuse may affect children's cognitive schemas in several ways. First, the cognitive schemas may become completely segregated from one another, leading to the formation of two separate schemas encapsulating two seemingly complete but different information pools (e.g., two separate child alters in our index patient, one who knows about dad abusing her, the other who just knows she has a wonderful father).

Second, the cognitive schemas may be partially severed from one another with both overlapping and disjunctive parts leading to a common information pool and one or more divergent pools. Two personalities may know that dad abused them (common information); however, one believes it was just physical abuse whereas the other knows about some of the sexual abuse (separate information).

Third, the cognitive schemas may be entirely severed in an imbalanced way, with one cognitive schema being replete with information while the other schema holds only minimal residual information. One adult alter has a schema that contains information surrounding who all family members are whereas a different adult alter, who prides herself in helping maintain the family together, reveals under further questioning that she really only remembers the maternal grandmother, who was one of the few people in her family who was truly kind.

Finally, the cognitive schemas may be entirely severed and forced into exact self-replication. In this particular patient, this type of dissociation of schema has not been found. It appears more commonly in MPD patients who experience event-based dissociative episodes.

Until research data are available to support or refute this perspective, it would be futile to argue which of these four possibilities predominates. Clinical experience suggests that all four affects may be observed within the cognitive structures of a single patient. Defective or imperfect schemas may remain operative. The risk then becomes the assimilation of flawed schemas to form distorted schemes. Another possibility is that if the cognitive schemas are extremely severed, then cognitive regression or cognitive shift to more stably functional schemas may be attempted to reestablish equilibrium.

Indeed, regardless of the mind's efforts to minimize the effects of dissociation on developing cognitive structures, the abuse may be such an ongoing element in the child's life that chaos and mayhem cannot be avoided. As a result, stable equilibria with unbalanced schemas may be established. This type of equilibration fosters adaptational schemes that are distorted and that may lead the individual to semantic mishaps and continued alienation because of errors in thinking. One could speculate that if equilibration remains unstable or does not occur, then regressing to a lower but perhaps better accommodated and more fully assimilated cognitive level is the child's attempt to renegotiate the environment and readapt. In that case, the child may continue to rely on immature, substituted, or less shattered cognitive schemas.

In their seminal chapter on the effects of trauma on the thinking of abused children, Fish-Murray et al. (1987) suggested that the children in their sample experience disruptions in the cognitive functions of conservation and reversibility. These functions are typically achieved at the concrete operational level (between 7 and 11 years old) and are central to later difficulties in inferential thinking and hypothesis testing. Do the present data on age of occurrence of abuse support Fish-Murray et al.'s views? Finkelhor's (1984) survey on the incidence of child sexual abuse reported a mean age of onset of abuse at 8.6 years. This corresponds to the period during which a child is attempting to master conservation and reversibility. On the other hand, in her nonpatient sample of incestuously abused women, Russell (1986) found that the most common time for the onset of abuse is between 10 and 13 years of age. Those mistreated at that age were abused at the concrete operational period and at the beginning of the stage of formal operations.

Schultz et al. (1986) studied an incestuously abused sample of MPD patients. Their patients had an onset of abuse at approximately 4 years of age, which corresponds to the preoperational stage of cognitive development. During this stage, the cognitive precursors to conservation and reversibility are likely to be disrupted, rather than conservation and reversibility proper. If cognitive regression occurs as a consequence of abuse, as postulated earlier, then concrete operational children may regress to preoperational functioning, and preoperational children may regress to sensorimotor functioning while renegotiating object permanence and object constancy.

The MPD subsample, more than any other group, has had their cognitive development interfered with at an earlier developmental stage. A disruption at this earlier level better explains some of the additional difficulties experienced by MPD patients, such as problems surrounding the concepts of time, space, and causality, the precursors of which are object constancy and object permanence (Langer 1969). Cognitive replication/substitution may be attempted. This "cloning" of cognitive schemas, although perhaps faulty and/or incomplete, is an attempt on the part of the organism to negotiate, in the present and at the appropriate developmental level, the meaning of the abuse.

IMPLICATIONS FOR TREATMENT

Although the bulk of this chapter is concerned with the effects of abuse on the thinking of incest victims, cognitive symptoms are rarely part of their presenting complaints. Most often incest victims present with affective problems. They are usually depressed (Kaufman et al. 1954; Weiner 1962) and feeling guilty, shameful, and unable to trust others (Brothers 1982; Butler 1978; Forward and Buck 1978). Without reopening the debate of which came first, the cognition (Beck 1976) or the affect (Zajonc 1980), established clinical evidence and numerous research findings (Gioe 1975; Rush et al. 1978; Shipley and Fazio 1973; Taylor and Marshall 1977) support the belief that how someone thinks will affect how that person feels, and, therefore, changing how someone thinks may change his or her affective picture. Incest survivors may have rigidly determined belief systems based on incomplete and/or tainted cognitive schemas assimilated into distorted cognitive schemes. These must be rectified to facilitate affective change. It is understood that some of the schemes have equilibrated in a way such that two, three, or more mutually exclusive opinions coexist within one patient (or even one personality); the situation becomes more perplexing to the therapist when she realizes that rather than approaching this circumstance with appropriate circumspection and confusion, the incest victim may respond with a degree of *la belle indifférence* to the illogical coexistence of contradictory alternatives.

The therapist's task is challenging. The therapist endeavors to establish a trusting working relationship with the patient as he or she progressively disrupts the cognitive distortions and disequilibrates the schemes in order to create cognitive dissonance; it is only at that point that work with the schemes will be addressed.

The Braun (1988) BASK model of dissociation offers the therapist a paradigm as well as a structure from which to disrupt the cognitions consistently. Challenging the cognition, the cognitive schema, or cognitive scheme through the Socratic method will facilitate dissonance and the necessary cognitive reframing. Braun's model will facilitate monitoring the change over time of both cognition and affect. The host personality of Elayne H—our index case—had formed an idealized view of the father based most definitely on his professional accomplishments; she clearly had no memory of him in any nonprofessional capacity. She was initially engaged by the therapist in reconsidering her view of her father by a very general dialogue:

> Therapist: So, many things make people what they are!
> Patient: Yeah, it's fairly remarkable!
> Therapist: It's truly effortful to juggle all the roles we have and keep them all balanced; some things we are just better at than others.
> Patient: Yes, . . . (then she gives examples from her life)
> Therapist: I guess we all struggle with that . . . your father must have too!
> Patient: What do you mean?
> Therapist: You have told me of all your father's accomplishments, he must have had some areas where . . . you mean he never hit his finger

> with a hammer instead of hitting the nail, he never scratched the car up, he never missed the golf ball or was late for dinner or had to rush to the office from home for an urgent business problem, etc. . . .

Patient: (looking puzzled) I don't know the relevance of this, I don't remember him . . . (pulls apart the silly examples) . . .

Therapist: Well, what does he do at home?

Patient: (very uneasy and looking increasingly panicked) I don't know.

Therapist: What do you mean, you don't know?

Patient: (patient tries to divert by saying) All therapists say what do you mean to the most obvious things!

Therapist: Why don't you know?

Patient: (angrily) I can't answer, because I don't remember him around the house.

Eventually after many such exchanges, the host personality acknowledged that it made no sense to her that she had such limited information about her father considering the fact that her parents had been happily married for so many years and that their home could only be a "haven for all." Nonetheless, she remained guarded about inquiring further.

Therefore, until cognitive dissonance is achieved and the patient has a different framework from which to understand her problem, focusing solely on the affect, although perhaps cathartic, may be more retraumatizing than helpful. It would not have been terribly helpful to the host personality described previously to have her experience, at this time, other personalities' feelings about the father and consequently overwhelm her. Although frustrated at times by the therapist's insistence and questioning of "obvious banalities," the patient was learning to review and challenge rigid schemes and (re-) learning how to think.

Many incest victims have lost their ability to learn from experience. If they remain untouched, their distorted cognitive schemes will condemn them to a position of continued helplessness rather than facilitate their recovery. An empathic and supportive educative stance on the part of the therapist may prove sufficient to enhance dissonance, but hypnotherapeutically facilitated interventions may be required. Incestuously molested MPD patients, for instance, may benefit from a time-limited blending of cognitive schemes through temporary merging of personalities to enhance learning and to foster mastery (Fine and Comstock 1989).

In her book, *The Secret Trauma: Incest in the Lives of Girls and Women*, Russell (1986) offered powerful testimony to the high prevalence of incest in our present society. Dissociative sequelae are common in these victims (Gelinas 1983). In this chapter, I have attempted to demonstrate that these phenomena have a pervasive impact. They permeate how incest survivors feel, how they behave, and even how they think. The thinking of victims of abuse is plagued by long-held faulty cognitions based on distorted schemes. These schemes are formed through the assimilation of potentially tainted accommodated schemas and represent the building blocks for the altered information processing that accompanies cognitive distortions. One of the treatment strategies is to foster cognitive dissonance in order to depotentiate maladaptive cognitive adaptations. Encouraging dissonance will engage the patient in de-equilibrating and re-equilibrating cognitive schemes to modify their intercategorical connotative meaning toward less distorted cognitive structures and processes. Once this is achieved, the victim of incest may become able to start learning from past experience and therefore decrease the likelihood of her subsequent revictimization (Kluft, Chapter 13, this volume).

REFERENCES

Allport F: Theories of Perception and the Concept of Structure. New York, John Wiley, 1955

Beck AT: Cognitive Therapy and the Emotional Disorders. New York, International Universities Press, 1976

Beck AT, Rush AJ, Shaw BF, et al: Cognitive Therapy of Depression. New York, Guilford Press, 1979

Braun BG: The BASK model of dissociation. Dissociation 1:4–23, 1988

Braun BG, Sachs RG: The development of multiple personality disorder: predisposing, precipitating, and perpetuating factors, in Childhood Antecedents of Multiple Personality. Edited by Kluft RP. Washington, DC, American Psychiatric Press, 1985, pp 37–64

Brothers D: Trust disturbances among rape and incest victims. Dissertation Abstracts International 43(4-B):1247, 1982

Butler S: Conspiracy of Silence: The Trauma of Incest. San Francisco, CA, New Glide, 1978

Cowan PA: Piaget With Feeling: Cognitive, Social and Emotional Dimensions. New York, Holt Rinehart & Winston, 1978

DeRobertis EDP, Nowinski WW, Saez FA: Cell Biology. Philadelphia, PA, WB Saunders, 1970

Despine A: De l'emploi du magnetisme animal et des eaux minerales dans le traitement des maladies nerveuses, suivi d'une observation tres curieuse de guérison de nevropathie. Paris, Baillere, 1840

Epstein S: The self-concept revisted: or a theory of a theory. Am Psychol 28:404–416, 1973

Epstein S: The ecological study of emotions in humans, in Advances in Communication and Affect, Vol 5. Edited by Pliner P, Blankstein KR, Spigel IM. New York, Plenum, 1979, pp

Fine CG: The work of Antoine Despine: diagnosis and treatment of a child with multiple personality disorder. Am J Clin Hypn 31:1, 1988

Fine CG, Comstock C: Completion of cognitive schemata and affective realms through temporary blending of personalities, in Dissociative Disorders 1989. Edited by Braun BG. Chicago, IL, Rush University, 1989, p 17

Finkelhor D: Child Sexual Abuse: New Theory and Research. New York, Free Press, 1984

Fish-Murray CC, Koby EV, van der Kolk BA: Evolving ideas: the effect of abuse on children's thought, in Psychological Trauma. Edited by van de Kolk BA. Washington, DC, American Psychiatric Press, 1987, pp 89–110

Forward S, Buck C: Betrayal of Innocence: Incest and Its Devastation. Los Angeles, CA, Tarcher, 1978

Frischholz EJ: The relationship among dissociation, hypnosis, and child abuse in the development of multiple personality disorder, in Childhood Antecedents of Multiple Personality. Edited by Kluft RP. Washington, DC, American Psychiatric Press, 1985, pp 100–126

Gelinas D: The persisting negative effects of incest. Psychiatry 46:312–332, 1983

Gioe VJ: Cognitive modification and positive group experience as a treatment for depression. Dissertation Abstracts International 36:3039B–3040B, 1975 (University Microfilms No 75-28, 219)

Goodwin J: Sexual Abuse: Incest Victims and Their Families. Littleton, MA, PSG Publishing, 1982

Grinker R, Spiegel J: Men Under Stress. Philadelphia, PA, Blakiston, 1945

Hartman M, Finn SE, Leon GR: Sexual abuse experiences in a clinical population: comparisons of familial and nonfamilial abuse. Psychotherapy 24:154–159, 1987

Henderson DJ: Incest, in Comprehensive Textbook of Psychiatry. Edited by Freedman AM, Kaplan HI, Sadock BJ. Baltimore, MD, Williams & Wilkins, 1975, pp 1530–1539

Herman J: Father-Daughter Incest. Cambridge, MA, Harvard University Press, 1981

Janet P: L'Automatisme psychologigue. Paris, Baillere, 1889

Janoff-Bulman R: The after-math of victimization: rebuilding shattered assumptions, in Trauma and Its Wake: The Study and Treatment of Post Traumatic Stress Disorder. Edited by Figley CR. New York, Brunner/Mazel, 1985, pp 15–35

Kaufman I, Peck AL, Taguiri CK: The family constellation and overt incestuous relations between father and daughter. Am J Orthopsychiatry 24:266–277, 1954

Kluft RP: Multiple personality in childhood. Psychiatr Clin North Am 7:1, 1984

Kluft RP: Childhood multiple personality disorder: predictors, clinical findings, and treatment results, in Childhood Antecedents of Multiple Personality. Edited by Kluft RP. Washington, DC, American Psychiatric Press, 1985, pp 167–196

Kluft RP: Making the diagnosis of multiple personality disorder, in Diagnostics and Psychopathology (Directions in Psychiatry Monograph Series). Edited by Flach F. New York, WW Norton, 1987, pp 207–225

Langer J: Theories of Development. New York, Holt Rinehart & Winston, 1969

Luborsky L: Principles of Psychoanalytic Psychotherapy: A Manual for Supportive-Expressive Treatment. New York, Basic Books, 1984

Nash J: Developmental Psychology: A Psychobiological Approach. Englewood Cliffs, NJ, Prentice-Hall, 1970

Neisser U: Cognition and Reality: Principles and Implications of Cognitive Psychology. San Francisco, CA, WH Freeman, 1976

Nemiah JC: Dissociative Disorders, in Comprehensive Textbook of Psychiatry, 3rd Edition. Edited by Kaplan H, Freedman A, Sadock B. Baltimore, MD, Williams & Wilkins, 1981, pp 1544–1561

Piaget J: The Child's Conception of Physical Causality. Totowa, NJ, Littlefield, Adams, 1960a

Piaget J: The Psychology of Intelligence. Totowa, NJ, Littlefield, Adams, 1960b

Piaget J: Development and learning, in Piaget Rediscovered: A Report of the Conference on Cognitive Studies and Curriculum Development. Edited by Ripple RE, Rockcastle VN. Ithaca, NY, Cornell University Press, 1964, pp 35–47

Piaget J: The Mechanisms of Perception. New York, Basic Books, 1969

Piaget J: Biology and Knowledge: An Essay on the Relations Between Organic Regulations and Cognitive Processes. Chicago, IL, University of Chicago Press, 1971

Putnam FW: Dissociation as a response to extreme trauma, in Childhood Antecedents of Multiple Personality. Edited by Kulft RP. Washington, DC, American Psychiatric Press, 1985, pp 65–97

Putnam FW, Guroff JJ, Silberman EK, et al: The clinical phenomenology of multiple personality disorder: review of 100 recent cases. J Clin Psychiatry 47:285–293, 1986

Rascovsky MW, Rascovsky A: On consummated incest. Int J Psychoanal 31:42–47, 1950

Rush AJ, Hollon SD, Beck AT, et al: Depression: must pharmacotherapy fail for cognitive therapy to succeed? Cognitive Therapy and Research 2:199–206, 1978

Russell DE: The Secret Trauma: Incest in the Lives of Girls and Women. New York, Basic Books, 1986

Schultz R, Kluft RP, Braun BG: The interface between multiple personality disorder and borderline personality disorder, in Dissociative Disorders 1986. Edited by Braun BG. Chicago, IL, Rush University, 1986, p 122

Shipley CR, Fazio AF: Pilot study for a treatment of psychological depression. J Abnorm Psychol 82:372–376, 1973

Spiegel D: Multiple personality as a post-traumatic stress disorder. Psychiatr Clin North Am 7:1, 1984

Spiegel D, Hunt T, Dondershine HE: Dissociation and hypnotizability in post traumatic stress disorder. Am J Psychiatry 145:301–305, 1988

Taylor FG, Marshall WL: Experimental analysis of a cognitive-behavioral therapy for depression. Cognitive Therapy and Research 1:59–72, 1977

Watkins JG, Watkins HH: Ego-state therapy, in The Newer Therapies: A Source Book. Edited by Abt LE, Stuart IR. New York, Van Nostrand Reinhold, 1982, pp 127–155

Weiner IB: Father-daughter incest: a clinical report. Psychiatr Q 36:607–631, 1962

Young W: Observations on fantasy in the formation of multiple personality disorder. Dissociation 1(3):13–20, 1988

Zajonc RB: Feeling and thinking: preferences need no inferences. Am Psychol 35:151–175, 1980

CHAPTER 9

Incest in the Borderline Patient

Michael H. Stone, M.D.

In this chapter, I will concentrate on three areas of relevance to the phenomenon of incest in populations of borderline patients: 1) the possibility of a causal significance between incest and subsequent development of borderline personality disorder (BPD) in cases where a history of incest was present; 2) the actual frequency of incest history in various populations of borderline patients; and 3) the delineation of a clinical picture, the "incest profile," whose presence may alert clinicians to an incest history.

Because of the embarrassment surrounding the topic of incest, mental health professionals often fail to inquire about it during the initial consultation. Patients who have been incest victims often omit mention of the fact altogether until someone serendipitously asks the right question. Such is the strength of the taboo that, until recently, incest was regarded as a phenomenon of surpassing rarity (Freud 1896; Henderson 1975; Malcolm 1984)—as something that "happened" now and then in the imagination of a Sophocles or an O'Neill, but hardly ever in real life.

Within the past 10 years, reticence about acknowledging an incest history has diminished (Forward and Buck 1978; Goodwin 1982; Herman 1981; Kempe and Kempe 1984). While distortion and falsification affect the validity of some purported incest cases, the veridicality of many revelations cannot be seriously doubted.

The author wishes to acknowledge with gratitude the generous help of Drs. Allan Unwin and Bronwin Beacham of Brisbane, Australia, in the study of incest histories among the borderline inpatients of the Belmont Hospital, and of Dr. Stephen Hurt of New York Hospital, Westchester Division, who evaluated statistically the results of the studies represented in Tables 9-1 through 9-7.

Thus far most of the studies that bear on the subject have been epidemiologic. Women are much more apt to have been incest victims than men. The work of Finkelhor (1984), based on interviews of college students, suggested that approximately 1 woman in 20 had experienced incest, if the latter were defined broadly and if both blood relatives and steprelatives were included. Russell's (1986) monograph reflected the large-scale project she and her colleagues carried out in San Francisco and reported an incest rate in females of 16%. Since Russell used female research assistants of the same ethnic stock (wherever possible) as the respondents, the accuracy is probably greater than in previous studies. All socioeconomic groups were represented, in proportions reflective of the San Francisco population. Russell used a broad definition with 18 descriptors (grouped into three levels of severity, from most severe [forced rape] to least [erotic kissing, fondling through clothes]. In the absence of other studies similar in scale, it is not clear what variability there might be from one locale to another.

Few reports deal with the incest rate, according to specific diagnostic subgroups, in a population of psychiatrically ill patients. Kluft (1985) noted the extraordinarily high incidence of incest in cases of multiple personality disorder. All 100 "multiples" alluded to in his book had been the victims either of incest, parental physical cruelty, or both. Elsewhere I noted (Stone 1981) that an incest history was common (30% or higher) in female borderline patients, particularly in those who had been hospitalized.

Interest has focused on this area not only because of the apparently high proportion of incest histories in female borderline patients, but also because of the possible etiologic significance of incest in generating some of the mental attitudes and behavioral characteristics that help define certain patients as borderline.

The following clinical vignette is illustrative:

A 26-year-old divorced woman had been hospitalized because of a serious suicide attempt (an overdose of hypnotics), reckless driving (with the hope of "ending it all" in a smashup) and wrist-cutting, all occurring within a 1-week interval following her dismissal from a part-time job. She had been living in a halfway house for a few months, following her release from a 3-year hospitalization on a unit devoted to long-term psychotherapy. That hospitalization had also been prompted by a series of suicidal acts. She was diagnosed as manifesting BPD.

Having been raised in an affluent home in the Northwest, she had been shy and timorous as a child but became, for no discernible reason, rebellious and impulsive as an adolescent. She ran away from home on two occasions. She had many brief sexual affairs with boys from the "wrong side of the tracks" socially. For a time she abused marijuana and alcohol and developed a penchant for self-injurious acts. These consisted at first of superficial wrist-cutting, but she progressed, on entering college at 18, to more serious acts, such as overdosing with hypnotics or breathing exhaust fumes in the family garage. She was hospitalized briefly on three such occasions before her long-term stay on the specialized unit. At 19 she married a man she had known only a few months.

She sought a divorce half a year later, citing sexual incompatibility. Several times she became panicky during sex for "unaccountable" reasons and would run out of the bedroom, hastily don an overcoat, and dash into the street.

During her most recent admission, the hospital staff requested a consultation. In the opinion of the consultant, her history appeared in keeping with the "incest profile" (as adumbrated later on in this chapter). Her coyness and evasiveness while being interviewed were also consonant with this picture.

For these reasons the consultant made discreet inquiry about the possibility of sexual molestation earlier in her life. The technique of interviewing has been sketched elsewhere (Stone 1989). The patient revealed that she had been repeatedly abused by her father from the time she was 5 or 6 until mid-adolescence. The ritual consisted of sitting in her father's lap, naked from the waist down. Her father would rub his penis against her buttocks, reaching orgasm and abjuring her never to tell anyone or he "couldn't guarantee what'd happen to her." Her "rebelliousness" in adolescence was in reaction to her becoming more aware that this secret life was socially condemned, especially by the teachers at her church. The conflict between these precepts and her strong attachment to her father was irresolvable and so intense as to make suicide the only "solution." She married on impulse, to get away from home, only to discover that her husband was fond of anal sex. His attempts to penetrate her in this fashion led to intolerable "flashbacks" of the sexual experiences with her father. These experiences were so terrifying that, in the past few years, she "swore off men" and avoided sex in any form. She felt condemned to a solitary life, which was no less intolerable to her than was intimacy with a man. As a result, she was determined to kill herself eventually. She regarded with a kind of bemused detachment the efforts of her therapist and of the hospital personnel to treat her, secure in her knowledge (if such it prove) that, once released, she would no longer waste her time with half-measures.

In an effort to assess the frequency of an incest history in cases of BPD, I have evaluated a number of samples, concentrating on hospitalized patients but also including one group of ambulatory patients. The largest series (the P.I.-500, described in the next section of this chapter) contained several male borderline patients with an incest history. Because the phenomenon is much less common among male than among female patients, however, I have presented my results only for the females for statistical purposes. The nature of the study and its results are described in the next section.

METHODS

Four patient samples were studied with respect to a past history of incest: 1) consecutively admitted patients to the Belmont Private Hospital, Psychodynamic Unit in Brisbane, Australia, 1984–1986; 2) consecutively admitted patients to the New York Hospital, Westchester Division, Unit 3-S, 1985–1986; 3) private patients in my office practice, 1966–1986; and 4) 550 consecutively admitted patients to the New York State Psychiatric Institute,

Intensive Psychotherapy Unit, 1963–1976 (referred to hereafter as the "P.I.-500").

The diagnosis of BPD was made according to DSM-III (American Psychiatric Association 1980) criteria.

Data were gathered by personal interviews or by interview of the therapists for all samples except the P.I.-500. In the latter, reliance was placed primarily on review of the old records, although this was supplemented in many cases by personal interview of the (former) patient or a relative or therapist in connection with the follow-up. At the time of this writing, 93% of the P.I.-500 have been traced (Stone 1987; Stone et al. 1987). Material is thus available from this sample on incest history and on 10- to 20-year outcome.

Of the private-practice sample, only female patients in therapy for at least 3 months were included, since data concerning an incest history were not consistently available for those seen only briefly or in consultation.

For definition and gradation of incest experience, the scale developed by Russell (1986) was used. In making the final tabulations, patients who had experienced any of the 18 varieties of incestuous acts were included as incest cases. Further compartmentalization into the three levels of severity was also made.

RESULTS

Frequency

The percentages of borderline females with a history of incest are shown in Table 9-1. All levels of severity are included in the final tally. The highest rates were noted in the two recent hospital surveys: 41% (7/17) in the Belmont Hospital unit and 36% (10/28) in the New York Hospital unit. Chi squares with Yates' correction achieved levels of significance only in these two samples—using the 16% incest rate in the base population, from Russell's (1986) study, as the comparison value. For those cases with an incest history, the levels of severity as well as the offending relatives are listed in Table 9-2.

Females with BPD in the P.I.-500 showed a rate of 19% (28/144). Females with BPD in the private practice series had an incest history in 26% of cases (7/27), whereas a similar number of females with neuroses in this series showed a rate of 8% (2/16).

Outcome

Systematic data on outcome were available only for the P.I.-500 patients. Table 9-3 shows global function as measured by the Global Assessment

Table 9-1.   Percentages of female patients with an incest history

Sample	Diagnosis	N	n with incest history	Percentage	χ^{2b}
San Francisco survey[a]	Normal population	930	152	16	—
Belmont Hospital (Brisbane, Australia)	Borderline personality disorder	17	7	41	5.3*
New York Hospital (White Plains, NY)	Borderline personality disorder	28	10	36	5.6*
P.I.-500	Borderline personality disorder	144	28	19	.068
Private practice	Borderline personality disorder	27	7	26	1.7
Private practice	Neuroses	26	2	8	1.12

[a]Russell (1986). [b]In relation to the Russell-study or reference standard.
*$p < .05$ (with Yates' correction).

Scale (GAS) (Endicott et al. 1976). This assessment was determined in relation to the 27 traced borderline females with an incest history. The offending relative or relatives are also indicated in the table as well as the level of severity relevant to each.

Table 9-4 shows GAS outcome scores in borderline patients who had experienced father-daughter incest. Scores are arranged by level of severity. Daughters who had better outcomes (GAS > 60) were significantly less likely to have been involved in the most severe forms of incestuous activity ($p = .035$, Fisher's exact test).

Table 9-5 shows GAS outcome scores for the patients who had experienced brother-sister incest but no sexual experiences with father or other older relatives. Although one-half of the brother-sister incest cases had a poor outcome (GAS ≤ 60) and nearly three-fourths of the father-daughter cases had a poor outcome, this difference was not statistically significant ($p = .38$, Fisher's exact test).

Comparison of long-term outcomes in females with borderline personality who were *not* known to have been incest victims with those who were is shown in Table 9-6. This table reflects six ranges within the continuum of outcome, beginning with "clinically recovered" (GAS > 70) and "good" (minimal symptoms; GAS 60–70). These two groups may be considered to constitute the portion of patients who are now "well." Below these levels are "fair" (GAS 51–60), marginal (GAS 31–50), and incapa-

Table 9-2. Incest histories in female inpatients with borderline personality
disorder

Case no.	Incest level[a]	Relative
Belmont Hospital[b]		
5	II	Brother
7	I	Brother
9	II	Father
10	I	Father
11	I	Father
16	I	Stepfather
17	III	Father
New York Hospital[c]		
1	II	Father
2	I	Father
5	III	Father
6	I	Grandfather
9	III	Father
11	III	Mother
12	I	Stepbrother
17	III	Father
22	III	Uncle
27	III	Father

[a]Incest level (Browning and Boatman 1977): I = most severe, II = severe, III = least
severe.
[b]1984–1986; average age, 29.7 years (range, 14–46 years).
[c]1985–1986; average age, 24.0 years (range, 18–33 years).

citated (GAS 1–30). Zero signifies a completed suicide. Borderline patients in the P.I.-500 *without* a history of incest were significantly more
likely to have a positive outcome (GAS > 60) than those who had a history
of incest (χ^2 = 3.93, 1 df, p < .048).

Table 9-7 shows the percentage of patients from the P.I.-500 with an
incest history and suffering from a retrospectively diagnosed psychotic
illness according to DSM-III criteria: schizophrenia, schizoaffective psychosis, bipolar disorder, and acute schizophreniform reactions (the latter
precipitated most often, in this series, by abuse of psychotomimetic drugs).

In the schizoaffective group, the incest rate was greater than that of
the BPD group. Two other schizoaffective patients reported near-incest
experiences (the father of one approached her sexually but did nothing;
another often witnessed her father masturbating).

DISCUSSION

The data presented in the previous section lend support to the contention
that an incest history is common in female patients with BPD, especially
in hospitalized series.

Table 9-3. P.I.-500 female borderline patients with an incest history: Global Assessment Scale score, level of severity, and offending relative(s)

Case no.	Global Assessment Scale score[a]	Level of severity[b]	Relative
1	75	?	Father
2	55	?	Father
3	37	I	Father
4	74	I	Father
5	85}	I	Brother
		II	Stepfather
6	69	III	Father
7	62	II	Father
8	55	I	Brother
9	30	I	Stepfather
10	70	I	Brother
11	55	?	Father
12	53	I	Father, Mother
13	80	III	Father
14	68	I	Brother
15	54	II	Father
16	88	I	Father
17	suicide	?	Father
18	untraced}	I	Stepbrother
		III	Stepfather
19	64	III	Father
20	31	I	Brother
21	82	II	Father
22	58	I	Father
23	suicide}	I	Brother
		I	Father
24	45	I	Father
25	71	II	Father
26	suicide	I	Brother
27	74	I	Brother
28	84	II	Father

[a]The Global Assessment Scale scores derive from the Global Assessment Scale of Endicott et al. (1976), now incorporated into DSM-III and DSM-III-R (American Psychiatric Association 1987).

[b]Levels of severity of incest relate to the hierarchically arranged list provided by Russell (1986). Level I corresponds to the "most severe" category (items 1–8), including acts ranging in severity from rape to nonforcible attempted fellatio. Level II (items 9–16) includes a range of behaviors from forced genital contact to nonforcible attempted breast contact. The least severe category, Level III (items 17 and 18), includes forced and nonforced sexual kissing.

Table 9-4. P.I.-500 Global Assessment Scale outcome scores of female borderline patients who had experienced father-daughter incest[a]

	Level of severity			
	---	---	---	---
Case no.	I	II	III	?
1				75
2				55
3	37			
4	74			
6			69	
7		62		
11				55
12	53			
13			80	
15		54		
16	88			
17				suicide
19			64	
21		82		
22	58			
23	suicide			
24	45			
25		71		
28		84		

Note. See note to Table 9-3 for explanation of levels of severity.
[a]Global Assessment Scale score >60 in I versus II + III: $p < .35$, Fisher's exact test.

Table 9-5. Global Assessment Scale outcome scores of female borderline patients who had experienced brother-sister incest but no father-daughter incest[a]

Case no.	Global Assessment Scale score
5	85
8	55
10	70
14	68
20	31
26	(suicide)
27	74

Note. See note to Table 9-3 for explanation of levels of severity.
[a]Level of severity was I in every instance. Brother-sister, Level I incest versus father-daughter, Level I incest: $p < .35$, Fisher's exact test.

Table 9-6. P.I.-500 Global Assessment Scale outcome scores of 144 female borderline patients with and without an incest history[a]

Global Assessment Scale outcome score range		BPD females, no incest history ($N = 116$)	BPD females, with incest history ($N = 28$)
Well	> 70 (recovered)	47	9
	60–70 (good)	34	5
Not well	51–60 (fair)	17	6
	31–50 (marginal)	6	3
	1–30 (incapacitated)	2	1
	0 (completed suicide)	7	3
Untraced		3	1
Total		116	28

[a]Well/not well: $\chi^2 = 3.93$, 1 df, $p < .048$.

Table 9-7. P.I.-500 incest history in female patients with a psychotic illness compared with patients with borderline personality disorder

Diagnostic subgroup	N	n with incest history	Percentage
Psychotic illness			
Schizophrenia	39	2	5.1
Schizoaffective psychosis	41	11	26.8
Manic-depressive illness (bipolar I & II, unipolar—combined)	15	1	6.7
Schizophreniform psychosis	9	0	0
Borderline Personality Disorder	144	27	19

Until the publication of Russell's (1986) monograph, the base rate among women was estimated at 5% in the United States (Finkelhor 1984). Even a rate of 16% to 20% (as noted in the BPD patients of the P.I.-500) would have appeared markedly increased and of unquestionable statistical significance. If an incest history is as common as Russell suggested, not only in the community where the study was carried out but elsewhere as well, then one cannot speak of a significantly greater likelihood of incest in women with BPD, unless a rate of perhaps 30% or more is observed (as, for example, in the recent New York and Queensland inpatient samples).

Even without other epidemiologic studies in Australia and in America, however, some meaning may still be extracted from the marked discrepancies between incest rates in neurotic versus borderline samples (as noted in Table 9-1) or between BPD versus schizophrenia samples (as noted in Table 9-7).

The higher rate in BPD when compared with schizophrenic women is of particular interest because of popular assumptions about chaotic conditions in the families of schizophrenic patients. It is probably nearer the truth to say that, while the families of some schizophrenic patients are grossly maladaptive and disrespectful of personal boundaries, the majority are not. Borderline patients, in contrast, often do report violence and inappropriate sexual behavior as characteristics of their original families. Elsewhere, evidence of affective illness in the close relatives of borderline patients has been presented (Stone et al. 1981). The overrepresentation of manic-depressive conditions in these families was understood as carrying etiologic significance: risk genes for manic-depression predisposed to the development of "borderline" conditions in early adult life. While I still believe that in certain families constitutional vulnerability to manic-depression does contribute to borderline development, in other families the decisive factors may be largely, at times entirely, environmental.

In my view, BPD would appear to be the final common pathway of several interacting pathogenic factors: predominantly heredofamilial in some cases, purely "psychogenic" in other cases, and a blend of the two in the majority. Problems in separation and individuation have been emphasized, in relation to the psychogenic factors, by some authors (Masterson 1981; Rinsley 1982). Incest and gratuitous corporal punishment may, in the families of some future borderline patients, loom even larger as etiologic factors. The influence of parental brutality, as distinct from sexual molestation, will be discussed in greater detail elsewhere (Stone 1990). Either incest or brutality appears capable of engendering serious deformation of personality; when both have been present, their action appears synergistic.

The high incest rate in the private-practice BPD patients compared to the comparatively lower rate in the neurotic patients may be an index of the pathogenicity of incest itself, since few of these patients had also experienced parental brutality. This pathogenicity may also have specificity—insofar as an incest history correlated with subsequent development of BPD and schizoaffective (or "atypical") psychosis but not with the other conditions we studied.

With respect to outcome, the picture is complex. Incest, particularly when committed by a relative of the older generation, may set in motion a series of reactions whose collective impact on the developing personality eventually crystalizes as a "borderline" condition. If the molestation had been especially severe and the child especially vulnerable, one may even see an "atypical" psychosis (Tsuang and Dempsey 1979). The latter may take a clinical form compatible with the diagnosis of "schizoaffective psychosis," implying severe disorders of cognition and of mood regulation at the same time. This type of disorder in an incest victim may represent a "phenocopy" of the more customary heredofamilial schizoaffective psychoses, whose principal etiologic factor is trauma rather than adverse genetic influences. Kolb's (1987) concept of the posttraumatic stress disorder is especially relevant in this context. Kolb advanced the hypothesis that "intense memories of aversive stimulation" (p. 994) may lead to functional change in neuronal and synaptic cortical processing, eventuating in impaired cognition, abnormal "release" phenomena (viz., irritability, nightmares), reactive affective states, avoidance behavior, and so on. Although Kolb based his observations on combat-induced posttraumatic stress victims, they would appear applicable as well to the most severely abused incest victims. The latter, if their reaction impairs reality sense severely, may manifest a (pseudo-) schizoaffective disorder; if reality testing remains intact, they may manifest a "borderline" disorder.

In this regard, molestation by a father is probably more serious than molestation by an uncle or brother, since society holds the father more accountable as protector and preserver of boundaries than it does other male relatives. Although I could not demonstrate a significant difference in outcome between brother-sister versus father-daughter incest in the borderline patients of the P.I.-500 sample, clinically some of the severe father-daughter cases among the "schizoaffective" patients led to suicide within brief intervals. Whether the nature of the relationship (e.g., father, brother, uncle) has a significant impact will have to be reevaluated in the light of a larger sample than was available here.

Although even a solitary episode may have a lasting effect, episodic or continuous incest is especially likely to engender lasting problems with impulsivity, guilt, sense of betrayal, simultaneous adoration and vilification of the abusing relative, and craving for revenge. All these attributes are typical of patients with BPD. In the samples alluded to in this chapter, incest victims were prone to adolescent running away, promiscuity, rage attacks, self-mutilation, fire setting, and other destructive attributes. Although some have done remarkably well, the life trajectories of borderline incest victims, on average, are less favorable than those of borderline patients who have not been incest victims.

I am also of the opinion that some of these patients lacked genetic or other "risk" and, apart from their incest experiences, might not have developed BPD in the first place.

The relatively good *average* outcome of the borderline patients with an incest history is itself somewhat deceptive. Many of the women who were constitutionally less vulnerable or who were molested in less serious ways have been able, over time, to make good adjustments. One-third of the patients in Table 9-3 now have GAS scores greater than 70 and are in the clinically recovered range. There were, however, two suicides and several poorly adjusted patients, whose morbidity was attributable in large part to their incest experiences. One of the suicides had been chronically molested by her father and forced repeatedly by two of her brothers into having intercourse. She became bulimic and suicidally depressed during adolescence, went through a series of hospitalizations, between which periods she abused drugs, was promiscuous, and prone to outbursts of rage, in one of which she set fire to her apartment. In other respects she was attractive and had been a talented dancer who showed promise of an excellent career. In her late 20s she impulsively married a man she had met while both were involved in a drug-rehabilitation program. Feeling despondent about ever being able to lead a stable and satisfying life, she committed suicide shortly after her wedding.

In contrast to the New York Hospital and P.I.-500 series, the borderline patients at Belmont Hospital in Brisbane had relatively little family history of manic depression or schizophrenia. Parental alcoholism was high in this as in all samples. Both physical and sexual abuse had been in the background of at least three of the Belmont patients. Here, the effects of each type of abuse are difficult to separate. The resulting clinical picture, in any event, was one of aggressive and destructive behavior, cynicism, and a disturbed sexual life. One patient, for example, molested on many occasions by her alcoholic father, had also witnessed similar molestation of her younger sisters. Now in her 30s, she has alternated between suicidal and assaultive outbursts. During heated arguments with her boyfriend, she has sometimes smashed his property and attacked his person. Of the four Belmont patients who were not abused physically, the clinical picture has been dominated by self-mutilation and suicide gestures, with relatively little aggression directed outwardly. In the New York Hospital series, as in the Belmont series, self-mutilation and suicide gestures were common in the female BPD patients; those with concomitant physical abuse were more apt to become assaultive or destructive of property at home or on the unit than were those who had not been beaten as children. A history of physical abuse was elicited from one-fourth of the patients in either series.

Disentangling the effects of physical versus sexual trauma is a difficult task, as may be gleaned from the histories of two borderline women, one hospitalized in Brisbane, the other in New York. The father of one woman forced cold water into his daughter's vagina when she was 8 years old. He did this to "teach" her about the evils of sex and the treachery of men. When she was 18 he impregnated her, drove her to an abortion clinic many miles away, and left her to get back home by hitchhiking. She had a brief psychotic episode and was hospitalized. The other woman was traumatized by her mother, a member of a fundamentalist religious sect, who took to "purifying" her daughter on Sundays by rubbing steel wool on her genitals. In these examples, sexual and physical abuse are completely intertwined.

SUMMARY: COMMENTS ON THE INCEST PROFILE

The Incest Rate in Borderline Patients

The incest rate in hospitalized patients with BPD was clearly elevated in those of the series cited in this chapter where specific questioning of the patients was possible during the height of their illness. The 35% rate noted in the New York Hospital sample and the 41% rate noted in the Brisbane sample are approximately twice that of the best available figures elicited from the general population in the United States (Russell 1986). The 19% rate mentioned in Table 9-1 for the BPD patients in the P.I.-500 stemmed primarily from review of charts, written in an era when incest histories were not routinely inquired about. The true figure for that group may well have been 10% higher, judging from the number of patients who showed the clinical profile in the absence of a "positive" chart or record.

I feel it is justified to claim that an incest history, especially where the sexual traumatization has been intense, prolonged, and accompanied by hostility or contempt on the part of the abuser, may contribute importantly to the subsequent deformation of personality development that we now categorize under the rubric of BPD. Concomitant physical abuse during childhood and/or adolescence intensified the traumatic effects of the incest.

The Incest Profile

Clinically, a profile emerges whose presence should alert diagnosticians and therapists to the likelihood of an incest history, especially in one's initial consultations with young female patients. Those who show many of the following characteristics at once will often have had such a history: seductiveness, impulsivity, coyness, secretiveness, self-mutilation, destructiveness, volatility, guardedness, and preoccupation with feelings of shame, revenge, cynicism, and mistrust. Destructiveness and revenge, if present, may be understood as reactions to childhood exploitation: victim becomes aggressor. Female incest victims tend also to be unconventional, to feel estranged from others (as though a "pariah"), and to have difficulties making friends with women their age.

The many components of the incest profile may, for heuristic purposes, be compartmentalized into abnormalities of emotion, behavior, or cognition, and into a number of discrete syndromes and other symptom pictures. These I have outlined in Tables 9-8 through 9-11.

As with other constellations in psychiatry, no one of these signs or traits is pathognomonic. It remains for the future to establish which features

Table 9-8. Symptoms noted with special frequency in female incest victims

Anxiety, fearfulness (10, 19, 55)

Depression, suicidal preoccupation and behavior (9, 10, 14, 19, 20, 28–30, 32, 34, 48, 50, 55, 66)

Dissociative tendencies (viz., psychogenic fugue, multiple personality disorder) (36)

Dysmorphophobia (60)

Extreme avoidance of gaze (63)

Impulse dyscontrol (viz., rage outbursts, substance abuse, antisocial behavior) (11, 34, 41, 50, 57)

Nightmares (63)

Self-mutilation (11, 20, 28, 32, 41, 48, 50, 57, 63)

Sexual dysfunction (viz., frigidity, extreme avoidance of sex; hypersexuality with nymphomania) (4, 5, 10, 20, 28, 31, 39, 40, 42, 44, 46, 47, 53, 55, 58, 60)

Note. Numbers refer to numbers in brackets in the reference list.

Table 9-9. Attitudes and personality traits found commonly in female incest victims

Anger, irritability (9, 62, 63)

Coyness (60)

Deceitfulness (63)

Dependency (63)

Emotional volatility (9, 62)

Hostility (52)

Irresponsibility, disregard for social rules and customs (63)

Jealousy (60, 62)

Low self-esteem (60)

Manipulativeness, exploitativeness (60)

Masochism (60)

Mistrust, suspiciousness (60, 62)

Secretiveness (32)

Seductiveness (32)

Shame (60)

Note. Numbers refer to numbers in brackets in the reference list.

Table 9-10.   Disturbances in object relations commonly encountered in female
incest victims

Ambivalence, with a tendency to oscillate between adoration and vilification (a manifestation of "splitting") (62)

Intense loyalty to abusing relative, especially to a father, with inability to form enduring attachment to any other male (63)

Primacy of the dominance/submission mode in intimate relationships, with impairment in the capacity for the (more mature) mode of cooperativeness (60)

Possessiveness (60)

Abnormalities in intimacy with either *avoidance of men* or (more commonly) *stormy relationships*, with a tendency to choose abusive partners reminiscent of the original offending relative (55, 62)

Infidelity (55)

Distorted attitudes toward sex: a tilting toward sex as a power-mechanism for enslavement or punishment of the partner, rather than as a pleasure and bonding mechanism; occasionally, a turning away from men altogether and toward homosexual object choice (especially where offending relative was cruel or humiliating); occasionally, an avoidance of specific sexual acts indulged in by the offending relative (26, 60)

In married women with daughters: a tendency to divorce husband when daughter reaches same age as when mother was first abused (60)

Note.   Numbers refer to numbers in brackets in the reference list.

are the most common and to work out the specificities and sensitivities, vis-à-vis an incest history, of the various features and their combinations.

Questions for the Future

Related to these issues are a couple of as yet unresolved questions. What is the power of a BPD diagnosis as a predictor of an incest history? What is the power of determining an incest history in a young person as a predictor of developing BPD in late adolescence or early adulthood? Some of the figures relevant to these calculations are already available from recent epidemiologic surveys; other percentages have not yet been established. The Bayesian equations that relate to this type of determination are shown, within the context of a clinical example, in the Appendix.

Summary

Long-term follow-up of incest victims with BPD in the P.I.-500 series suggests that clinical recovery is possible in a reasonable proportion of such patients, but that serious and persistent damage occurs in many instances. Most often the damage manifests itself as a gross inability to

Table 9-11.   Other phenomena that may be associated with an incest history

Primarily behavioral	Primarily cognitive
Acting-out (9)	Boundary blurring (32, 52)
Aggressive behavior (10, 34)	Identity disturbance (14, 33, 47)
Alcohol abuse (55)	Learning problems (19, 34)
Child abuse (22)	Motherhood, fears about (29)
Drug abuse (20, 30, 34, 41, 55)	Power over men, fantasies of (vengeful fantasies) (29)
Homosexuality (26)	
Prostitution (24, 38, 51, 69)	Posttraumatic psychosis (1, 3, 37, 63, 68)
Pseudomaturity (52)	
Separation problems (41)	Role confusion (52)
Social skills, impaired social withdrawal, suicidal feelings, gestures (52)	Self-image problems (29, 32)
	Trust, diminished capacity for (29, 52)
Affective	Conditions and syndromes
Covert hostility (52)	Borderline personality disorders (8, 12, 18, 21, 25, 49, 63)
Fearfulness (9, 10)	
Guilt (9, 32, 58, 66)	Developmental failure (52)
Isolation, feelings of (29, 55)	Chronic pain (9)
Repressed anger (52)	Somatic symptoms (7, 9, 14, 19, 23, 34, 47)
Anger toward women (29)	
	Multiple personality disorder (6, 36)

Note.   Numbers refer to numbers in brackets in the reference list.

trust sexual partners, with a corresponding disturbance in close relationships. In a few cases, avoidance of men was total and object-choice was homosexual. Incest history also appears to heighten the risk of suicide.

REFERENCES

American Psychiatric Association: Diagnostic and Statistical Manual of Mental Disorders, 3rd Edition. Washington, DC, American Psychiatric Association, 1980 [1]

American Psychiatric Association: Diagnostic and Statistical Manual of Mental Disorders, 3rd Edition, Revised. Washington, DC, American Psychiatric Association, 1987 [2]

Numbers in brackets refer to numbers in Table 9-8, 9-9, 9-10, and 9-11.

Bender L, Grugett A: A follow-up report on children who had atypical sexual experiences. Am J Orthopsychiatry 22:825–837, 1951 [3]

Berry GW: Incest: some clinical variations on a classical theme. J Am Acad Psychoanal 3:151–161, 1975 [4]

Bess B, Janssen Y: A pilot study. Hillside J Clin Psychiatry 4:39–52, 1982 [5]

Bliss EL: Multiple Personality, Allied Disorders and Hypnosis. New York, Oxford University Press, 1986 [6]

Brooks B: Incidence of incest among borderline patients: data from New York Hospital-Westchester Division. Unpublished manuscript, 1980 [7]

Brooks B: Incest and identity: an Eriksonian dilemma. Paper presented at the annual meeting of the American Psychological Association, Anaheim, CA, 1983 [8]

Browning DH, Boatman B: Incest: children at risk. Am J Psychiatry 134:69–72, 1977 [9]

DeFrancis V: Protecting the child victim of sex crimes committed by adults. Denver, CO, American Humane Association, 1969 [10]

DeYoung M: Self-injurious behavior in incest victims: a research note. Child Welfare 61:577–584, 1982 [11]

Emslie GJ, Rosenfeld A: Incest reported by children and adolescents hospitalized for severe psychiatric problems. Am J Psychiatry 140:708–711, 1983 [12]

Endicott J, Spitzer RL, Fleiss JL, et al: The Global Assessment Scale. Arch Gen Psychiatry 33:766–771, 1976 [13]

Fibel B: A family systems approach to incestuous relations: the incest victim versus the oedipal victor. Paper presented at the annual meeting of the American Psychological Association, Toronto, 1978 [14]

Finkelhor D: Child Sexual Abuse. New York, Free Press, 1984 [15]

Forward S, Buck C: Betrayal of Innocence: Incest and Its Devastation. Harmondsworth, England, Penguin, 1978 [16]

Freud S: The aetiology of hysteria (1896), in The Standard Edition of the Complete Psychological Works of Sigmund Freud, Vol 3. Translated and edited by Strachey J. London, Hogarth Press, 1962, pp 191–221 [17]

Friedman RC, Hurt SW, Clarkin JF, et al: Sexual histories and premenstrual affective syndrome in psychiatric inpatients. Am J Psychiatry 139:1484–1486, 1982 [18]

Geiser RL: Incest and psychological violence. International Journal of Family Psychiatry 2:291–300, 1981 [19]

Gelinas DJ: Identification and treatment of incest victims, in Women and Mental Health. Edited by Howell D, Bayes E. New York, Basic Books, 1981 [20]

Gelinas DJ, Carr A, Goodman B, et al: Prevalence, sequelae and recognition of undisclosed incest in a general inpatient psychiatric population. Unpublished manuscript, 1983 [21]

Goodwin J: Sexual Abuse: Incest Victims and Their Families. Littleton, MA, PSG Publishing, 1982 [22]

Greenacre P: The prepuberty trauma in girls, in Trauma, Growth and Personality. Edited by Greenacre P. London, Hogarth Press, 1953, pp 204–223 [23]

Greenwald H: The Call Girl: A Social and Psychoanalytic Study. New York, Ballantine Books, 1958 [24]

Gross RJ, Doerr H, Caldirola D, et al: Borderline syndrome and incest in chronic pelvic pain patients. Int J Psychiatry Med 10:79–96, 1980 [25]

Gunderson JG, Zanarini MG: Current overview of the borderline diagnosis. J Clin Psychiatry 48 (suppl 8):5–11, 1986

Grundlach RH: Sexual molestation and rape reported by homosexual and heterosexual women. J Homosex 2:367–384, 1977 [26]

Henderson DJ: Incest, in Comprehensive Textbook of Psychiatry, 2nd Edition. Edited by Kaplan HI, Sadock BJ. Baltimore, MD, Williams & Wilkins, 1975, p 1532 [27]

Herman JL: Father-Daughter Incest. Cambridge, MA, Harvard University Press, 1981 [28]

Herman J, Hirschman L: Families at risk for father-daughter incest. Am J Psychiatry 138:967–970, 1981a [29]

Herman J, Hirschman L: Incest between fathers and daughters, in Women and Mental Health. Edited by Howell E, Bayes E. New York, Basic Books, 1981b [30]

Hersko M, et al: Incest: a three-way process. Journal of Social Therapy 7:22–31, 1961 [31]

Justice B, Justice R: The Broken Taboo. New York, Human Sciences Press, 1979 [32]

Katan A: Children who were raped. Psychoanal Study Child 28:208–224, 1973 [33]

Kaufman I, Peck AL, Tagiuri CK: The family constellation and overt incestuous relations between father and daughter. Am J Orthopsychiatry 24:266–277, 1954 [34]

Kempe RS, Kempe CH: The Common Secret: Sexual Abuse of Children and Adolescents. New York, WH Freeman, 1984 [35]

Kluft RP (ed): Childhood Antecendents of Multiple Personality. Washington, DC, American Psychiatric Press, 1985 [36]

Kolb LF: A neuropsychological hypothesis explaining post-traumatic stress disorders. Am J Psychiatry 144:989–995, 1987 [37]

Kubo S: Researchers and studies on incest in Japan. Hiroshima J Med Sci 8:99–159, 1959 [38]

Landis J: Experiences of 500 children with adult sexual deviants. Psychiatr Q (Suppl) 30:91–109, 1956 [39]

Lukianowicz N: Incest. Br J Psychiatry 120:201–212, 1972 [40]

Lustig N, Dresser J, Spellman S, et al: Incest: a family group survival pattern. Arch Gen Psychiatry 14:31–40, 1966 [41]

Magal V, Winnick HZ: Role of incest in family structure. Israel Annals of Psychiatry and Related Disciplines 6:173–189, 1968 [42]

Malcolm J: In the Freud Archives. New York, Random House, 1984 [43]

Masters WH, Johnson VE: Human Sexual Inadequacy. Boston, MA, Little, Brown, 1970 [44]

Masterson JF: The Narcissistic and Borderline Disorder. Northvale, NJ, Jason Aronson, 1981 [45]

Medlicott RW: Parent-child incest. Aust N Z J Psychiatry 1:180–187, 1967 [46]

Meiselman KC: Incest: A Psychological Study of Causes and Effects With Treatment Recommendations. San Francisco, CA, Jossey-Bass, 1978 [47]

Molnar G, Cameron P: Incest syndromes: observations in a general hospital psychiatric unit. Canadian Psychiatric Association Journal 20:373–377, 1975 [48]

Nielsen G: Borderline and Acting-Out Adolescents: A Developmental Approach. New York, Human Sciences Press, 1983 [49]

Perlmutter LH, Engel T, Sager CJ: The incest taboo: loosened sexual boundaries in remarried families. J Sex Marital Ther 8:83–96, 1982 [50]

Peters JJ: Children who are victims of sexual assault and the psychology of offenders. Am J Psychother 30:298–341, 1976 [51]

Porter FC, Blick LC, Sgroi SM: Treatment of the sexually abused child, in Handbook of Clinical Intervention in Child Sexual Abuse. Edited by Sgroi SM. Lexington, MA, Lexington Books, 1982, pp 109–146 [52]

Rascovsky MW, Rascovsky M: On consummated incest. Int J Psychoanal 31:42–47, 1950 [53]

Rinsley DB: Borderline and Other Self Disorders. Northvale, NJ, Jason Aronson, 1982 [54]

Rosenfeld A: Incidence of a history of incest among 18 female psychiatric patients. Am J Psychiatry 136:791–795, 1979 [55]

Russell DEH: The Secret Trauma: Incest in the Lives of Girls and Women. New York, Basic Books, 1986 [56]

Shapiro ER: Research on family dynamics: clinical implications for the family of the borderline adolescent, in Adolescent Psychiatry, Vol 6. Edited by Feinstein SC, Giovacchini PL. Chicago, IL, University of Chicago Press, 1978, pp 360–376 [57]

Sloan P, Karpinski E: Effects of incest on the participants. Am J Orthopsychiatry 12:666–673, 1942 [58]

Stone MH: Borderline syndromes: a consideration of subtypes and an overview: directions for research. Psychiatr Clin North Am 4:3–24, 1981 [59]

Stone MH: Disturbances in sex and love in borderline patients, in Contemporary Aspects of Sexuality. Edited by DeFries Z, Friedman RC, Korn R. Westport, CT, Greenwood Press, 1985, pp 159–186 [60]

Stone MH: Psychotherapy of borderline patients in light of long term follow-up. Bull Menninger Clin 51:231–247, 1987 [61]

Stone MH: The borderline domain: the "inner script" and other common psychodynamics, in Modern Perspectives in Clinical Psychiatry. Edited by Howells JG. New York, Brunner/Mazel, 1988, pp 203–234 [62]

Stone MH: Individual psychotherapy with victims of incest. Psychiatr Clin North Am 14:237–255, 1989 [63]

Stone MH: The Fate of Borderline Patients. New York, Guilford Press, 1990

Stone MH, Kahn E, Flye B: Psychiatrically ill relatives of borderline patients: a family study. Psychiatr Q 53:71–84, 1981 [64]

Stone MH, Hurt SW, Stone DK: The PI-500: long-term follow-up of borderline inpatients meeting DSM III criteria. Journal of Personality Disorders 1:291–298

Tsai M, Wagner N: Therapy groups for women sexually molested as children. Arch Sex Behav 7:417–427, 1978 [66]

Tsuang MT, Dempsey GM: Long-term outcome of major psychoses, II: schizoaffective disorder compared with schizophrenia, affective disorders and a surgical control group. Arch Gen Psychiatry 36:1302–1304, 1979 [67]

Wahl CW: The psychodynamics of consummated maternal incest: a report of two cases. Arch Gen Psychiatry 3:188–193, 1960 [68]

Weinberg SK: Incest Behavior. New York, Citadel, 1955 [69]

APPENDIX

The following example demonstrates the Bayesian method of determining conditional probabilities relative to the possible interrelationship between borderline personality disorder (BPD) and an incest history.

Among women, suppose we know two events: "A_1," that 16% are incest victims and "A_2," that (by mutual exclusion) 84% are not, that is, the probability (PR) of $A_1 = 0.16$; of $A_2 = 0.84$.

Suppose further that 15% of incest victims go on to develop BPD whereas only 3% of nonincest victims develop BPD. This may be notated:

$B|A_1$ (likelihood of BPD, given an incest history) $= 0.15$

$B|A_2$ (BPD, given *no* incest history) $= 0.03$

a. What is the chance a woman will have *both* BPD *and* an incest history? This is represented by

PR $(A_1 \times B)$, which equals

PR $(B|A_1) \times$ PR $(A_1) = (0.15)(0.16) = 0.024$

b. What is the chance a woman will *not* have an incest history but *will* have BPD?

$=$ PR $(A_2 \times B) =$

PR $(B|A_2) \times$ PR $(A_2) = (0.03)(0.84) = 0.0252$

c. What is the chance of *BPD*? BPD can develop in two mutually exclusive ways, that is, with and without an incest history.

PR (BPD) $=$ PR (B) $=$ PR $(A_1 \times B) +$ PR $(A_2 \times B)$

$= 0.024 + 0.0252 = 0.0492$

d. With the knowledge that a woman exhibits BPD, what is the chance she has been an incest victim?

$$\text{PR } (A_1|B) = \frac{\text{PR } (A_1 \times B)}{\text{PR } B} = \frac{0.024}{0.0492} = 0.4878$$

That is, a woman manifesting the features of BPD would have, in this example, a 48.8% chance of having been an incest victim; she would be about three times as likely to have an incest history as would a nonborderline woman.

The weak links in the chain of logic here are, of course, the percentages of incest victims and of nonincest victims who go on to develop BPD. Epidemiologic surveys addressing these issues have not as yet been carf6d out. The estimates in the above example derive from impressions of Gunderson and Zanarini (1987) and others that about 4% or 5% of women might show a clinical picture compatible with BPD. Since not all BPD cases have an incest history, I chose arbitrarily the 3% figure for $(B|A_2)$ and a figure for $(B|A_1)$ that yielded a percentage for total borderlines in the 5% range (4.92%, in the actual example). The above example uses a value for $(B|A_1) = 15\%$. This figure implies that 15% of incest victims later develop BPD—a "guesstimate," but not unrealistic. Further epidemiologic work of the sort carried out by Russell and her co-workers (1986) should be able to provide a more precise measure for this correlation.

CHAPTER 10

Symptoms of Posttraumatic Stress and Dissociation in Women Victims of Abuse

Philip M. Coons, M.D., Coral Cole, M.A.,
Terri A. Pellow, M.D., and Victor Milstein, Ph.D.

This study grew out of our interest in abused women, posttraumatic stress disorder (PTSD), and the dissociative disorders, particularly multiple personality disorder (MPD). The presence of six women with MPD, five with either psychogenic amnesia or atypical dissociative disorder, and numerous others with posttraumatic flashbacks within the population of a women's counseling clinic led us to undertake a more ambitious study of the clinic population. We wanted to know the extent of abuse suffered by the women patients and the extent to which they suffered from symptoms of posttraumatic stress and dissociation.

Prior to describing the study further, however, the literature regarding child abuse, wife abuse, and rape will be reviewed. This review will be followed by a brief review of the two major groups of disorders investigated in this study, PTSDs and the dissociative disorders, both of which are intimately related to trauma.

The three major types of abuse perpetrated by men against women are physical, sexual, and emotional abuse. When abuse occurs during childhood, it is called child abuse. Child abuse can be divided into sexual

A revision of a paper originally presented at the Third International Conference on Multiple Personality/Dissociative States, Chicago, IL, October 1986.

abuse, physical abuse, emotional abuse, and neglect. Sexual abuse can be subdivided into incestuous and nonincestuous types, depending on the relationship of the perpetrator to the victim. When a sexual assault includes sexual intercourse against the victim's will, it is called rape. Rape can occur both in childhood and adulthood and may be accompanied by physical assault. Wife abuse is abuse perpetrated against a wife by her husband and can include physical, sexual, and emotional forms.

Precise figures concerning the prevalence of these various types of abuse have begun to emerge only during the last 10 years because child abuse, rape, and wife abuse have been seriously underreported to both mental health professionals and law enforcement officials. In all studies to date the abuse rate for clinical populations has been higher than the rate for nonclinical populations (Jacobson et al. 1987).

Two major studies of nonclinical populations have reported on different types of sexual abuse of women. In Finkelhor's (1979) survey of 800 students enrolled in six Eastern colleges, 19.2% of the women described at least one coercive sexual experience with an adult before the age of 13 years. The prevalence of paternal incest in this study was 1%. Russell (1986) reported that 16% of 930 San Francisco women had been sexually abused by a relative prior to the age of 18 years. Of these women, 4.5% had been sexually abused by their fathers. Extrafamilial sexual abuse involving petting or genital sex prior to age 18 had occurred in 31%.

The prevalence of abuse among clinical populations varies according to the population surveyed. Carmen et al. (1984) reported that 53% of women psychiatric inpatients had histories of either physical or sexual abuse. In 190 consecutive outpatient evaluations, Herman (1986) found that one-third of female patients had been victims of either physical or sexual violence. Jacobson and Richardson (1987) found the following prevalence figures for four major types of physical and sexual assault in 50 women psychiatric inpatients: childhood physical abuse, 44%; childhood sexual abuse, 22%; adult physical abuse, 64%; and adult sexual abuse, 38%. Bryer et al. (1987) found that 72% of 66 women psychiatric inpatients had experienced a history of abuse at some time during their lives. Prior to the age of 16, 21% reported sexual abuse only, 15% reported physical abuse only, and 23% reported both types of abuse. At age 16 or after, 14% reported sexual abuse, 24% reported physical abuse, and 20% reported both types of abuse. The prevalence of childhood sexual abuse among women with MPD varies from 75% to 90% (Bliss 1984; Coons and Milstein 1986; Putnam et al. 1986). In Stone's (Chapter 9, this volume) review of female borderline personality disorder patients, incest rates varied between 8% and 41%.

The prevalence of incest among female psychiatric patients also varies according to the population surveyed. Lukianowicz (1972) reported a prevalence of 4%, but suggested that many cases may have been missed among the 650 psychiatric inpatients and outpatients surveyed. Rosenfeld (1979) reported that 33% of 18 consecutive outpatients had a history of incest. Husain and Chapel (1983) found that 14% of female adolescent inpatients reported a history of incest. Emslie and Rosenfeld (1983) found that 35% of 26 consecutively admitted female psychiatric patients ages 9 to 17 years had suffered from incest. Sansonnet-Hayden et al. (1987) reported that 38% of 29 consecutively admitted adolescent female psychiatric patients had been sexually abused. Of 26 chronically hospitalized female psychiatric patients on two units of a Massachusetts state hospital, 46% reported histories of childhood incest (Beck and van der Kolk 1987). In another group of psychiatric inpatients, Goodwin et al. (1988) found that 70% of the women reported incestual experiences.

Like incest, the incidence of rape has been vastly underreported. In 1982 the incidence of rape was 33.6 per 100,000 women in the United States (Federal Bureau of Investigation 1982). Hilberman (1976) estimated that 50% to 90% of all rapes go unreported. Kilpatrick and Veronen (1984) surveyed a random sample of 2,004 women residents of Charleston, South Carolina, and found that 5% had been victims of rape and that 4% had been victims of attempted rape. Both Carmen et al. (1984) and Katz and Mazur (1979) reported a high prevalence of rape in psychiatric populations, although they did not specify exact rates. The prevalence of rape and sexual assault among patients with MPD ranges from 35% to 48% (Coons and Milstein 1984; Putnam et al. 1986).

Like child abuse and rape, the prevalence of wife abuse is considerably underreported. Rounsaville and Weissman (1977–1978) reported that 3.8% of women who presented to an emergency room trauma service and 3.4% of women who presented to an emergency psychiatric service were battered. However, when Stark et al. (1979) analyzed new data from the same emergency service, they concluded that approximately 25% of the women patients had been battered. In a large national sample of married women, Straus (1978) found that 28% had experienced wife battery at some point in their marriages. Of 600 couples in the process of divorce, Levinger (1966) found that 40% of the lower-class women and 23% of the middle-class women had experienced wife battery.

Exact figures for the prevalence of PTSD are unknown (American Psychiatric Association 1987). The prevalence rises, however, during wartime or after natural disasters. One study reported the following rates of chronic PTSD for Vietnam combat veterans: active duty veterans, 5.1%; reservist veterans, 10.9%; and civilian veterans, 32% (Stretch, unpublished manuscript, 1984). Another study (Boulanger 1985) found that 26% of servicemen in heavy combat, 17% of servicemen in average combat, and 7% of noncombatants and nonwar-zone veterans had PTSD. In the civilian sector, both Kilpatrick et al. (1985) and Frank and Anderson (1987) reported that most (approximately 70%) rape victims meet the criteria for PTSD.

Of 26 adult women psychiatric patients who had experienced childhood incest, Donaldson and Gardner (1985) found that 25 experienced symptoms of PTSD. Finally, there is increasing recognition that all sorts of severe trauma—such as rape, natural disasters, severe accidents, incest, childhood physical abuse, assault, and torture—can result in PTSD (American Psychiatric Association 1987; Coons and Milstein 1984; Eth and Pynoos 1985; Goodwin 1984; Kilpatrick et al. 1985).

The prevalence of the dissociative disorders such as psychogenic amnesia, psychogenic fugue, or MPD is also unknown, but most were thought to range from "rare" to "extremely rare," except during wartime or natural disasters (American Psychiatric Association 1980). However, more recent reports indicate that MPD is more common than previously thought (American Psychiatric Association 1987; Bliss and Jeppsen 1985; Coons 1986; French 1984). MPD is linked etiologically to severe childhood trauma, particularly sexual abuse (Coons and Milstein 1986; Greaves 1980; Putnam et al. 1986; Saltman and Solomon 1982).

The literature describing the symptoms of PTSD (American Psychiatric Association 1987; Horowitz 1986) and the dissociative disorders (Coons 1980; Greaves 1980; Kluft 1985; Putnam et al. 1986) has been previously reviewed and will not be repeated in detail here. It is important to recognize, however, that most of the symptoms of these disorders are not generally evaluated in the routine psychiatric evaluation (Arnold 1985; Jacobson et al. 1987; Kluft 1985). Symptoms of PTSD include intrusive recollections of the trauma, recurrent dreams of the trauma, avoidance of activities reminiscent of the trauma, flashbacks, numbing, hyperalertness, sleep disturbance, decreased interest, constricted affect, trouble concentrating, and survivor guilt (American Psychiatric Association 1987). Symptoms of the major dissociative disorders include difficulty with recent memory, difficulty with remote memory, blank spells, depersonalization, derealization, depression, discontinuity of time, disorientation, fugue, auditory hallucinations, personality changes ranging from perplexity to the assumption of a new identity, and various psychophysiologic symptoms including headaches and conversion (American Psychiatric Association 1987).

Tests to measure the extent of dissociation and posttraumatic stress have been developed. Bernstein and Putnam (1986) developed a Dissociative Experiences Scale, which they used to assess the extent of dissociation across different psychiatric populations. Although symptoms of dissociation were low in normal controls, alcoholic patients, and agoraphobic patients, there was an increased incidence of dissociation in adolescents and schizophrenic patients and an even higher incidence in individuals with PTSD and MPD. Keane et al. (1984) developed a 49-item Minnesota Multiphasic Personality Inventory (MMPI) (Hathaway and McKinley 1967) subscale for the diagnosis of PTSD. This subscale was 82% to 90% congruent with PTSD diagnosed by structured interviews and histories.

In this study we examine the incidence of symptoms of posttraumatic stress and dissociation in women victims of abuse and compare the results to a control group of bulimic women. Four representative case studies are presented, followed by a discussion of the highlights of the study. We include in an appendix the questionnaire utilized to collect the data for this study so that it might be utilized by other clinicians.

METHODS

The subjects were 46 women who were outpatients of the Julian Center, a women's counseling clinic. This clinic is staffed exclusively by women therapists, and the therapy covers a wide range of women's issues, including identity formation, marriage and the family, career counseling, incest, rape, and wife battery. Sixteen subjects were undergoing therapy at the time of the survey; 30 were undergoing assessment prior to beginning therapy. The study group included nearly all of the patients seen at the center during a 2-month period. Less than 10% of the patients at the clinic chose not to be a part of the study, but these individuals did not give reasons for their nonparticipation.

A control group also was evaluated and consisted of 20 consecutive bulimic outpatients who were attending an eating disorders outpatient clinic in a state psychiatric hospital. Bulimic patients were chosen to serve as a control group because they were outpatients with similar socioeconomic backgrounds to the patients from the women's center. This particular control group was also chosen because a controlled study indicated that the incidence of incest in bulimic patients was similar to that of a general psychiatric population (Finn et al. 1986).

In addition to the regular clinical assessment provided by clinicians at the Julian Center and the psychiatric hospital outpatient clinic, the subjects and controls were given a questionnaire, including questions about demographic data, previous abuse, previous psychotherapy, previous psychiatric diagnoses, and symptoms of posttraumatic stress (10 items) and dissociation (10 items). A revised version of this questionnaire, which is now used as a screening device and guide to clinician inquiries at the Julian Center, is included in the Appendix. Although not all of the women attending the women's clinic underwent formal psychiatric evaluations by the authors, the patients attending the eating disorders clinic were evaluated and diagnosed according to the DSM-III (American Psychiatric Association 1980) criteria in use at the time the study was begun.

The study and control groups were compared statistically by means of χ^2 or t tests. A probability level of .05 was used to determine a level of statistical significance.

RESULTS

The demographic data for the study and control groups are shown in Table 10-1. Although the study group tended to be somewhat more advanced in occupational status, this difference was not statistically significant except for the semiskilled group.

The previous diagnoses (by patient report) are listed in Table 10-2. Of the 46 women in the study group, 78% had been in therapy previously. Interestingly, 60% of this group felt comfortable only with a woman therapist. (No corresponding data are available for the control group.)

Table 10-3 shows the types of abuse or trauma suffered by patients in both groups. The groups differed significantly in that 56% of the study group had suffered childhood sexual abuse compared with 10% of the control subjects. Conversely, only 13% of the women in the study group

Table 10-1. Demographic data

	Women's clinic group (N = 46)		Bulimia control group (N = 20)	
	n	%	n	%
Sex				
Female	46	100	19	95
Male	0	0	1	5
Race				
Caucasian	43	94	20	100
Black	2	4	0	0
Hispanic	1	2	0	0
Occupation				
Professional	9	20	1	5
Managerial	5	11	1	5
Skilled	9	20	5	25
Semiskilled*	14	30	1	5
Unskilled	1	2	3	15
Homemaker	4	9	4	20
Student	1	2	3	15
Unemployed	3	6	2	10
Marital status				
Single	18	39	11	55
Married	13	28	8	40
Divorced*	15	33	1	5
	Years	Range	Years	Range
Mean age	30	19–50	26	18–38
Mean education	13	9–18	13	12–18

*$p < .025$.

Table 10-2. Previous psychiatric diagnoses (by patient report)

Diagnosis	Women's clinic group (N = 46)		Bulimia control group (N = 20)	
	n	%	n	%
Depressive disorder	36	78	12	60
Anxiety disorder*	28	61	5	25
Alcohol abuse	9	20	1	5
Drug abuse	6	13	0	0
Major psychosis	5	11	1	5
Multiple personality	4	9	0	0
Eating disorder*	2	4	20	100

*$p < .005$.

Table 10-3. Types of abuse or trauma

Type	Women's clinic group (N = 46)		Bulimia control group (N = 20)	
	n	%	n	%
Any type of abuse or trauma*	40	87	6	30
Childhood sexual abuse*	26	56	2	10
Childhood physical abuse	15	33	2	10
Adult rape	11	24	1	5
Wife battery	11	24	1	5
Childhood neglect	10	22	1	5
No abuse or trauma*	6	13	14	70

*$p < .005$.

had not experienced abuse or trauma as compared with 70% of the control subjects. Of the women in the study group, 63% had experienced some type of child abuse. While 52% of the patients in the study group had experienced more than one type of abuse, this was true of only 10% of the patients in the control group. Although the patients in the bulimia control group suffered less trauma or abuse in all categories, this was not always statistically significant.

The incidence of symptoms of posttraumatic stress for both groups is shown in Table 10-4. Those symptoms indicative of present concern and involvement with the traumatic event, such as recurrent dreams, flashbacks, and intrusive thoughts of the trauma, significantly differentiated the study and control groups.

The incidence of symptoms of dissociation for both groups is shown in Table 10-5. There were six symptoms that were not experienced by the control group subjects. However, only two symptoms, depersonalization

Table 10-4. Symptoms of posttraumatic stress

Symptom	Women's clinic group (N = 46)		Bulimia control group (N = 20)	
	n	%	n	%
Recurrent dreams of trauma*	24	52	5	25
Certain events reminiscent of trauma**	24	52	4	20
Numbing or detachment	23	50	8	40
Avoidance of activities reminiscent of trauma	23	50	5	25
Easily startled	23	50	10	50
Decreased concentration	22	48	11	55
Insomnia	22	48	9	45
Flashbacks of trauma***	21	46	1	5
Intrusive thoughts of trauma*	21	46	4	20
Loss of interest	20	43	9	45

*$p < .05$. **$p < .025$. ***$p < .005$.

Table 10-5. Symptoms of dissociation

Symptom	Women's clinic group (N = 46)		Bulimia control group (N = 20)	
	n	%	n	%
Inability to remember recent events	15	33	2	10
Depersonalization**	13	28	0	0
Inability to remember remote events	12	26	5	25
Amnesia not associated with substance abuse	12	26	5	25
Blank spells	11	24	2	10
Inner voices*	10	22	0	0
Fugue	6	13	0	0
Recognized by unfamiliar people	5	11	0	0
Finding unfamiliar possessions	3	6	0	0
Called by unfamiliar names	1	2	0	0

*$p < .025$. **$p < .01$.

and inner voices, significantly distinguished the control from the study group. Although symptoms involving defective memory occurred far more commonly in the study group, the differences fell short of statistical significance.

CASE HISTORIES

The following case histories, drawn from the women's clinic population, will serve to familiarize the reader with the spectrum of dissociative and posttraumatic stress symptoms experienced by these patients. All of these women were personally seen by one of the authors (P.C.) for a diagnostic evaluation. This evaluation usually extended over a 3- to 4-week period of extensive history gathering and observation. Old records were obtained and collateral sources were interviewed.

Case 1

A 37-year-old divorced nurse was seen because her 17-year-old son had sexually molested her foster daughter. The mother had been sexually molested by both an uncle and brother when she was a child in addition to having been physically abused by her father. Her memory for childhood and adolescence was characterized by considerable amnesia. For example, she could not recollect details of some of the child abuse, a family reunion, her best friend in high school, or her wedding day and honeymoon. She had experienced no episodes of amnesia in adulthood. She had abused medically prescribed narcotic pain medication in the past year, but had experienced no memory loss from this drug abuse. She denied symptoms of PTSD and careful observation and exploration failed to reveal MPD.

> Diagnosis: Psychogenic amnesia (selective) and mixed substance abuse.
> Comment: Other dissociative disorders that should be considered in the dif-
> ferential diagnosis include MPD and dissociative disorder not oth-
> erwise specified (DDNOS) since psychogenic amnesia is not generally
> selective or recurrent. For example, the patient may have had MPD
> when she was younger but might not have dissociated for a long
> time. Further observation over a considerable period of time is
> definitely warranted.

Case 2

A 36-year-old separated woman had experienced amnesic episodes since childhood in addition to recent amnesic episodes, which included periods when she was driving her car and when she had dinner with her estranged husband. She indicated that she had been sexually abused by her step-father from age 5 until age 10. She had been battered by her first two husbands. She heard voices that gave her advice and had seen a vision of a "black spirit," which repeatedly appeared and tried to touch her. She felt if she touched the apparition that she would die. She also had pre-monitions of certain events. Her mental status examination revealed in-appropriate affect, blocking, and loose associations. At no time was she observed to dissociate into alter personality states. The MMPI revealed a classic paranoid schizophrenic profile. Her Draw-A-Person test (Mach-over 1949) also appeared psychotic due to humanoid creatures with big eyes and distorted body parts. Although she denied posttraumatic flashbacks, she experienced intrusive recollections of her childhood abuse and felt that the whippings provided by her first two husbands were punishment for her "sin" of having been abused.

Diagnosis: Paranoid schizophrenia and psychogenic amnesia.

Comment: Another diagnostic possibility is MPD with an atypical psychosis. Occasionally patients with MPD decompensate into brief psychoses (Coons 1984). Further observation is definitely indicated.

Case 3

A 50-year-old separated woman had been severely abused during childhood by her psychotic mother. The abuse consisted of the mother's repetitive attempts to kill her in rather bizarre fashions, such as trying to pour kerosene down her throat. She and her siblings were removed to different foster homes. She was subsequently sexually molested by both a foster sister and a foster father. Although she eventually married, she was battered by her husband. She had difficulty remembering events in childhood and had lost an entire 2 years after her foster father's death. She often found herself in strange or dangerous situations, such as driving toward a bridge abutment or awakening in a large basement furnace. She spoke of herself as existing in parts including an "outer person" and "parts" that "hurt or have anger," but further exploration and observation failed to reveal evidence of multiple personalities. Symptoms of posttraumatic stress included intrusive recollections, flashbacks, nightmares, numbing, survivor guilt, and avoidance of activities that reminded her of the abuse.

Diagnosis: Atypical dissociative disorder (now DDNOS) and PTSD, chronic.

Comment: This patient could also have MPD since dissociation may not have occurred during the diagnostic evaluation. Further observation is necessary.

Case 4

A 38-year-old married woman was sexually abused by her maternal grandfather, who also had abused his daughters and other granddaughters. In addition, she had been battered by her first two husbands. She experienced repeated amnesic episodes lasting 30 minutes or longer, depression, headaches, and other psychosomatic complaints, and talked of herself in the third person. Further exploration revealed two distinct personalities. One personality was depressed and suicidal, abhorred sex, and was a "homebody." Her alter personality was outgoing, enjoyed sex, and held a responsible job. Symptoms of posttraumatic stress included intrusive recollections, nightmares, flashbacks, numbing, survivor guilt, and avoidance of activities that reminded her of the abuse.

Diagnosis: MPD and PTSD, chronic.

Comment: As this patient continued in therapy, a third personality emerged. An initial integration failed because of the emergence of a large group of previously unsuspected personalities.

DISCUSSION

Both the study and control groups were composed of predominantly white, fairly well-educated working women. The demographic data of both groups were remarkably similar, except that significantly more women in the study group were divorced. This may have been related to their slightly older age, but also may have been due to the difficulty that this group had with male interpersonal relationships, especially those of a sexual nature. The background of sexual abuse and/or battery, which was significantly higher in the study group, may tend to inhibit these women from forming more intimate personal relationships with men.

The study group as a whole tended to be higher in occupational status than the control group. This difference was near statistical significance in the upper end of the occupational spectrum and significant in the semi-skilled category. This difference is probably because the Julian Center serves a slightly more well-to-do clientele than the state psychiatric outpatient clinic.

Although both the study and control groups were located in or near large inner-city black neighborhoods, blacks were underrepresented in both groups. Since black women are certainly not abused less frequently than white women (Goodstein and Page 1981), this cannot account for the underrepresentation. We speculate that the underrepresentation of black women in both groups occurred because blacks often seek help from family or friends and prefer not to utilize professional caregivers because of cultural differences, financial expense, lack of knowledge of community resources, distrust of authorities, and reluctance to seek care except in cases of emergency or very serious illness.

We were surprised at the high incidence of previous abuse in our study population. In retrospect, it probably should not have been unexpected since the women's center has gained a community-wide reputation for work with victims of incest, rape, and wife battery.

Symptoms of posttraumatic stress and dissociation were more frequent in the study group. This is understandable since the study group experienced considerably more abuse and battery than did the control group. After all, by definition, PTSD is related to traumatic experiences. Further, all of the dissociative disorders have recently been linked to various types of trauma (Putnam 1985).

Certain symptoms of posttraumatic stress are similar to those found in depression. These include decreased concentration, detachment, insomnia, and loss of interest. Both groups reported moderate levels of such symptoms. This is not unexpected since significant depressive symptoms, such as decreased self-esteem, guilt, self-blame, and disturbed sleep, have been reported in bulimic patients (Hudson et al. 1982; Johnson and Stuckey 1982; Pyle et al. 1981) and in groups of abused women such as those with MPD (Bliss 1984; Coons and Milstein 1986; Putnam et al. 1986) or those who have experienced rape (Becker et al. 1984; Burgess and Holstrom 1974) or child abuse (Blumberg 1981; Tsai and Wagner 1978).

We were particularly interested to observe the amount of dissociation and sexual abuse in the control group of bulimic patients since previous reports have indicated a relationship between hypnotizability (which some experts feel to be dissociative in nature) and bulimia (Pettinati et al. 1985); a possible relationship of dissociation and eating disorders (Torem 1986); a possible relationship of sexual abuse and eating disorders, particularly anorexia nervosa (Sloan and Leichner 1986; Torem 1986); but a lack of a relationship of bulimia and incest (Finn et al. 1986). Unfortunately, the Finn et al. study did not have enough anorexic patients to confirm or disconfirm a relationship between sexual abuse and anorexia nervosa.

Our data indicate that dissociative symptoms do occur in bulimic patients, but at a lower rate compared to the women victims of abuse in our study. Further, histories of childhood sexual abuse do occur in 10% of bulimic patients, but this is no more than one would expect in a general psychiatric population. The relationship of eating disorders, dissociative disorders, and sexual abuse deserves further research.

The high incidence of symptoms of posttraumatic stress and dissociation experienced by the study group is in agreement with conclusions from previous reports that incest (Gelinas 1983), dissociative disorders (Kluft 1985), and PTSD (Arnold 1985) are underdiagnosed. Such findings highlight the need for more thorough questioning of patients regarding histories of abuse or trauma. The routine history and mental status examination should also contain questions about symptoms of dissociative disorders and PTSD, especially if a history of abuse or trauma is uncovered. As Gelinas suggested, if attention is not paid to these matters and incest is left hidden, then its negative effects are not recognized and made accessible to treatment. At the women's clinic, routine use of our questionnaire is now made to assess the incidence of abuse and symptoms of posttraumatic stress and dissociation in newly admitted patients. Hopefully, early recognition of dissociative disorders and PTSD will result in lessened morbidity.

From our data it appears that at least 10 patients (22%) from the study group had enough symptoms to fulfill the criteria for PTSD and an additional four patients (9%) had symptoms strongly suggestive of MPD. In fact, two of these latter patients had already been diagnosed as having MPD in previous psychiatric evaluations. We are rather cautious about making such conclusions about diagnosis because, with the exception of the two patients with previously diagnosed MPD and the patients presented in our case histories, most of the others had not had the benefit of a psychiatric evaluation to confirm their diagnoses. In addition, since some symptoms of PTSD overlap with those of depression, we may be overestimating the incidence of PTSD.

This study has several shortcomings. It would have been preferable to have clinically examined all of the patients in the Julian Center study group, but this was not attempted due to time constraints on the authors and the possible reluctance of this population to be studied with full psychiatric evaluations. Our study instrument, the questionnaire, deserves comment also. As of yet, it remains unvalidated. Another shortcoming is that it cannot differentiate between symptoms of depression and symptoms of PTSD. This must still be done on clinical grounds. A final shortcoming is that histories of abuse often cannot be picked up early in the course of evaluation and treatment of patients with significant dissociation because they cannot be remembered yet. Thus we may have underestimated the extent of abuse in both study and control groups. Future studies with similar problems should address these needs.

Further study is required to assess the extent of symptoms of posttraumatic stress and dissociation across different psychiatric populations. Our assessment instrument needs to be refined and validated. Other easily administered assessment instruments to screen both for PTSD (Keane et al. 1984) and dissociation (Bernstein and Putnam 1986) have now been developed. Eventually an MMPI subscale may be developed to assess dissociation just as one has been devised to assess PTSD. Finally, we hope that the Structured Clinical Interview for the DSM-III will be revised to include a section on the dissociative disorders, just as it now contains a section on PTSD (Spitzer and Williams, unpublished manuscript, 1983). At the present time, work is proceeding on a structured clinical interview for DSM-III-R (American Psychiatric Association 1987) dissociative disorders (Steinberg 1990). Such work will ensure more accurate diagnosis of MPD and PTSD in the future.

SUMMARY

To assess the symptoms of posttraumatic stress and dissociation, a questionnaire was administered to a group of 46 women attending a women's clinic and a control group of 20 female bulimic outpatients. Although the demography of both groups was quite similar, the patients from the women's clinic suffered from a significantly higher incidence of traumatization than did the bulimic patients in the control group. Such trauma included child abuse, rape, and wife battery. The incidence of dissociative and posttraumatic symptoms was significantly higher in the study group, although the control group also experienced low levels of both types of symptoms. The high incidence of dissociative and posttraumatic symptomatology in groups of individuals who have experienced child abuse, rape, or wife battery suggests that special attention is required to avoid the underdiagnosis of both PTSD and the dissociative disorders.

REFERENCES

American Psychiatric Association: Diagnostic and Statistical Manual of Mental Disorders, 3rd Edition. Washington, DC, American Psychiatric Association, 1980

American Psychiatric Association: Diagnostic and Statistical Manual of Mental Disorders, 3rd Edition, Revised. Washington, DC, American Psychiatric Association, 1987

Arnold AL: Diagnosis of posttraumatic stress disorder in Vietnam veterans, in The Trauma of War: Stress and Recovery in Vietnam Veterans. Edited by Sonnenberg SM, Blank AS, Talbott JA. Washington, DC, American Psychiatric Press, 1985, pp 99–123

Beck JC, van der Kolk B: Reports of childhood incest and current behavior of chronically hospitalized women. Am J Psychiatry 144:1472–1476, 1987

Becker JV, Skinner LJ, Abel GG, et al: Depressive symptoms associated with sexual assault. J Sex Marital Ther 10:185–192, 1984

Bernstein MA, Putnam FW: Development, reliability, and validity of a dissociation scale. J Nerv Ment Dis 174:727–735, 1986

Bliss EL: A symptom profile of patients with multiple personality disorder, including MMPI results. J Nerv Ment Dis 172:197–202, 1984

Bliss EL, Jeppsen EA: Prevalence of multiple personality among inpatients and outpatients. Am J Psychiatry 142:250–251, 1985

Blumberg ML: Depression in abused and neglected children. Am J Psychother 35:342–355, 1981

Boulanger G: Posttraumatic stress disorder: an old problem with a new name, in The Trauma of War: Stress and Recovery in Vietnam Veterans. Edited by Sonnenberg SM, Blank AS, Talbott JA. Washington, DC, American Psychiatric Press, 1985, pp 13–29

Bryer JB, Nelson BA, Miller JB, et al: Childhood physical and sexual abuse as factors in adult psychiatric illness. Am J Psychiatry 144:1426–1430, 1987

Burgess AW, Holstrom LL: Rape trauma syndrome. Am J Psychiatry 131:981–986, 1974

Carmen EH, Risher PP, Mills T: Victims of violence and psychiatric illness. Am J Psychiatry 141:378–383, 1984

Coons PM: Multiple personality: diagnostic considerations. J Clin Psychiatry 41:330–336, 1980

Coons PM: The differential diagnosis of mutiple personality: a comprehensive review. Psychiatr Clin North Am 7:51–67, 1984

Coons PM: The prevalence of multiple personality disorder. Newsletter of the International Society for the Study of Multiple Personality and Dissociation 4:6–8, 1986

Coons PM, Milstein V: Rape and posttraumatic stress in multiple personality. Psychol Rep 55:839–845, 1984

Coons PM, Milstein V: Psychosexual disturbances in multiple personality: characteristics, etiology, and treatment. J Clin Psychiatry 47:106–110, 1986

Donaldson MA, Gardner R: Diagnosis and treatment of traumatic stress among women after childhood incest, in Trauma and Its Wake: The Study and Treatment of Posttraumatic Stress Disorder. Edited by Figley CR. New York, Brunner/Mazel, 1985, pp 356–377

Emslie GJ, Rosenfeld A: Incest reported by children and adolescents hospitalized for severe psychiatric problems. Am J Psychiatry 140:708–711, 1983

Eth S, Pynoos RS (eds): Post-Traumatic Stress Disorder in Children. Washington, DC, American Psychiatric Press, 1985

Federal Bureau of Investigation: Uniform Crime Reports for the United States. Washington, DC, U.S. Government Printing Office, 1982

Finn SE, Hartman M, Leon GR, et al: Eating disorders and sexual abuse: lack of confirmation for a clinical hypothesis. International Journal of Eating Disorders 51:1051–1060, 1986

Finkelhor D: Sexually Victimized Children. New York, Free Press, 1979

Frank E, Anderson BP: Psychiatric disorders in rape victims: past history and current symptomatology. Compr Psychiatry 28:77–82, 1987

French O: The prevalence of multiple personality disorder, in Proceedings of the First International Conference on Multiple Personality/Dissociative States. Edited by Braun BG. Chicago, IL, Rush-Presbyterian-St. Luke's Medical Center, 1984, p 97

Gelinas D: The persisting negative effects of incest. Psychiatry 46:312–332, 1983

Goodstein RK, Page AW: Battered wife syndrome: overview of dynamics and treatment. Am J Psychiatry 138:1036–1044, 1981

Goodwin J: Incest victims exhibit posttraumatic stress disorder symptoms. Clinical Psychiatry News 12:13, 1984

Goodwin J, Attias R, McCarty T, et al: Routine questions about childhood sexual abuse in psychiatry inpatients. Am J Psychiatry 145:1183, 1988

Greaves GB: Multiple personality 165 years after Mary Reynolds. J Nerv Ment Dis 168:577–597, 1980

Hathaway SR, McKinley JL: Minnesota Multiphasic Personality Inventory (revised edition). New York, Psychological Corporation, 1967

Herman JL: Histories of violence in an outpatient population. Am J Psychiatry 65:137–141, 1986

Hilberman E: The Rape Victim. New York, Basic Books, 1976

Horowitz MJ: Stress-response syndrome: a review of posttraumatic stress and adjustment disorders. Hosp Community Psychiatry 37:241–249, 1986

Hudson JI, Leffer PS, Pope HG: Bulimia related to affective disorder by family history and response to the dexamethasone suppression test. Am J Psychiatry 139:685–687, 1982

Husain A, Chapel JL: History of incest in girls admitted to a psychiatric hospital. Am J Psychiatry 140:591–593, 1983

Jacobson A, Richardson B: Assault experiences of 100 psychiatric inpatients: evidence of the need for routine inquiry. Am J Psychiatry 144:508–513, 1987

Jacobson A, Koehler JE, Jones-Brown C: The failure of routine assessment to detect histories of assault experienced by psychiatric patients. Hosp Community Psychiatry 38:386–389, 1987

Johnson CL, Stuckey MK: Bulimia: a descriptive survey of 316 cases. International Journal of Eating Disorders 2:3–16, 1982

Katz S, Mazur MA: Understanding the Rape Victim: A Synthesis of Research Findings. New York, John Wiley, 1979

Keane TM, Malloy PF, Fairbank JA: Empirical development of an MMPI subscale for the assessment of combat-related posttraumatic stress disorder. J Consult Clin Psychol 52:888–891, 1984

Kilpatrick DG, Veronen LJ: Treatment of fear and anxiety in victims of rape (Final report NIMH grant no HMH29602). Rockville, MD, National Institute of Mental Health, 1984

Kilpatrick DG, Veronen LJ, Best CL: Factors predicting psychological distress among rape victims, in Trauma and Its Wake: The Study and Treatment of Posttraumatic Stress Disorder. Edited by Figley CR. New York, Brunner/Mazel, 1985, pp 113–141

Kluft RP: Making the diagnosis of multiple personality disorder (MPD). Directions in Psychiatry 5:1–10, 1985

Levinger G: Sources of marital dissatisfaction among applicants for divorce. Am J Orthopsychiatry 36:803–807, 1966

Lukianowicz N: Incest. Br J Psychiatry 120:301–313, 1972

Machover K: Personality Projection in the Drawing of the Human Figure. Springfield, IL, 1949

Pettinati HM, Horne RL, Staats JM: Hypnotizability in patients with anorexia nervosa and bulimia. Arch Gen Psychiatry 42:1014–1016, 1985

Putnam FW: Dissociation as a response to extreme trauma, in Childhood Antecedents of Multiple Personality. Edited by Kluft RP. Washington, DC, American Psychiatric Press, 1985, pp 65–97

Putnam FW, Guroff JJ, Silberman SK, et al: The clinical phenomenology of multiple personality disorder: a review of 100 recent cases. J Clin Psychiatry 47:285–293, 1986

Pyle RL, Mitchell JE, Eckert ED: Bulimia: a report of 34 cases. J Clin Psychiatry 42:60–64, 1981

Rosenfeld AA: Incidence of a history of incest among 18 female psychiatric patients. Am J Psychiatry 136:791–795, 1979

Rounsaville B, Weissman MM: Battered women: a medical problem requiring detection. Int J Psychiatry Med 8:191–202, 1977–1978

Russell DEH: The Secret Trauma: Incest in the Lives of Girls and Women. New York, Basic Books, 1986

Saltman V, Solomon RS: Incest and multiple personality. Psychol Rep 50:1127–1141, 1982

Sansonnet-Hayden H, Haley G, Marriage G, et al: Sexual abuse and psychopathology in hospitalized adolescents. J Am Acad Child Adolesc Psychiatry 26:753–757, 1987

Sloan G, Leichner P: Is there a relationship between sexual abuse or incest and eating disorders? Can J Psychiatry 31:656–660, 1986

Stark E, Flitcraft A, Frazier W: Medicine and patriarchal violence: the social construction of a private event. Int J Health Serv 9:461–493, 1979

Steinberg M, Rounsaville B, Cicchetti D: The Structured Clinical Interview for DSM-III-R dissociative disorders: preliminary report on a new diagnostic instrument. Am J Psychiatry 147:76–82, 1990

Straus MA: Wife beating: how common and why? Victimology 2:443–458, 1978

Torem M: Dissociative states presenting as an eating disorder. Am J Clin Hypn 29:137–142, 1986

Tsai M, Wagner WN: Therapy groups for women sexually molested as children. Arch Sex Behav 7:417–427, 1978

APPENDIX: QUESTIONNAIRE ON SYMPTOMS OF POSTTRAUMATIC STRESS AND DISSOCIATION

1. Age _____ years

2. Sex   (Check one)
   - A. Male   ( )
   - B. Female   ( )

3. Marital status   (Check one)
   - A. Never married   ( )
   - B. Married   ( )
   - C. Separated   ( )
   - D. Divorced   ( )
   - E. Widowed   ( )
   - F. Remarried   ( )

4. Educational level   (Check one)
   - A. Less than 6 grades ( )
   - B. Completed 6th grade ( )
   - C. Completed 9th grade ( )
   - D. High school diploma ( )
   - E. College diploma   ( )
   - F. Masters degree   ( )
   - G. Doctoral degree   ( )
   - H. Postdoctoral degree ( )

5. Race   (Check one)
   - A. White   ( )
   - B. Black   ( )
   - C. American Indian   ( )
   - D. Hispanic   ( )
   - E. Oriental   ( )
   - F. Other _____ ( )

6. Occupation   (Check one)
   - A. Professional   ( )
   - B. Managerial   ( )
   - C. Skilled   ( )
   - D. Semiskilled   ( )
   - E. Unskilled   ( )
   - F. Unemployed   ( )
   - G. Homemaker   ( )
   - H. Student   ( )

7. I have experienced the following types of abuse or trauma (Check any that apply)
   - A. Child abuse
     1. Physical   ( )

    2. Sexual ( )
    3. Emotional ( )
    4. Neglect ( )
  B. Severe accident ( )
  C. Natural disaster ( )
  D. Wife abuse ( )
  E. Rape ( )
  F. War related ( )
  G. Hostage ( )
  H. Other _____ ( )

8. I have been previously diagnosed as having the following (Check any that apply)
  A. Depression ( )
  B. Anxiety ( )
  C. Phobia ( )
  D. Posttraumatic stress ( )
  E. Anorexia nervosa ( )
  F. Bulimia ( )
  G. Obesity ( )
  H. Schizophrenia ( )
  I. Mania ( )
  J. Multiple personality ( )
  K. Amnesia ( )
  L. Epilepsy ( )
  M. Alcohol abuse ( )
  N. Drug abuse ( )
  O. Concussion ( )
  P. Senility ( )
  Q. Other _____ ( )

9. I suffer from the following problems or symptoms (Check any that apply)
  1. Unwanted or intrusive thoughts about abuse or trauma ( )
  2. Unfamiliar people seem to know me ( )
  3. I have been told that I do things I don't remember ( )
  4. Bad dreams or nightmares about abuse or trauma ( )
  5. I can't recall doing or saying things others tell me about ( )
  6. Often it seem as if I'm in a dream or a fog ( )
  7. I have flashbacks of previous abuse or trauma ( )
  8. I can't stop myself from doing things ( )

9. Certain events remind me of abuse or
   trauma   ( )
10. Sometimes I find myself in strange places
    at some distance from where I live or work   ( )
11. Sometimes I feel controlled by some force   ( )
12. I try to avoid thoughts or feelings which
    remind me of the abuse or trauma   ( )
13. I hear voices inside my head   ( )
14. I feel like I'm split into different parts   ( )
15. I avoid activities which remind me of abuse
    or trauma   ( )
16. Blank spells   ( )
17. I experience sudden and unexpected mood
    changes   ( )
18. I can't remember some abuse or trauma   ( )
19. People call me by unfamiliar names   ( )
20. I do things out of character for me   ( )
21. Loss of interest in formerly pleasurable
    activities   ( )
22. I find things which I don't remember
    purchasing   ( )
23. My memory for some things is much bet-
    ter than for most people   ( )
24. I have feelings of detachment   ( )
25. I have trouble with memory even when
    I'm not drinking or using drugs/medica-
    tion   ( )
26. I have difficulty trusting others   ( )
27. I feel numb or unable to express feelings   ( )
28. I feel outside my body watching myself
    do things   ( )
29. I blame myself for bad things which have
    happened to me   ( )
30. I have difficulty sleeping   ( )
31. I have recurrent fantasies which seem
    real   ( )
32. I try to forget or ignore trauma or abuse   ( )
33. I have unexplained irritability or out-
    bursts of anger   ( )
34. I was often accused of lying but don't
    remember lying   ( )
35. I often feel like I want to run away or
    escape   ( )
36. I have decreased concentration   ( )

37. People or objects around me often seem
    unreal   ( )
38. I have the uncanny ability to predict the
    future   ( )
39. I am always on guard or fearful that harm
    will occur   ( )
40. I can often ignore pain   ( )
41. Sometimes parts of my body seem strange
    or like they don't belong   ( )
42. I am easily startled   ( )
43. I have found drawings or writing which
    I don't remember doing   ( )
44. I am unable to talk about traumatic events   ( )
45. I can't remember events in grade school
    or childhood   ( )

CHAPTER 11

Dissociative Disorders as Sequelae to Incest

Bennett G. Braun, M.D.

Multiple personality disorder (MPD) is one of the incest-related syndromes of adult dissociative psychopathology, but the causative relationship may lie with a constellation of child abuse rather than with incest per se (Braun 1987). While incest may be involved in child abuse that underlies 96% to 98% of MPD cases, the more important factor may be that the abuse is administered unpredictably by an adult who is a nurturing relative at other times. The severity of dissociation and MPD is more directly related to abuse that is administered by parents or other family members who are also able to give the child love and protection. The child with an inborn ability to dissociate is likely to respond to abuse by dissociating, setting the stage for subsequent dissociations if the abuse is perpetuated. The 3-P model of Braun and Sachs (1985) predicts that the MPD victim must have the biopsychological predisposition to dissociate defensively, that there must be a precipitating traumatic event that triggers dissociation, and that perpetuating traumas chain the dissociations affectively. In diagnosis and treatment of MPD, the alert therapist will focus not only on clues that point toward incest, but will suspect the possibility that incest may be a clue to a more extensive constellation of child abuse.

Adult-child incest is not understood or defined in any human culture as an expression of love. The adult who performs a sexual act with son, daughter, niece, nephew, etc., commits a form of child abuse, whether or not coercive physical violence is used (Braun 1989b). Unfortunately for the child victim, the abusing adult may be a "nurturing" relative at other times, and the child must deal psychodynamically with unpredictable infliction of abuse versus expression of love. When the state of affairs is overwhelming, psychic defenses must be erected. For those with biopsychological capacity to dissociate, the defenses are erected at a cost for which the victim may later pay in some form of adult dissociative psychopathology.

To dissociate is to sever the association of one thing from another. In psychiatry, dissociation is a defensive process that can intercede between affective states and/or thoughts to separate them from the mainstream of consciousness; between parts of behavioral chains; or between affects, behaviors, and/or thoughts. Dissociation may affect or distort the input level of perception (Braun 1984, 1985a, 1988a).

In abused persons with an inborn biopsychological capacity to dissociate, the predominant psychological/behavioral defense may be dissociation used as a fragmentation or compartmentalization process. The "price" paid for the use of this defense in later life may be MPD, dissociative disorder not otherwise specified (NOS), and related dissociative psychopathology. The prevalence of posttraumatic stress disorder (PTSD) among child-abuse victims may strengthen arguments to include PTSD among the dissociative disorders (Braun 1988a).

MPD is, in fact, one of the major sequelae of severe child abuse. Five major studies totaling over 1,000 patients have made the etiologic relationship clear: in patients with MPD, child abuse was found to be an etiologic factor in 98% (Schultz et al. 1989), 97.4% (Schultz et al. 1986), 97% (Putnam et al. 1986), 96% (Braun 1984), and 95.2% (Braun and Gray 1986). These five studies also indicated that more than 80% of patients had suffered sexual abuse. Only in the Braun and Gray study, however, were any data collected as to whether the sexual abuse was incestuous. In that study, 41% of the MPD patients who were sexually abused had incestuous abuse from a father. (This is unusually low; most current work is showing 60% or more by a father.) In addition, 23% had incestuous abuse from a mother, 17% from a male sibling, and 2% from a female sibling. Many were abused by more than one family member. Braun and Gray found that 15% had been sexually abused by both father and mother (50% by either parent).

Braun and Gray (1986) found indications that more than half of all MPD patients are victims of parental incest and that 25% of the abusing adults were first-degree female relatives. In these instances, fondling was not accepted as abuse; report of oral, anal, or vaginal penetration was required to define sexual abuse adequately. No previous literature on female incest-abusers was found, and the reasons may be the same ones that kept Freud, Kinsey, and other investigators under intellectual blinders regarding the profusion of incest: we just do not want to accept the fact that mothers (women) can be sexual abusers.

Although MPD and dissociation are being emphasized in this chapter, most of the dissociative disorders have been associated with incest. The only exception I know of is fugue. I have not seen a case nor do I know of a case where incest played a role in the creation of a fugue state, although it certainly would be a logical outcome.

So as not to burden the student of this area with repetition, I have limited this chapter to cases of MPD. Cases of PTSD, psychogenic amnesia, and dissociative disorder NOS are published elsewhere (Braun 1989b). Depersonalization related to incest and/or incest rape (especially) is most often reported in these patients when they are being treated for major depressive disorder (recurrent), which is common in victims of incest.

Identification of incest as one form of child abuse leaves open the question of whether incest-abuse predisposes toward dissociative disorders in a manner different from other forms of abuse. Seven types of child abuse contributing to MPD and dissociation may be identified, although the types are usually mixed (e.g., collateral physical, sexual, and psychological abuse): 1) severe neglect, physical and psychological; 2) physical abuse, often by family members; 3) sexual and physical abuse, not incestuous; 4) sexual abuse, incestuous; 5) physical abuse and presumed sexual abuse; 6) sexual abuse, pornography, incest; and 7) ritual, satanic abuse, family members often involved.

Experience indicates that the more severe and/or ritualistic the abuse suffered as a child, the more fragmented is the adult patient's personality and thinking. Victims of satanic abuse are likely to exhibit polyfragmented atypical dissociative disorder (ADD) (dissociative disorder NOS) or polyfragmented MPD. Some victims of incest may not exhibit any exaggerated or special dissociative psychopathology. The discovery of incest in the history of a patient with a dissociative disorder, however, should be taken as an indicator that "something worse" *may* have happened to account for the psychopathology. Case histories presented later in this chapter will illustrate the point. First, however, the phenomenology of MPD is summarized as a paradigm of dissociative pathology, with special emphasis on the etiologic relationship of child abuse and dissociative disorders.

MULTIPLE PERSONALITY DISORDER

MPD is a dissociative disorder characterized by the disruption of memory and identity. The ability to dissociate appears to be a necessary but not sufficient predisposing factor in MPD. The fact that the person "predisposed" to MPD is also usually highly hypnotizable and often artistically creative appears to provide support for the hypothesis that "ability to dissociate" is important in the pathogenesis of MPD.

Braun (1980, 1984) described MPD as the demonstration in one person of two or more personalities, each of whom possesses identifiably distinctive, consistently ongoing characteristics and a relatively separate memory of individual life history. Executive control of the body is transferred from one personality to another, but the total individual is never out of touch with reality. Some or all of the personalities frequently experience periods of amnesia, time loss, or blackouts.

Amnesia for thoughts or actions of other personalities often occurs for the host personality (Braun 1986a), the one that has executive control of the body the greatest percentage of the time during a given time period.

Braun (1985a, 1988a) proposed dissociative disorders as a continuum, placing automatism and hypnosis at one end and MPD at the opposite end. Braun (1988a) suggested that the complex phenomenon of dissociation can be conceptualized by a model in which behavior, affect, sensation, and knowledge (B-A-S-K) function along a time line. In the BASK model, hypnosis induced to create an anesthesia is seen as dissociation in affect and sensation, and MPD as dissociation in all four BASK elements.

The ability to dissociate is necessary for "splitting," the creation of a separate personality or fragment. A split-off personality has a full range of consistent and ongoing response patterns, whereas a fragment may exist only for limited, special purposes (Braun 1986a). Special-purpose fragments make up the bulk of the large numbers of "personalities" exhibited in some dramatic, highly publicized MPD patients; no more than 2 to 10 full personalities may exist in such patients.

The 3-P Model of Multiple Personality Disorder

Two predisposing factors appear to be necessary to the development of MPD: 1) biopsychological capacity to dissociate, usually identified with high responsiveness to hypnosis; and 2) repeated exposure to an inconsistently stressful environment (e.g., receiving love and abuse from the same person or persons at unpredictable times, as one might find in an abusive family environment). Both predisposing factors are necessary for MPD to develop. Neither is sufficient.

The 3-P model of MPD (Braun and Sachs 1985) (Figure 11-1) hypothesizes that predisposing, precipitating, and perpetuating factors are all necessary, and together are sufficient for the development of MPD.

The precipitating event in the 3-P model is almost always a specific overwhelming traumatic episode to which the potential MPD patient responds by dissociating. If such events are not common in the environment of a person with dissociative capacity, the result may be a discrete dissociative episode (e.g., fugue). Many persons who have had dissociative episodes in response to great trauma did not develop MPD.

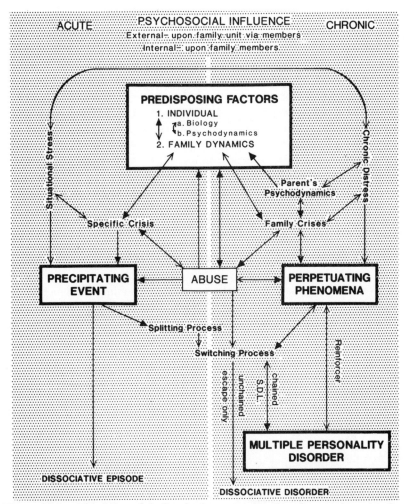

Figure 11-1. The 3-P model of multiple personality disorder: predisposing factors, precipitating events, and perpetuating phenomena. *Solid arrowheads* indicate a greater degree of influence than do *open arrowheads*. Reprinted from Kluft R: Childhood Antecedents of Multiple Personality. Washington, DC, American Psychiatric Press, 1985, p. 53, with permission from American Psychiatric Press.

The final necessary condition is the impact of perpetuating phenomena, which results in a linkage of the dissociative episodes by a common affective theme and/or neurophysiologic state (Braun 1984). The perpetuating phenomena associated with development of MPD are interactive behaviors, usually between the abuser(s) and abused. They result in separated memories for each dissociative episode, which the patient ultimately links together by common affective themes (state-dependent learning).

After continuous exposure to situations that are inconsistently abusive, the patient begins to experience unique life histories associated with each "file" of separate memories. Continued unpredictable trauma reinforces the chaining of memories and associated response patterns, and gradually the different adaptive response patterns become functionally separated by amnestic barriers. Thus the patient's personality is "split." The patient may suspect but not be aware of the extent to which he or she exhibits inconsistent behavior as personalities A, B, C, and so on function with individual life histories. An amnestic barrier more or less prevents each personality from knowing fully about the lives led by the others.

Incest and Incest/Rape in MPD

Does the incest and incest/rape victim with MPD or other dissociative disorder present uniquely different diagnostic and management problems for his or her therapist? When the question is examined in selected case histories, the answer appears to be that incest is associated with MPD and other dissociative psychopathology because incest is part of a diathesis of abuse.

Case Histories

Case 1: Severe Neglect and Psychological Abuse. RP is a middle-aged, married, white female referred to me by the psychiatrist whom she had originally consulted, at the age of 48, for the treatment of agoraphobia. This problem developed acutely after she had been treated with hypnosis for smoking. Over time, the original psychiatrist came to suspect that the patient suffered MPD because she frequently referred to "other parts" of herself. I confirmed the diagnosis of MPD 6 years after the patient first sought treatment.

RP had no signs or symptoms of organic disease. She had no history of serious physical illness. She was the mother of four adult children and had several grandchildren. Her husband of 25 years was very supportive of RP's therapy; he is a member of a positive and nurturing family. Except for times when he was away on business trips, Mr. RP drove his wife to therapy sessions. He waited for her during the early phase of therapy, when she was agoraphobic and most needed his support.

RP is one of three sisters who underwent similar experiences of neglect and psychological abuse. RP has documented MPD. Her older (4 years) sister, also seen by me at the recommendation of RP, has been diagnosed as suffering from ADD with features of MPD (now called dissociative disorder NOS), and recurrent major depressive disorder. The oldest sister occasionally suffers from depression; she is a neurotic, manipulative woman with excessive convictions of entitlement, but no history of dissociation. All three sisters are fully functional socially; the youngest two are married to successful businessmen and the oldest sister's husband is retired.

In the case of RP, at least, it is known from standard tests that she is highly hypnotizable and, therefore, has a biopsychological capacity to dissociate. Thus she demonstrates the primary predisposing factor for development of MPD.

There is a clearly defined precipitating factor in the family history. When RP was 7 years old, her mother, then 48 years of age, suddenly and unexpectedly died of pneumonia. Three days earlier, although suffering from a cold, RP's mother had taken the little girl into town on a trolley car to buy her a dress for her first Holy Communion. The following day, the mother was too ill to attend the Communion ceremony. Two days after that, the mother was dead. RP learned of her mother's death when she came home from school to eat lunch and saw her mother's body carried out of the house.

Family reaction to the death was chaotic and hysterical. RP was ignored or even "pushed aside"; she distanced herself and dissociated the death and ensuing events. Her personality split, and while one part denied her mother's death, another part went to the funeral and feared being pulled into the grave by her mother.

Perpetuating factors also were clearly present in this patient's family history (i.e., factors that began, repetitively, to chain dissociative episodes with common affective themes). RP's father, who could not accept his wife's death, began to drink heavily. He subsequently became a chronic alcoholic. He was otherwise a caring man, and RP loved him, but his severe alcoholism and a physical injury, both of which required repeated hospitalizations, made him more and more inaccessible. During the same period after their mother's death, the three sisters were sent to live with a paternal aunt and uncle. There, the girls were ostracized as unwanted outsiders and were psychologically and literally abandoned. Their father appeared occasionally, often heavily intoxicated, and was never able to give emotional support.

The 3rd major split in RP's personality was at age 13 when a newly created personality "killed" the father by denying that she knew who her father had been. In later school and social environments, other personalities were created to compartmentalize anger, loneliness, and sadness. One of the personalities dated and eventually married and remained basically compartmentalized until she underwent hypnotic treatment for smoking cessation.

RPs MPD reexpressed itself when she was 48 years old, the age of her mother's death. RP began to decompensate psychologically and exhibited

expectations of dying. Subsequent therapy discovered five full personalities and 20 fragments or special-purpose fragments in RP's constellation.
RP never exhibited any self-mutilative or suicidal behaviors. She has
achieved full integration but remains in follow-up and supportive therapy.

Case 2: Physical Abuse by Family, Sexual Abuse by Strangers. Miss KM
is a 47-year-old, single, black female who has been in some form of
psychotherapy most of her adult life. She was diagnosed as suffering from
MPD about 6 years ago, after 15 years in the mental health system. Until
MPD was recognized, Miss KM and her constellation of personalities was
usually diagnosed as bipolar. She always has been fully functional in
society; in appearance, she is an often striking woman who frequently
dressed with a high sense of style.

Miss KM is an insulin-dependent diabetic. It is now recognized that
some of her personalities exhibit singular metabolic as well as psychological characteristics; these include variable responses to insulin and change-
able blood pressure, which have caused her to be hospitalized occasionally.

She is highly hypnotizable. Although at this point her personal and
family history do not reveal when the first split in personality occurred
(definitely by age 4½), given the presence of dissociation as a predisposing
factor, there are an abundance of precipitating and perpetuating factors
in the history. Miss KM was abandoned by her father in infancy and was
raised by her mother and maternal grandmother. Both women manifest
signs and symptoms of MPD. Both also raised Miss KM in an emotionally
equivocal environment of love, fundamentalist religious piety, and physical abuse. Mother and grandmother beat the child with sticks, rods, and
a doubled electrical cord to enforce their religiously colored mandate of
"goodness." However, both women also had men friends who dropped
in from time to time to have sexual intercourse, sometimes in view of the
child. The religiously fanatic grandmother demanded "goodness" from
Miss KM but also instructed the child to "sit on it, Honey, because it
will sell when corn and cotton won't."

Sexual encounters were present in Miss KM's childhood. At the age
of 4 years, she was sexually assaulted by a male stranger and forced to
perform fellatio. Throughout her early childhood, she slept in the same
room with several male cousins; no sexual experiences are recalled. Miss
KM had several personalities with male-protector characteristics. In later
childhood, Miss KM's mother married a very supportive man with whom
Miss KM had a loving father-daughter relationship. In high school, she
had what was probably her first love relationship with a male, a fellow
student. The boy was killed by an automobile one evening while he was
bicycling to her home to visit her. Twice during her adult life she was
raped at gunpoint by male strangers, during which she split off fragments

to cope. These were easily integrated after processing the incidents therapeutically.

In psychotherapy, Miss KM was found to have 10 personalities plus a dozen fragments or special-purpose fragments. Most of the personalities represented different ages or stages of life (from childhood through adolescence to adulthood), or forms of protection. Several of the personalities and fragments were organized around Miss KM's use of sex to act out and to gain advantage over men. When a love affair with a professional athlete proved unsatisfactory to "prim" Miss KM, another personality had serial intercourse with the boyfriend's entire team.

Miss KM never married but has, as a single parent, adopted a daughter. On one occasion, Miss KM requested hospitalization because she feared that she had or would beat her daughter with a belt as a punishment. Over her years of treatment, she has fled from therapy several times. During one period when she appeared near integration, her insulin requirements began to fluctuate dangerously; she was hospitalized medically, and psychotherapy was temporarily suspended. At another time after a major integration, her insulin requirement decreased dramatically, from 100+ units (50 NPH and 40–60 regular, sliding scale) to 25 units of NPH. During the course of therapy, Miss KM has not made any suicide attempts, reported any suicidal behavior, or exhibited any evidence of self-mutilation. She appears calmer, near final integration, with only two personalities remaining, and has been able to be controlled on oral hypoglycemic agents alone despite her weight remaining approximately the same.

Case 3: Sexual and Physical Abuse, Not Known To Be Incestuous. Mrs. BD is a 33-year-old white woman, married for 14 years to an alcoholic man. At times he became physically abusive. Her husband is a therapist in a state psychiatric hospital. They have no children, by their mutual decision. She works for a small newspaper as a graphic artist.

Mrs. BD has currently been in psychotherapy for 18 months, but first saw her psychotherapist 24 months earlier when her husband induced her to seek marital counseling. The first visit was unsatisfactory because she felt coerced into it by her husband. Six months later, she returned for individual therapy, citing her unhappy marriage, a volatile lesbian affair, problems with a verbally abusive male employer, and suicidal feelings. She has been chronically suicidal since entering therapy, and occasionally claims she has homicidal feelings directed at her boss. Destructive feelings have been managed by frequent telephone contacts with her psychotherapist and by frequently renewed contracts to do no harm to herself or to others (Braun 1986b). Financial restrictions limit the intensity of her psychotherapy.

Multiple "parts" were acknowledged by Mrs. BD early in her therapy;

MPD was confirmed after various personalities and fragments were identified in later sessions. One of the parts is known to have existed prior to
adolescence. Very little of Mrs. BD's early life history has been recovered
in detail for several reasons: her limited access to psychotherapy, her
suicidal and homicidal urges, and the consequent inability to deal psychodynamically with memories and trauma. It is known that both of her
parents are living and healthy and that Mrs. BD has two older brothers,
one of whom is homosexual. There are partially recovered memories of
concurrent sexual abuse. At age 4 years a "grandfatherly" neighbor sexually abused her, then warned her not to tell anyone of the incident. At
age 5 she escaped a repeat of the abuse, but saw and heard her close
friend, a 5-year-old boy, being sexually abused. Between the ages of 10
and 12 years, she was sexually abused regularly by another male authority
figure, her pediatrician, who also warned her not to tell. At age 18 she
was the victim of a "date rape," after which she began to abuse drugs
and alcohol seriously. She used chemical dissociation daily from ages 18
to 22, and often thereafter.

Easily hypnotizable in therapy, Mrs. BD has demonstrated the ability
to dissociate as a predisposing factor. Sexual abuse in childhood by male
authority figures may be identified as a precipitating factor. Sex with the
pediatrician, date rape at age 18, increased dependence on chemical
dissociation to control anxiety, and continuing problems with abusive
males have probably been perpetuating factors for MPD. Mrs. BD has
no serious organic illness. Her medical problems are panic disorder,
nicotine dependence, polysubstance abuse, and premenstrual syndrome.

She has a history of physical abuse from her husband when both of
them are drinking. She may also precipitate his violence.

There are documented incidents of violence initiated by Mrs. BD in
early adulthood. Several years ago, Mrs. BD threw a female co-worker
against a wall when she believed the woman was taking advantage of her.
Earlier, as a young adult in college, while under the influence of alcohol,
she tried to strangle a classmate who also was her lesbian lover, then
made two apparent suicide attempts. At that time she was in a college
counseling program, withdrawing "cold turkey" from abuse of mescaline,
marijuana, THC (tetrahydrocannabinol), LSD (lysergic acid diethylam-
ide), and other drugs.

Six personalities or fragments have been identified. Although it is not
certain that it was the first split, one part is known to have been created
in response to the abuse of her friend, which occurred when Mrs. BD
was 5 years old. Two other parts are impulsive and sexually promiscuous
and abuse drugs and alcohol. One of these has been identified as being
responsible for the attack on Mrs. BD's lesbian lover in college.

In addition, a part known as "artist" is responsible for maintaining Mrs.
BD's professional life. All six of the parts that have so far been identified
are able to "meet" at a table set with seven chairs. The owner of the

seventh chair has not been identified. Mrs. BD is at a fairly early stage in psychotherapy, and I expect that there are several fragments yet to be uncovered. Mrs. BD has attempted suicide on two occasions earlier in treatment and has reported a few periods of suicidal ideation. Although she has abused alcohol and other substances, she has not mutilated herself in any way during her current psychotherapy.

Case 4: Sexual Abuse: Incestuous, Nonviolent. Miss HT is a 35-year-old, single, white female hypnotic virtuoso who entered psychotherapy for treatment of obesity. She fled therapy when frightening material began to emerge, but returned after experiencing a dream of being stabbed by two naked women. After her return, psychotherapy eventually led to a diagnosis of MPD. Miss HT has had three bouts of very severe suicidal ideation, one prior to beginning therapy and two for which she required hospitalization. She has experienced intermittent suicidal ideation, but no self-mutilatory behaviors. Miss HT has been in therapy for several years and appears to be near a final stable integration. In fact, as of this writing she has been fully integrated for 7 months, during which she has suffered no dissociative episodes. She is becoming much more functional socially. Although she is an excellent, accurate typist, she had had difficulty with the social skills needed to hold a job. She is currently working as an executive secretary.

As an only child, Miss HT was coerced into performing fellatio on her father from approximately the age of 2 years to about age 3. When she was 3 years old, he ejaculated into her mouth; this apparently frightened him and he abruptly ended the fellatio. It was never repeated, and he refused to demonstrate any physical affection for her from that time on. Miss HT had enjoyed the close, loving relationship with her "perfect" father, who also was later used as the model for her "perfect lover." She could not understand why her relationship with her father had ended. It appears possible that Miss HT's mother had discovered the sexual relationship, but did not intervene. Miss HT's mother also suffered MPD (observed by me), and her father, by history, may also have had the condition.

The father became very distant emotionally. He would talk to Miss HT, but would not touch her. When she was 9 years old, her father and mother began to have serious family fights. Miss HT began to gain the weight that would eventually become gross obesity. She felt that this was done in part to keep her parents together.

Miss HT has proven to be exquisitely hypnotizable; thus the capacity to dissociate is demonstrated as a probable predisposing factor in her MPD, as is the family history of dissociation. Incest contributed to a deteriorating family dynamic, but incest per se was not the probable precipitating factor in this instance. Rather, it was rejection by her father that initiated a pattern of rejection: her father rejected her emotionally, then both of her parents were behaving inconsistently and neglected her over a period of many years of bitter fighting. Finally, when she was 27 years old, her father died and she lost the one person she felt had loved her most in her life.

Just a few years prior to the death of her father, Miss HT also experienced rejection in her first sexual relationship. Her first employer seduced her and, a month later, fired her. The rejection was made worse by the fact that she had recently moved away from her parents for the first time and was living alone.

When she was first diagnosed in therapy, Miss HT had six personalities and 14 fragments. Several of the personalities used sex to act out and to control men. Even though she was obese, Miss HT attracted men and was able to enter into sexual relationships consistently.

Integrated, Miss HT is again living with her mother, primarily for sharing expenses. Her mother has entered therapy. She and Miss HT have explored their mutual jealousy over the father's attentions. The mother has shown indications of MPD in interviews I had with her, and family history indicates MPD in her father and in her maternal grandmother.

Case 5: Physical and Sexual Abuse.   Miss CL is a single, white female in her mid-40s whose MPD psychodynamics are rooted in her history as the adopted child of abusive parents. Her life in this family may have been the major predisposing factor for developing MPD. The specific precipitating factor is not known, but there are indications that it may have been sexual abuse in infancy. Life in her family environment was a series of perpetuating factors, additionally reinforced by two incidents of sexual abuse from persons outside the nuclear family. At age 10 she was sexually fondled several times in a public pool; as a teenager she was forced to perform fellatio on an uncle. Neither of these incidents resulted in intercourse.

Miss CL is functioning in society, usually managing to control her potential for violence against others. She has urges to inflict harm even when she has not been attacked first. Nevertheless, she is highly motivated in therapy, despite a stormy course that has included several hospitalizations. The first of these hospitalizations was precipitated by the anniversary of her father's death and a vacation by her psychotherapist. The second was triggered by inappropriate behavior and abandonment by her outpatient psychotherapist, a social worker. She has been in therapy for MPD for 8 years; she was in the mental health system for 7 years prior to her diagnosis as suffering from MPD. She is a very good hypnotic subject.

Nothing is known of Miss CL's natural parents. Miss CL was available for adoption in infancy and apparently was placed with at least 10 different families over a 6-month period. During this time her records were "lost" so she could be moved to another state and be adopted by a wealthy family that already had several children.

The family had significant psychopathology. The adoptive father was alcoholic. Both parents were psychologically abusive, and the mother was physically abusive as well. Miss CL was continuously terrorized and physically abused by two adoptive brothers, of whom one is alcoholic and one bipolar. Three of her adoptive sisters were bed wetters until they were married.

Miss CL's lack of identity as a child, her chaotic early life, the abuse within her foster family, and the family's psychopathology seem to be factors that would perpetuate dissociation precipitated by the abuse. Miss CL is, in fact, polyfragmented with five principal systems of personalities and many fragments. She has been doing well in therapy, but requires large doses of medication to maintain control. Although she has exhibited no self-mutilatory behaviors and has not made any suicide attempts, on two occasions she required hospitalizations for severe suicidal ideation and once was hospitalized for obsessive homicidal ideation.

Case 6: Sexual Abuse, Pornography, Incest.   Miss MM, a single, white female, presented herself for psychiatric counseling at age 35. Her case demonstrates common findings in the background of MPD patients: that the condition is transgenerational (Braun 1985b), causally linked with child abuse, and takes the most severely fragmented forms in those persons who were most severely abused in childhood.

She had no organic disease. There are some indications that she had sought psychotherapy previously, but her excessive secrecy about herself makes such information difficult to obtain. Miss MM has never been arrested despite a long involvement in a child pornography ring operated by her family and despite her working as a prostitute for many years.

Between the ages of 1 and 12 years, Miss MM was forced by her family to take part in sadomasochistic child pornography films. On camera, her mother beat her and forced her to perform fellatio on her older brother. Her mother beat her with a whip at other times to make her submit to performing other sex acts with a variety of other children and adults and animals. She may have been forced to observe several murders that were committed during acts of sex in "snuff" movies. Off camera, she was beaten frequently and severely by her mother, father, and brother. Her brother and men associated with the pornography ring raped her a number of times.

While attending Catholic elementary school, Miss MM once told nuns about her desperate situation at home. When the nuns called Miss MM's mother to verify the story, the mother convinced them it was not true. Subsequently, she beat and choked her daughter into unconsciousness.

As a young woman, Miss MM already had a number of personalities and an even greater number of fragments. One full personality was an expensive call girl who had only wealthy, important men as clients and refused to perform any sadomasochistic or perverse sexual acts. Fragments could perform these acts, but they were otherwise only marginally able to relate to men, except in abusive situations. They were sometimes abusive to men and put themselves in situations where they would be raped and beaten. A special-purpose fragment (Braun 1986a) appeared only to perform fellatio. When this fragment was present in therapy, Miss MM's somatic memory reproduced on her body the red stripes and welts associated with the beatings inflicted by her mother during the filming of child pornography. Somatic memory is the reproduction of physical symptoms similar or identical to those experienced at a previous (often traumatic) time.

In therapy, nine full personalities and hundreds of fragments and special-purpose fragments were discovered. They were organized into seven systems of personalities and complementary fragments. Miss MM suffers polyfragmented MPD, as one would expect to find in a victim of such severe child abuse. Nevertheless, as one sees more often than not in MPD sufferers, Miss MM is intelligent, highly hypnotizable, and creative. She holds an advanced degree in the sciences, won at great effort on her part.

Therapy helped Miss MM retrieve the memory of being involved in child pornography. The recalled memory led her into compulsive visits to adult bookstores, where one day she found a picture of herself as a child pornography performer. The experience affected her deeply. She ran screaming into the street, certain that other patrons could recognize her even though she was now an adult, 18 inches taller, and 120 pounds heavier than when she was exploited in child pornography. Miss MM is an outpatient but has had long periods of inpatient therapy as a result of several suicide attempts and frequent suicidal ideation. She has not been integrated. Family history and interviews document that her entire family is subject to dissociative disorders: her father has documented fugues, and her mother and brother exhibit a full range of MPD signs and symptoms. Her sister has dissociative disorder NOS, and her niece has MPD. Both her sister and her niece have been seen in psychotherapy with me. Her brother is alleged to have committed a number of violent acts that may include several murders.

Case 7: Ritual, Satanic Physical and Sexual Abuse and Incest. Mrs. WM is a 40-year-old, married, white female who also manifests the rule of thumb that "the more ritualistic and severe the abuse, the more fragmented the victim's personality." Mrs. WM is one of the most fragmented and disturbed patients ever seen by the author. She appears to be close to a polyfragmented MPD; however, an earlier working diagnosis was polyfragmented ADD.

Alcoholism was Mrs. WM's primary diagnosis during 12 years in the mental health system prior to her referral to the author. The "blackouts" that she reported after drinking two or three beers were unrecognized dissociative episodes. During some of these "blackouts," she would awaken to find herself driving naked down a highway, or in bed with a man whom she could not recall ever having seen before. She also had been diagnosed as manic-depressive and put on a regimen of lithium. She was referred after she failed to respond to pharmacotherapy and still had "alcoholic blackouts" despite her no longer consuming alcohol.

At the time of referral, Mrs. WM was unable to function socially. A few years earlier, she had held a job as a teacher. Now she could not hold three consecutive thoughts; her writing consisted of page after page of words without punctuation or capitalization. She was unable to make any statements about sex or to use words that named or described sexual organs. At this point, her working diagnosis was polyfragmented ADD, based in part on the rapid "switching" observed by her therapists.

Because large doses of propranolol have been useful in decreasing switching and fragmentation in other patients, propranolol was added to her regimen of benzodiazepines after a trial of clonidine failed due to excessive sedation. At 300 mg of propranolol per day, some improvement began to appear. At 360 mg per day, results were significant enough to permit the beginning of psychotherapy. Throughout most of the course of therapy she received 240 mg of propranolol. As of this writing she is functioning well as an outpatient, is gainfully employed, and is no longer taking any psychotropic medications.

Sand tray therapy (Braun 1986b; Sachs and Braun 1986) was used psychotherapeutically to help the patient organize and stabilize her thought processes. Psychotherapy then began to identify fragments, which became meaningful in terms of the memories that Mrs. WM was able to recover.

Mrs. WM had been ritually and incestuously abused by both of her parents and by other members of her family throughout her infancy and childhood. The ritual abuse was both physical and sexual and was part of the satanic cult activities in which her entire family was involved. She was also extensively involved in pornography, including "snuff" films, with children, adults, and animals. Cult members practiced human sacrifice and cannibalism. Mrs. WM was forced to be an observer and was forced to participate, but later participated voluntarily. The ritual abuse did not end until Mrs. WM was hospitalized, and she and her therapists recognized what had been happening.

Mrs. WM has made numerous suicide attempts and has experienced many incidents of self-mutilation. Some of her multiple suicide attempts have been due to programming she received from the cult to commit suicide at specific ages or if she remembered too much or revealed secrets (Braun 1989a). Mrs. WM probably dissociated defensively amost as soon as her ritual abuse began. The predisposing factors were high hypnotizability, inconsistent love and abuse, and cult training from infancy. Precipitating and perpetuating events were so numerous as to defy counting and occurred all her life into adulthood.

SUMMARY

In a series of case histories, we see the adult psychopathologic outcomes of severe child abuse (Table 11-1). In some instances, the abuse is psychological, as in extreme neglect and ostracism; in other cases, the abuse is physical, or sexual, or both. At the far end of the abuse spectrum are cases of sadomasochistic and satanic ritual abuse administered by the victim's own families. In all of the cases presented, the victims responded to the abuse diathesis with the ultimate development of MPD. Child abuse has been shown to be the most common underlying cause of MPD.

Whether or not the abuse is incestuous does not appear to be relevant to the subsequent development of MPD, nor does it significantly change the treatment approach (Braun 1986b, 1988b, 1989b). However, the greater the terror and force used, the greater was the damage. The 3-P model predicts that the MPD victim must have the biopsychological predisposition to dissociate defensively in the face of trauma, and that there must be a precipitating traumatic event that triggers dissociation, followed by perpetuating traumas that chain the dissociations affectively. The child with an inborn ability to dissociate is likely to respond to abuse by dissociating, setting the stage for subsequent dissociations if the abuse is perpetuated. If the child does not have the capacity to dissociate, severe, repeated abuse may ultimately result in a type of PTSD, recurrent depression, or psychosis. PTSD is a likely response to single incidents of incest/ rape. Recurrent depression and suicidal behavior are sometimes clues to ongoing incest in children, in adolescents, and in some adults.

While incest may be involved in child abuse that underlies MPD, the more important factor may be the unpredictable nature of the abuse. The severity of dissociation and MPD is most directly related to abuse that is administered by parents or other family members who, at other times, are able to give the child love and protection. The abuser may be a mother, a father, or both. Abusing parents also are likely to have been abused as children; the transgenerational nature of both child abuse and MPD have been documented (Braun 1985a; Coons 1985; Gelles 1987; Kluft 1985). Thus abusers may be incestuous, but their causative relationship with MPD may not lie in the incest per se (granted the closer one's relationship to the abuser, the greater the traumatic effect) but the whole constellation

Table 11-1. Adult psychopathologic outcomes of severe child abuse in seven case histories

Case no.	Suicidal ideation	Suicide attempts	Self-mutilation	Polyfragmented	Personalities (n)	Fragments (n)
1. Neglect; physical/psychological	Rare/passive	None	None	No	5	20
2. Physical abuse, often by family members	3	None	None	No	10	12
3. Sexual and physical abuse, not incestuous	Few	2	None	No	7	Several
4. Sexual abuse, incestuous	3	1	None	No	6	14
5. Physical abuse and sexual abuse	2 severe	None	None	5 principal systems	10	60+
6. Sexual abuse, pornography, incest	Frequent	Several	None	7 principal systems	9	100+
7. Ritual, satanic abuse, family members often involved	Frequent	Numerous	Numerous	4+ principal systems	10	100+

of traumas. The more severe and prolonged the trauma, the more severe the fragmentation.

Severity and the ritual nature of abuse has a significant causative relationship with polyfragmentation in ADD and/or in MPD. Ritual, satanic abuse is usually administered by parents and other family cult members, and incest is of necessity involved. Incestuous abuse is not necessarily related to the most severe, polyfragmented forms of MPD; however, ritual abuse, with or without incest, is the most common underlying cause of polyfragmentation for MPD or dissociative disorders NOS.

In summary, MPD is one of the incest-related syndromes of adult psychopathology. Dissociation, dissociative disorders, and nondissociative pathologies are also seen. The alert therapist focuses not only on the clues that encourage him or her to suspect incest, but also the the unsettling possibility that the discovery of incest, however reprehensible, may be the clue that still more has occurred, that it may be the "tip of the iceberg" of the most severe abuse imaginable. The therapist should never lose sight of the fact that even deep pathologies based in severe abuse may still be treatable (Braun 1989b; Kluft 1984).

REFERENCES

Braun BG: Hypnosis for multiple personalities, in Hypnosis in Clinical Medicine. Edited by Wain HR. Chicago, IL, Year Book Medical, 1980, pp 209–217

Braun BG: Towards a theory of multiple personality and other dissociative phenomena. Psychiatr Clin North Am 7:171–194, 1984

Braun BG: Dissociation: behavior, affect, sensation, knowledge, in Dissociative Disorders 1985: Proceedings of the Second International Conference on Multiple Personality/Dissociative States. Edited by Braun BG. Chicago, IL, Rush University, 1985a, p 6

Braun BG: The transgenerational incidence of dissociation and multiple personality disorder: a preliminary report, in Childhood Antecedents of Multiple Personality. Washington, DC, American Psychiatric Press, 1985b, pp 128–150

Braun BG: Introduction, in Treatment of Multiple Personality Disorder. Edited by Braun BG. Washington, DC, American Psychiatric Press, 1986a, pp xi–xxi

Braun BG: Issues in the treatment of multiple personality disorder, in Treatment of Multiple Personality Disorder. Edited by Braun BG. Washington, DC, American Psychiatric Press, 1986b, pp 1–28

Braun BG: Dissociative disorder as a sequel to childhood incest. Paper presented at the annual meeting of the American Psychiatric Association, Chicago, IL, 1987

Braun BG: The BASK model of dissociation. Dissociation 1:4–15, 1988a

Braun BG: The BASK model of dissociation, part II: treatment. Dissociation 1:16–23, 1988b

Braun BG: Programmed suicide. Paper presented at the 22nd Annual Conference of the American Association of Suicidology, San Diego, CA, April 1, 1989a

Braun BG: Psychotherapy of the survivor of incest with a dissociative disorder. Psychiatr Clin North Am 12:2, 1989b, pp 307–324

Braun BG, Gray GT: Report on the 1985 questionnaire on multiple personality disorder, in Dissociative Disorders 1986: Proceedings of the Third International Conference on Multiple Personality/Dissociative States. Edited by Braun BG. Chicago, IL, Rush University, 1986, p 111

Braun BG, Sachs RG: The development of multiple personality disorder: predisposing, precipitating, and perpetuating factors, in Childhood Antecedents of Multiple Personality. Edited by Kluft RP. Washington, DC, American Psychiatric Press, 1985, pp 37–64

Coons PM: Children of parents with multiple personality disorder, in Childhood Antecedents of Multiple Personality. Edited by Kluft RP. Washington, DC, American Psychiatric Press, 1985, pp 151–165

Gelles RJ: The family and its role in the abuse of children. Psychiatric Annals 17:229–232, 1987

Kluft RP: Treatment of multiple personality disorder. Psychiatr Clin North Am 7:9–29, 1984

Kluft RP: Childhood multiple personality disorder: predictors, clinical findings, and treatment results, in Childhood Antecedents of Multiple Personality. Edited by Kluft RP. Washington, DC, American Psychiatric Press, 1985, pp 167–196

Putnam FW, Guroff JJ, Silberman EK, et al: The clinical phenomenology of multiple personality disorder: 100 recent cases. J Clin Psychiatry 47:285–293, 1986

Sachs RG, Braun BG: The use of sand trays in the treatment of multiple personality disorder, in Dissociative Disorders 1986: Proceedings of the Third International Conference on Multiple Personality/Dissociative States. Edited by Braun BG. Chicago, IL, Rush University, 1986, p 61

Schultz R, Braun BG, Kluft RP: Creativity and the imaginary companion phenomenon: prevalence and phenomenology in multiple personality disorder, in Dissociative Disorders 1985: Proceedings of the Third International Conference on Multiple Personality/Dissociative States. Edited by Braun BG. Chicago, IL, Rush University, 1985, p 103

Schultz R, Braun BG, Kluft RP: Multiple personality disorder: phenomenology of selected variables in comparison to major depression. Dissociation 2:45–51, 1989

Schultz R, Kluft RP, Braun BG: The interface between multiple personality disorder, in Dissociative Disorders 1986: Proceedings of the Third International Conference on Multiple Personality/Dissociative States. Edited by Braun BG. Chicago, IL, Rush University, 1986, p 112

CHAPTER 12

Trauma, Dissociation, and Hypnosis

David Spiegel, M.D.

In this chapter, I explore the importance of dissociation as a defense during trauma and as a part of the symptomatology of posttraumatic stress disorder (PTSD). I describe the nature of hypnotic phenomena related to dissociation and present evidence that there is spontaneous mobilization of hypnotic-like experience during and after traumatic events. Severe dissociative disorders such as multiple personality disorder (MPD) can be interpreted as chronic PTSDs. The effects of adult trauma on three patients with such chronic disorders are reviewed. These patients' past use of dissociative defenses against repeated traumatic experiences profoundly influenced their response to the adult trauma. In two of the three cases, dissociation was used not so much as a defense against the present trauma but as a means of reinforcing the patients' self-hatred and irrational self-blame for traumatic events inflicted on them by others earlier in life. The importance of the identification and use of phenomena related to hypnosis in the psychotherapy of such patients is discussed.

HYPNOTIC PHENOMENA

What do hypnosis, dissociation, and trauma have in common? Hypnosis is controlled dissociation elicited in a structured setting. It has three main

Development of this chapter was supported by the John D. and Catherine T. MacArthur Foundation.

components: in addition to the dissociation, it is comprised of absorption and suggestibility. Hypnosis is a state of aroused, attentive focal concentration with a relative suspension of peripheral awareness (Spiegel and Spiegel 1978). This state involves a narrowing of the focus of attention. Hypnotic concentration differs from ordinary concentration in somewhat the same way that a telephoto lens in a camera differs from a wide-angle lens. A hypnotized individual focuses on one perception, image, or idea with great intensity at the expense of peripheral awareness. Indeed, studies have shown that individuals who report that they frequently have such intense, self-altering experiences, such as getting so absorbed in a good movie or book that they lose awareness of their surroundings, are indeed more hypnotizable (Tellegen 1981; Tellegen and Atkinson 1974). This means that hypnosis is an altered and intensified form of concentration, and that hypnotizable individuals use their capacity spontaneously in the course of everyday life.

Dissociation can be conceptualized as a complementary aspect of absorption. Individuals intensely absorbed in one thing will be paying less attention to other events that normally occur in consciousness. A common example is "highway hypnosis," in which a person engaged in intense conversation with a passenger will not notice that he has driven past his exit on a highway. He is clearly driving and executing all the complex activities necessary to keep the car in the proper lane, and yet the procedures required for driving seem to be performed outside of conscious awareness. Processes that would ordinarily be considered conscious, such as driving the car, now seem unconscious, and furthermore, the bemused driver has no memory of having driven for the recent period of time, although obviously he or she has. Barriers are set up between aspects of consciousness. This is one of the most interesting aspects of hypnosis in that it seems possible to change the boundaries between conscious and unconscious experience. The more intensely one focuses on one aspect of experience, the more the remaining peripheral awareness is dissociated and unconscious. During hypnosis there is less connection among various aspects of experience. Events are thus dissociated.

The third component of hypnosis is suggestibility, enhanced responsiveness to instructions (Orne 1959). While hypnotized individuals are not deprived of their will and are able to refuse suggestions, they are less likely to do so because their critical scrutiny is relatively suspended. We modulate our tendency to act on our ideas by editing them, for example, reminding ourselves of what happened the last time we did something like the action we are contemplating, or questioning the motivation of the person who suggests it. Hynotized individuals are so intensely focused on one idea that they are less likely to critique or judge it. Indeed, some hypnotized individuals are unaware of the source of an idea, a phenomenon called "hypnotic source amnesia" (Evans 1979). An idea suggested to them by someone else may seem to them as though it had come from within.

TRAUMA THEORY AND DISSOCIATION

Defense mechanisms have customarily been viewed as psychological processes that provide protection against painful memories and unacceptable wishes rather than against painful experiences. The reasons for a given individual's use of one particular defense mechanism rather than another have always been considered rather mysterious (Freud 1946). More recently, attention has been directed toward the mobilization of defense mechanisms as a process of protection against the overwhelming experience of trauma as it is inflicted. There has been growing recognition that patients with severe dissociative disorders, of which MPD is an increasingly well-studied example, have been victims of severe physical abuse in childhood, and that their dissociative capacities were spontaneously mobilized to help them cope psychologically with the repeated assaults that they endured (Frischholz 1985; Putnam 1985; Spiegel 1984). It certainly makes sense that individuals capable of profound dissociation and of achieving the analgesia associated with high hypnotizability might well mobilize such defenses during an episode of physical trauma.

The study of dissociation began with observations of overlapping phenomena in hypnosis and patients with MPD (Nemiah 1985). Hysterical patients prone to dissociative symptoms have been found to be highly hypnotizable (Bliss 1980; Spiegel 1984; Spiegel and Fink 1979; Steingard and Frankel 1985) and are likely to use their dissociative capacities in the face of stress: "Hysterical patients . . . have an exaggerated, perhaps inborn, tendency toward mental dissociation that provides them with a ready-made mechanism of defense for dealing with emotionally painful events" (Nemiah 1985, p. 947). Janet (1920) emphasized dissociation as the primary mechanism of defense; Freud (1933) acknowledged dissociation but emphasized repression. The major distinction between the two defense mechanisms can be understood in terms of the relationships among the material that is kept out of conscious awareness. In dissociation, specific memories and associated feelings contain rules excluding other memories and feelings from conscious awareness, although these rules are not absolute and the boundaries can be breached (Frischholz 1985). In repression, similar material may be kept out of awareness to exclude the uncomfortable affects that accompany it, but there is no presumption that one set of material necessitates the exclusion of others.

Freud (1933) was troubled about the relationship between his general theory that repression served as a means of keeping unacceptable wishes out of consciousness and traumatic neuroses. Why would trauma be repressed when it was not wished for? His repression model fits the development of and conflicts engendered by oedipal fears and wishes better than it does the mind's response to trauma. Much has recently been made of Freud's abandonment of the trauma theory as the general explanation for the neuroses. Of more interest is the possibility that different defenses (e.g., dissociation) are mobilized by trauma rather than by long-standing conflicts and warded-off wishes (e.g., repression).

Most of the symptoms associated with PTSD in the DSM-III-R (American Psychiatric Association 1987) have a dissociative flavor: the reexperiencing of a traumatic event through intrusive recollections, nightmares, or flashbacks; emotional numbing with feelings of detachment or isolation; stimulus sensitivity (including the avoidance of environmental cues that are associated with recollections of the traumatic events); survivor guilt; and difficulty concentrating. The phenomenon of dissociation implies that an isolated set of interacting affects and memories has become segregated from the mainstream of an individual's psychological life and the store of readily available mental contents, but can be reactivated. They are both sequestered and recovered more or less as a unit, consistent with evidence in cognitive psychology for state-dependent memory (Bower 1981). Bower has shown that mental content can be retrieved more accurately when the mood state in the retrieval process is congruent with that in which the material was learned. Memories laid down in the company of strong affect might therefore be available only if the person were able to tolerate reexperiencing the associated intense affect. Such experiences are defensively avoided, and thus the memories and the affects associated with them are dissociated.

Furthermore, there is another kind of state besides affect that can influence memory retrieval. It is the state of consciousness itself. For individuals who have developed a pattern of responding to trauma by dissociating, the experience of dissociation itself becomes contaminated with the affective content of trauma. Numerous patients with MPD and some with other dissociative disorders respond in an idiosyncratic way to a standard hypnotic induction procedure. Within a few seconds of the initial induction, and prior to any intervention that might request, inquire after, or otherwise cue a recollection or revivification of painful material, they slip into a dissociative state and respond as if they were being traumatized. Thus the dissociation itself has become contaminated with the experience of trauma, a different kind of state-dependent memory.

One woman who suffered hysterical pseudoseizures that were unresponsive to phenytoin and other antiseizure medications started to have one of these seizures shortly after commencing administration of the Hypnotic Induction Profile (Spiegel and Spiegel 1987), a brief test of hypnotizability. Asked later to visualize an earlier traumatic scene, she pictured a time when she had been held, along with her dog, against her will and beaten. Toward the end of this scene, her head started to move in the same way it did during her seizures. These phenomena then were understood and successfully treated as a dissociative conversion reaction related to her PTSD.

The Dissociative Response to Trauma

Trauma can be understood as the experience of being made into an object: the victim of someone else's rage, of nature's indifference, or of one's own physical or psychological limitations. Along with the pain and fear associated with rape, combat trauma, or natural disaster comes a marginally bearable sense of helplessness, a realization that one's own will and wishes become irrelevant to the course of events, leaving either a view of the self that is damaged; contaminated by the humiliation, pain, and fear that the event imposed; or a fragmented sense of self. There is an understandable desire to escape psychologically when one cannot escape physically. Since the literature on absorption has demonstrated that hypnotic-like dissociative experiences can occur in pleasant situations (e.g., at the movies), it would be strange indeed if individuals faced with overwhelming helplessness and fear did not utilize such resources to escape psychologically from events that are physically inescapable. The preexisting personality attempts to carry on as though nothing at all had happened. However, the need for the dissociation implies that pain and humiliation were, in fact, inflicted, and the person only partially reconsolidates, left with a sense that the real truth is the dissociated and warded-off self that was humiliated and damaged.

Indeed, it is not uncommon for victims of rape to find themselves floating above their own body, feeling sorry for the person beneath them who is being assaulted. One accident victim, who was so badly injured that he eventually lost one leg, found himself imagining that he was fishing on a pond with his father. He had been able to walk on his badly damaged legs to get off the highway and felt pain only several hours later in the hospital emergency room. Many victims at the time of trauma have a sense of unreality—"This is not happening to me." They dissociate the experience; they treat it as though it were happening to someone else, somewhere else.

This dissociative ability then comes to influence the nature of the PTSD that may follow. PTSD is often comprised of a polarization of consciousness, a sense of numbing and loss of pleasure in usually enjoyable activities, alternating with intrusive recollections of the event. These intrusive recollections take the dissociated form of reliving the event as though it were occurring in the present, or of extreme sensitivity to contemporary stimuli that remind the victim of the traumatic event. This on-off quality is very much like a hypnotic state. In hypnotic age regression, individuals do not merely remember previous events; they relive them as though they were occurring in the present, just as some trauma victims relive the traumatic experience when reminded of it (Spiegel et al. 1988). The numbing or loss of pleasure in usual activities seen in PTSD is a consequence of the fragmentation that a traumatic dissociation produces. Such victims feel that there is some hidden truth about themselves, even if they are not consciously aware of the trauma or its aftermath. They cannot fully enjoy present experience because a part of them has been fundamentally damaged by the traumatic occurrences and is not available to participate in present relationships and experiences.

Given this connection between trauma and dissociation, the most extreme form of pathologic dissociation, MPD, can be understood as a chronic form of PTSD. These patients have a history of childhood incest and physical violence (Coons and Milstein 1986; Kluft 1985; Kluft et al. 1984; Putnam et al. 1986). Many such patients report that the first experience they had of dissociating into another personality was the first time a parent or other caretaker beat or sexually asaulted them. One patient put it this way: "Blue said to me, 'You don't want to be with that so-and-so; you come and be with me.' " Patients report that these personalities initially comfort them and allow them to get through terrifying experiences without any sense of physical pain. Unfortunately, as the actual physical abuse is discontinued, these same personalities often turn on the patient, inflicting psychological and sometimes physical pain on the patients in a kind of identification with the aggressor that allows patients to feel that they had some control over catastrophic events during which, in fact, they were actually quite helpless.

The experience of involuntariness may be the link among hypnosis, dissociation, and trauma. The importance of involuntariness in hypnosis has been emphasized by Weitzenhoffer (1980). As discussed above, the kinds of events that mobilize discussion as a defense also seem to be those in which the patient's voluntary will is physically overridden. Thus the natural involuntariness associated with hypnosis can be viewed as a repetition of an experience in which patients literally have involuntariness imposed on them.

CLINICAL EVIDENCE: TRAUMA AND DISSOCIATION

Dissociation has been reported to occur during traumatic experiences (Spiegel 1988; Spiegel et al. 1987), and it may be that hypnotic-like abreactions in which the person relives rather than remembers a traumatic event owe some of their intensity to the fact that the patient was in a dissociated state during the trauma and is thus in a similar mental state while reliving it. The importance of imagery in posttraumatic symptomatology noted early by Breuer and Freud (1893) has been reemphasized (Brett and

Ostroff 1985). Theories of traumatic symptomatology differ, some emphasizing cognitive breakdown and withdrawal, with amnesia as a focal symptom (Horowitz 1976; Kardiner and Spiegel 1947), others emphasizing intrusive recollections and images (Horowitz 1976). DSM-III-R criteria include both types of symptoms: numbing of responsiveness on the one hand, and intrusive responses, sudden reliving of the traumatic events, and stimulus sensitivity on the other. Both observations may be fundamentally correct. What may occur in response to trauma is a polarization of experience in which trauma victims alternate between intense, vivid, and painful memories and images associated with the traumatic experience, and a kind of pseudonormality in which they avoid memory by traumatic amnesia, other forms of dissociation, or repression or by a complex combination of these mechanisms with a consequent constriction in adaptive ability and the availability of the full range of affective response. This polarization of consciousness can be seen in the hypnotic state, in which intense absorption in the hypnotic focal experience (Tellegen 1981; Tellegen and Atkinson 1974) is accomplished via the dissociation of experience at the periphery (Hilgard 1977; Spiegel and Spiegel 1987). Like the hypnotic experience, traumatic imagery is either intense or intensely avoided. Thus a more frequent use of dissociative defenses with their sharp cognitive boundaries would be especially likely among victims of severe trauma.

There have been few studies of the association between hynotizability and trauma that would provide some evidence regarding the link between trauma and dissociation (Nemiah 1985). Hypnotizability testing can be quite helpful to differential diagnosis, since dissociation is evoked and measured (Lavoie and Sabourin 1979). Those who are hypnotizable often use the capacity spontaneously (Spiegel 1974). Breuer (Breuer and Freud 1893) described dissociation as a "hypnoidal" state. The fundamental capacity to express dissociation in a structured setting (i.e., hypnotizability) should be high if extreme dissociative symptoms such as amnesia, fugue, hysterical psychosis, or MPD occur (Bliss 1980; Spiegel 1984; Spiegel and Fink 1979; Steingard and Frankel 1985). Hilgard (1970) observed a correlation ($r = .30$) between physical punishment inflicted during childhood and later high hypnotizability in a population of 187 normal college students. She speculated:

> A possible tie between punishment and hypnotic involvement might come by way of dissociation. . . . Although we have no direct evidence, some of our case material . . . suggests that reading or other involvements may sometimes be an escape from the harsh realities of a punitive environment (p. 221).

When Frischholz (1985) reanalyzed these data, he found that a multiple correlation combining imaginative involvement and punishment yielded a significantly higher correlation ($r = .4$) with hypnotizability than either variable had alone, suggesting that the two variables (and presumably others) contribute independently to the development or preservation of hypnotizability. This association between abuse and hypnotizability has been confirmed more recently by Nash et al. (1984).

Two studies have shown a positive relationship between symptoms of PTSD and hypnotizability. Stutman and Bliss (1985) divided 26 Vietnam combat veterans into high and low groups on the basis of posttraumatic symptoms. Those with high symptoms were found to be significantly more hypnotizable on the Stanford Hypnotic Susceptibility Scale, Form C (Weitzenhoffer and Hilgard 1962). Spiegel et al. (1988) compared the hypnotizability of 65 patients with DSM-III (American Psychiatric Association 1980) PTSD to that of four other patient samples. At a mean ($\pm$ SD) of 8.04 ± 2.24, their Hypnotic Induction Profile scores were significantly higher than those of all the patient groups studied and a nonpatient control sample. Analysis of covariance indicated a significant main effect for diagnosis ($F = 12.3$, $\frac{1}{5}$ df, $p < .001$). There was a significant main effect for age ($F = 7.17$, $\frac{1}{256}$ df, $p < .008$), but this did not account for the differences observed.

Thus there is evidence from several studies that the presence of symptoms of PTSD is associated with higher than normal hypnotizability. It is as though these people are forced to resort to their dissociative capacities to cope with trauma as it is inflicted, and this in turn makes dissociative symptoms a major component of the syndrome that follows the trauma. Having used dissociation to defend against the loss of physical control during the trauma, they now lose mental control in the wake of the traumatic experience, despite having regained physical control. The helplessness is now symbolized as an inability to control their state of mind, hence the intrusive recollections, startle reactions, and flashbacks.

EFFECTS OF TRAUMA INFLICTED ON PATIENTS WITH ESTABLISHED DISSOCIATIVE DISORDERS

The observations in this study are based on an analysis of 14 consecutive cases of MPD, of whom three had experienced rape as adults (i.e., subsequent to their development of dissociative symptoms), two of the three, during the course of their psychotherapy. One of the three developed a classic dissociative defense to the trauma. During the rape she formed a new "personality" named "No One." None of the other personalities had any memory for the rape, including one who had been aware of experiencing considerable trauma at the hands of her father. The choice of name for this new personality was rather interesting, since she was made to feel like a "nobody" by the rapist, yet she could reflect that "No One was raped."

The other two patients also had DSM-III-R features of MPD, were raped in adulthood by strangers, and yet were, interestingly enough, unable to mobilize dissociative defenses during the rape. They had painful conscious memories of the fear and humiliation they experienced, made worse by the fact that this episode reactivated additional memories of earlier sexual and physical abuse by parents. Given their well-developed dissociative capacities, why did they not use them as a means of coping with this new trauma?

One explanation is the myth of invulnerability that these patients construct as a means of coping with assault. They fundamentally blame themselves for the attacks inflicted on them by their parents or other abusers, a point of view that is amply reinforced by those who mistreated them, who rationalize the attacks as a punishment for some real or imagined misdeed. Indeed, one of these patients, Barb (in an alternate personality), would deliberately provoke an attack by her father to distract his attention from her younger sisters. She viewed this as an obligation and a price she had to pay as well as a means of rationalizing the misery that she endured. Most of the time she was able to maintain a dissociated state and reported feeling no pain, although occasionally her father would catch on to her apparent insensitivity and attempt to hurt her so severely that she could not eliminate the pain. She had promised herself when she left home that no one would ever do anything like that to her again. That is, she felt relatively invulnerable because of 1) her ability to manage her pain and emotional presence at the time of the assault, and 2) her unconscious fantasy that she could stop the assaults since she engaged in behavior that she thought provoked them. One of the major tasks of psychotherapy was helping her to face her fundamental helplessness at the hands of sadistic parents. Thus her history of victimization had left her with a compensatory fantasy of invulnerability.

When, during the course of her psychotherapy, she was raped by a stranger, she predictably blamed herself for inviting the assault by walking alone on a heavily traveled street at nine o'clock in the evening. Furthermore, she insisted that she should have been able to stop the assailant, a heavily muscled man with a knife, or die in the attempt. He made explicit threats to kill her and overpowered her physically before raping her. It had not occurred to her until it was brought up in the therapy a year after the rape that even had she tried to fight to the death with him, he might have chosen to rape rather than murder her. Several months after this event, she reported that a stranger approached her from behind and grabbed her. This time, an alternative personality (named Barbara) emerged, kicked him hard in the knee, and he ran away. Using hypnosis, I inquired of this alternative personality why she had not helped during the first assault. With an air of hostile detachment, she said, "I just thought I would let Barb handle it; I don't care much for her anyway. I'm trying to get rid of her and I thought this would speed the process." That is, a dissociated personality took a stance of identification with the aggressor and maintained her fantasy of invulnerability. Such was not the case in the second assault, either because she had been sensitized to the danger of attack by the first assault or because a successful physical defense was possible.

What these cases show is that while dissociation can be mobilized in the event of physical trauma, and often is, it is a complex choice, made more difficult by the embedded history linking dissociation to trauma that the patient experienced earlier in life. Since such patients often feel that they provoked and even deserved the abuse they suffered in childhood, later trauma reactivates these painful thoughts. Simply "allowing" the attack to proceed while the patient dissociates may seem to someone with a previous history of sexual assault as though it were an implicit choice to yield passively not only to the current assault but to the previous ones. A dissociative defense thus may be less acceptable to a person with a history of abuse than it is to someone without such prior experience of earlier physical abuse. Clearly, an assault, which is traumatic enough anyway, constitutes a major setback for a patient who is attempting to work through a history of previous sexual trauma. In these patients, the frequency and severity of spontaneous dissociation increased substantially after the rape episodes and set back the slow process of integrating the disparate personalities.

Thus while dissociation serves the function of defending consciousness from the immediate experience of painful events—physical pain, fear, anxiety, and helplessness—it then becomes an entrenched part of the overall view of the self. Once divided in a powerful way, the experience of unity becomes problematic, since ordinary self-consciousness is no longer synonymous with the entirety of self and personal history. Rather, consciousness of self becomes associated with the unconscious awareness of some warded-off tragedy, the moment of humiliation and fear, the act of cowardice, the sense of having been degraded. The person comes to feel that there is an inauthentic self that carries on the everyday functions of life but experiences them as filtered through numbness, with a lack of genuine pleasure in otherwise pleasurable activities. The unconscious, warded-off memories exert censorship on conscious experience. The process of dissociation becomes part of the patient's identity, to be remobilized in the face of subsequent stress or even imagined situations reminiscent of this stress. Thus for a patient with a history of trauma-induced dissociation to enter a dissociated state seems almost to create and accept the assault rather than to defend against it.

An important issue in the psychotherapy of such patients is teaching them to transform their experience of dissociation. One teenage girl who had spontaneous hypnotic age regressions (Spiegel and Rosenfeld 1984; Spiegel and Spiegel 1985) initially dissociated to the age of 4, when her father had thrown her across the room. As she relived this experience, she started to cry and was fearful that I would assault her as well. I reassured her that I would not and told her that some terrible things had happened but that they would not happen any more. I complimented her for being a brave little girl for trying to protect her mother from her father. She began to cry and said, "Nobody ever called me brave before." She learned to use the self-hypnotic state to picture on the one hand these moments of fear and pain, and on the other hand how she had tried to protect herself or other members of her family during such episodes. She practiced this regularly, and her spontaneous dissociations to the age of 4 ceased. Of special interest is the fact that she, on her own, came to experience the dissociative state as a "protective light" that surrounded her, making her feel safe and comfortable. Her uncoupling of the experience of dissociation from the fantasy of acquiescence to, or at least defense against, the experience of physical assault was an important step in the psychotherapy.

It is of some interest that the same dissociated personality states that appear to be quite self-destructive and hostile to the primary personality are often reported to have started out for the purpose of helping protect the person from assault as a child. Later, usually shortly after the physical abuse stops, such alternative personalities "take over" and inflict lacerations on the patients' bodies, leaving the primary personalities to "wake up and discover" the mutilation. Why does this change occur?

One possibility is that while the destruction is being inflicted by the parent, dissociation serves primarily as a defense against the immediate pain and fear. When the patient finally escapes from the parent, the defensive task is internalized. Protection is required not against the external physical threat but rather against the memories associated with assault and the associated uncomfortable affect, ranging from sadness and fear to rage. The problem is then symbolized by the identification of the alternative personality with the aggressor. This defense gives these patients the fantasy that they controlled a situation over which they were, in fact, helpless. Indeed, these alternative aggressor personalities often relish pain inflicted on the patient. When Barb was raped, the second alter (Barbara, the aggressor personality) said:

> She is such a fool. She trusts people. That will teach her a lesson not to trust anyone. She is always wasting her time trying to do good for people. Who ever did any good for her? When things like this happen, it just convinces her to go away. That's what I want. I just want to get rid of her.

This rationalization that pain inflicted is somehow deserved and even educational is, of course, the excuse abusing parents frequently employ. The patient thus internalizes and recapitulates the pain inflicted on her.

Indeed, the dissociation, along with identification with the aggressor, can represent the tragic double-bind these patients experienced as children (Spiegel 1984, 1987). The double-bind theory (Bateson et al. 1956) died an appropriate death in regard to schizophrenia. Abundant genetic and biochemical evidence makes it highly unlikely that family communication patterns result in schizophrenia. Indeed, the disordered family communication patterns may result from schizophrenia or schizotypal symptoms in a child (Spiegel 1982). However, abusing parents often literally impose a double-bind. They tell the child that he or she should be absolutely perfect, indeed spend all of his or her time caring for the parents' needs and, at the same time, with cruel and erratic punishment, convey exactly the opposite message, that the child is a horrible little person deserving of nothing but punishment. Children are, of course prohibited from commenting on the injustice or paradox of the situation into which they are thrust. Such a child may respond by becoming an impoverished collection of people, one of them pathetically attempting to serve others, and another, cruel and vindictive, even to the self.

Furthermore, these individuals internalize the cruel paradox of blaming themselves for their victimization by parents and other adults. The badness inflicted on them comes to be within them. Thus the hostile destructiveness learned by identification with the aggressor becomes part of their own internal, if fragmented, identity. In her primary personality, Barb was terribly afraid of demonstrating any assertiveness at all in her relationships with others because of her fear that to do so would make her "just like" her alcoholic and abusive father. She saw no middle ground. Her alternative personality, Barbara, was contemptuous of compassion for other people. Although critical of her father's physical abuse of her, she considered any sense of moral standards mere foolishness; hence, her stance of disinterest and even glee in the demoralizing effects of rape during adulthood on her alternative personality. Thus her identification with sadistic aggression only served to confirm her in her belief that she deserved the abuse she experienced as a child. The explanation is modulated from her being a "bad girl" to being naive and foolish. Nonetheless, she thereby maintains a myth of invulnerability and avoids a confrontation with her fundamental helplessness at the hands of a sadistic victimizer.

CONCLUSION

The experience of extremes of physical violence is so psychologically devastating that rather extreme defenses are mobilized to deal with it. Such experiences are doubly traumatic when they reopen memories of similar trauma inflicted in childhood. Victims of PTSD are indeed especially sensitive to subsequent trauma. Even comparatively minor events such as traffic accidents can trigger a catastrophic reaction related to the original trauma as state-dependent memories are activated.

The experience of dissociation, which occurs as a normal and even pleasant experience, has been contaminated for these patients by its repeated use to defend against trauma. Mobilizing it again in adulthood as a defense against trauma is thus a conflict-laden experience, connoting to the patient not only acquiescence to the assault, but resubmission to previous assaults. Psychotherapeutic work with these patients requires great sensitivity to the enforced mingling of past and present pain (Krystal 1971). The transference is contaminated with images of parents who either inflicted misery on the patient or observed it without interfering. Addressing the material directly may provoke feelings of being assaulted once again, but ignoring it arouses a sense of abandonment to the assailant. Using techniques like hypnosis to help the patient control access to traumatic memories can help in defining boundaries to the grief work necessary to put the trauma into perspective, but attention to the patient's ability to control such memories and dissociative states is critical (Spiegel 1981, 1986). The fact that dissociation helped the patient at the time of trauma makes it an ambivalently held state, contaminated by memories and fantasies of assault. For this reason, it is not uniformly available during subsequent assault, and it must be employed carefully in the psychotherapy of past and recent trauma.

REFERENCES

American Psychiatric Association: Diagnostic and Statistical Manual of Mental Disorders, 3rd Edition. Washington, DC, American Psychiatric Association, 1980

American Psychiatric Association: Diagnostic and Statistical Manual of Mental Disorders, 3rd Edition, Revised. Washington, DC, American Psychiatric Association, 1987

Bateson G, Jackson D, Haley J, et al: Toward a theory of schizophrenia. Behav Sci 1:251–264, 1956

Bliss EL: Multiple personalities: a report of 14 cases with implications for schizophrenia and hysteria. Arch Gen Psychiatry 37:1388–1397, 1980

Bower GH: Mood and memory. Am Psychol 36:129–148, 1981

Brett EA, Ostroff R: Imagery and posttraumatic stress disorder: an overview. Am J Psychiatry 142:417–424, 1985

Breuer J, Freud S: Studies on hysteria (1893), in The Standard Edition of the Complete Psychological Works of Sigmund Freud, Vol 2. Translated and edited by Strachey J. London, Hogarth Press, 1955, pp 1–322

Coons P, Milstein V: Psychosexual disturbances in multiple personality: characteristics, etiology, and treatment. J Clin Psychiatry 47:106–110, 1986

Evans FJ: Phenomena of hypnosis, 2: posthypnotic amnesia, in Handbook of Hypnosis and Psychosomatic Medicine. Edited by Burrows GD, Dennerstein L. New York, Elsevier North-Holland, 1979, pp 85–104

Freud A: The Ego and Mechanisms of Defense. New York, International Universities Press, 1946

Freud S: New introductory lectures on psychoanalysis (1933), in The Standard Edition of the Complete Psychological Works of Sigmund Freud, Vol 22. Translated and edited by Strachey J. London, Hogarth Press, 1964, pp 5–182

Frischholz EJ: The relationship among dissociation, hypnosis, and child abuse in the development of multiple personality disorder, in Childhood Antecedents of Multiple Personality. Edited by Kluft RP. Washington, DC, American Psychiatric Press, 1985, pp 99–126

Hilgard ER: Divided Consciousness: Multiple Controls in Human Thought and Action. New York, John Wiley, 1977

Hilgard JR: Personality and Hypnosis: A Study of Imaginative Involvement. Chicago, IL, University of Chicago Press, 1970

Horowitz MJ: Stress Response Syndromes. Northvale, NJ, Jason Aronson, 1976

Janet P: Psychological Healing: A Historical and Clinical Study (2 Vols) (1920). Translated by Paul E, Paul C. New York, Arne, 1976

Kardiner A, Spiegel H: War Stress and Neurotic Illness. New York, Paul Hoeber, 1947

Kluft RP: Childhood multiple personality disorder: predictors, clinical findings, and treatment result, in Childhood Antecedents of Multiple Personality. Edited by Kluft RP. Washington, DC, American Psychiatric Press, 1985, pp 167–196

Kluft RP, Braun BG, Sachs RG: Multiple personality, intrafamilial abuse, and family psychiatry. International Journal of Family Psychiatry 5:283–301, 1984

Krystal H, Niederland WG: Psychic Traumatization. Boston, MA, Little, Brown, 1971

Lavoie G, Sabourin M: Hypnosis and schizophrenia: a review of experimental and clinical studies, in Handbook of Hypnosis and Psychosomatic Medicine. New York, Elsevier North-Holland, 1979, pp 377–420

Nash MR, Lynn SJ, Givens DL: Adult hypnotic susceptibility, childhood punishment, and child abuse: a brief communication. Int J Clin Exp Hypn 32:6–11, 1984

Nemiah J: Dissociative disorders, in Comprehensive Textbook of Psychiatry, Vol 4. Edited by Kaplan HI, Sadock BM. Baltimore, MD, Williams & Wilkins, 1985, pp 942–957

Orne MT: The nature of hypnosis: artifact and essence. Journal of Abnormal and Social Psychology 58:277–299, 1959

Putnam FW: Dissociation as a response to extreme trauma, in Childhood Antecedents of Multiple Personality. Edited by Kluft RP. Washington, DC, American Psychiatric Press, 1985, pp 65–97

Putnam FW, Guroff JJ, Silberman ED, et al: The clinical phenomenology of multiple personality disorder: 100 recent cases. J Clin Psychiatry 47:285–293, 1986

Spiegel D: Vietnam grief work using hypnosis. Am J Clin Hypn 24:33–40, 1981

Spiegel D: Mothering, fathering, and mental illness, in Rethinking the Family: Some Feminist Questions. Edited by Thorne B, Yalom M. New York, Longman, 1982, pp 95–110

Spiegel D: Multiple personality as a post-traumatic stress disorder. Psychiatr Clin North Am 7:101–110, 1984

Spiegel D: Dissociating damage. Am J Clin Hypn 29:123–131, 1986

Spiegel D: Dissociation, double binds, and post-traumatic stress in multiple personality disorder, in The Treatment of Multiple Personality. Edited by Braun BG. Washington, DC, American Psychiatric Press, 1987, pp 61–77

Spiegel D, Fink R: Hysterical psychosis and hypnotizability. Am J Psychiatry 136:777–781, 1979

Spiegel D, Rosenfeld A: Spontaneous hypnotic age regression. J Clin Psychiatry 45:522–524, 1984

Spiegel D, Spiegel H: Hypnosis, in Comprehensive Textbook of Psychiatry IV. Edited by Kaplan HI, Sadock BJ. New York, Williams & Wilkins, 1985, pp 1389–1402

Spiegel D, Detrick D, Frischholz E: Hypnotizability and psychopathology. Am J Psychiatry 139:431–437, 1982

Spiegel D, Hunt T, Dondershine HE: Dissociation and hypnotizability in post-traumatic stress disorder. Am J Psychiatry 145:301–305, 1988

Spiegel H: The grade 5 syndrome: the high hypnotizable person. Int J Clin Exp Hypn 22:303–319, 1974

Spiegel H, Spiegel D: Trance and Treatment: Clinical Uses of Hypnosis. Washington, DC, American Psychiatric Press, 1978

Steingard S, Frankel FH: Dissociation and psychotic symptoms. Am J Psychiatry 142:953–955, 1985

Stutman RK, Bliss EL: Posttraumatic stress disorder, hypnotizability and imagery. Am J Psychiatry 142:741–743, 1985

Tellegen A: Practicing the two disciplines for relaxation and enlightenment: comment on "Role of the Feedback Signal in Electromyograph Biofeedback: The Relevance of Attention" by Qualls and Sheehan. J Exp Psychol 110:207–226, 1981

Tellegen A, Atkinson G: Openness to absorbing and self-altering experiences ("absorption"), a trait related to hypnotic susceptibility. J Abnorm Psychol 83:268–277, 1974

Weitzenhoffer AM: Hypnotic susceptibility revisited. Am J Clin Hypn 22:130–146, 1980

Weitzenhoffer AM, Hilgard ER: Stanford Hypnotic Susceptibility Scale: Form C. Palo Alto, CA, 1962

CHAPTER 13

Incest and Subsequent Revictimization: The Case of Therapist-Patient Sexual Exploitation, With a Description of the Sitting Duck Syndrome

Richard P. Kluft, M.D.

The study described in this chapter explores the incest victim's general vulnerability to revictimization by exploring therapist-patient sexual exploitation as a specific example and paradigm of revictimization. It describes findings in 12 incest victims who later experienced sexual contact with one or more therapists. It was inspired as I sat in the audience of a symposium during which Nanette Gartrell, Judith Herman, and Silvia Olarte described the results of their landmark National Study of Psychiatrist-Patient Sexual Contact (see Gartrell et al. 1986; Herman et al. 1987). As I listened, I associated to the patients in my practice who had had such experiences and was disconcerted to realize that each victim of therapist-patient sexual exploitation with whom I had worked or with whom I was working currently had been an incest victim. I determined to explore this coincidence further. Since I first presented this material, I have interviewed over two dozen patients with similar backgrounds (i.e., incest victims who had been sexually exploited by psychotherapists). However, since most were mental health professionals or their relatives, and read the literature of this field avidly, I have decided against expanding this article's data base.

Many incest victims are people whose lives seem to progress from crisis to crisis. There is widespread consensus among those who treat incest victims that, as a group, they are particularly vulnerable to revictimization. Although most studies do not distinguish between incest survivors and those who have suffered other types of sexual abuse, a problem noted by Schetky (Chapter 3, this volume), it is apparent that those who have suffered childhood sexual abuse are differentially vulnerable to rape after age 18 (Craine et al. 1988), to masochistic behavior (Kaufman et al. 1954; Katlan 1973; Sloan and Karpinski 1942; Summit and Kryso 1978), to sexual dysfunction (Tsai et al. 1979), to involvement with abusive men (Briere 1984; Fritz et al. 1981; Russell 1986; Tsai and Wagner 1978), to participation in prostitution (Harlan et al. 1981; James and Myerding 1977; Silbert and Pines 1981), to substance abuse (Benward and Densen-Gerber 1975; Herman 1981; Peters 1976), and to becoming psychiatric inpatients (Bryer et al. 1987; Carmen et al. 1984; Enslie and Rosenfeld 1983; Husain and Chapel 1983; Mills et al. 1984). Evidence is beginning to amass to suggest that once incest victims enter the mental health system, they are at greater risk for long hospital courses, even chronic institutionalization (Beck and van der Kolk 1987; Carmen et al. 1984; Sansonnet-Hayden et al. 1987).

Not only does the incest victim experience revictimization throughout the course of her life. When she turns to the mental health professions for surcease of her suffering and for assistance in correcting her maladaptive behavioral patterns, it is clear that she is differentially vulnerable to renewed exploitation in the context of sexual misuse by her therapist. The recent rise in attention to the unconscionable prevalence of therapist-patient misadventures—exemplified in the work of Gartrell and her colleagues (e.g., Gartrell et al. 1986) and Pope and his colleagues (e.g., Pope and Bouhoutsos 1986)—has made frequent incidental mention of the high incidence of incest victims among those sexually exploited by therapists. DeYoung (1981) explored this problem directly in a pioneering study.

Marmor (1972) drew many analogies between therapist-patient sex and incest. Voth (1972) studied a love affair between doctor and patient and observed that the patient had been molested by her stepfather. Stone (1976) studied boundary violations between therapists and patients and remarked on the high incidence of father-daughter incest among those patients who had become sexually involved with their therapists. Dujovne (1983) observed that not only was therapist-patient sex incestuous dynamically, but it often represented a reenactment. Feldman-Summers and Jones (1984) found that the strongest predictor of sexual contact with a treating professional was prior sexual victimization.

Summarizing their extensive experience in researching therapist-patient sex, Pope and Bouhoutsos (1986) determined that incest victims were in the group at highest risk for therapist-patient misadventures: "Although we have no large-scale empirical evidence as yet concerning the pre-morbid personalities of the high-risk group, there appears to be a large percentage of these women who, as children, experienced incestuous relationships" (p. 53). They observed that incest victims develop a repertoire of behaviors that helps them survive the incest, but leaves them at risk for future exploitation. They learn to take the blame for what has happened, exonerate the offender, and keep the situation a secret. Consequently:

> The therapist is assured of a pliable, often pathetically naive, needy patient, who will not tell and will not blame the therapist, but who *will* frequently remain in the therapeutic relationship for years, paying for the damage and feeling guilty for causing the inevitable abuse and neglect by the therapist. Even with substantial understanding and support, such women may find it almost impossible to admit to themselves that victimization has occurred. (1986, p. 53)

DeYoung (1981) offered the only study to date that focuses specifically on the sexual exploitation of incest victims by helping professionals. Three members of a 10-women incest support group proved to have had sexual liaisons with their therapists, She noted that these women had been reluctant to tell their therapists about the incest. They had withheld mention of it for some time. Their encounters with their therapists had been uniformly negative and were experienced as reminiscent of their incest. It was striking that the sexual contact was initiated shortly after the incest was revealed. DeYoung cited the work of Summit and Kryso (1978), who had observed that the incest victim may be perceived as dangerously attractive and, having been "publicly deflowered," may no longer be seen as deserving respect and/or protection.

BACKGROUND OF THE STUDY

Despite the fact that the prohibition against sexual contact between healer and patient has been an intrinsic aspect of the ethical code of every helping profession from the era of Hippocrates to the most recent statement of ethical principles by the American Psychiatric Association (1985), breaches have been far from infrequent, and the discipline of offenders has often been lax (Moore 1985; Stone 1983). Davidson (1977) described it as "psychiatry's problem with no name." Marmor (1972) described an anecdotal history of the practices of those few who have tested the boundaries of these principles in the name of therapy.

Notwithstanding the landmark efforts of Gartrell et al. (1986), and Herman et al. (1987), and parallel efforts within psychology (summarized in Pope and Bouhoutsos 1986), the true dimensions of the problem remain unknown. The available surveys provide conservative estimates at best.

Despite the best efforts of the investigators, it remains problematic whether the nonresponders contain a larger percentage of exploitive therapists then the responders. Also, it is possible that some exploiters will deny their behavior even in the context of an anonymous questionnaire. In addition, estimates of the percentage of a group that behaves inappropriately do not necessarily speak to the prevalence of the problem since they may neither assess the degree to which the respondents are repeat offenders, nor speak to the issue of their ongoing behavior after the survey instrument is completed.

These latter concerns are not merely theoretical. Some practitioners are rather energetic in their misadventures. To cite an egregious example, McCartney (1966), who defended a number of rather extreme practices as "overt transference," said that 30% of 825 female patients sat on his lap, held his hand, or hugged and kissed him, while about 10% "found it necessary to act out extremely, such as mutual undressing, genital manipulation, or coitus" (p. 236). Although such "Typhoid Marys" of unprofessional behavior may be relatively uncommon, less extreme exemplars are not, and the overall problem is widespread.

Marmor (1972) noted that he made his remarks against therapist-patient sexual relationships "in full knowledge that a number of prominent psychiatrists and psychoanalysts have married former patients" (p. 7). Greenacre (1954) cautioned that although accounts of "grosser overstepping of the transference limits" and the establishment of a sexual relationship either within or shortly after an analysis were often discounted or dismissed as the patient's fantasy, "that this is not so infrequent as one would wish to think becomes apparent to anyone who does many reanalyses" (p. 683).

Kardener et al. (1973) found that 10% of 114 male psychiatrists engaged in erotic behaviors with their patients and that half of that 10% had engaged in intercourse with their patients. Holroyd and Brodsky (1977) found that 5.5% of male and 0.6% of female psychologists had had intercourse with patients they were treating, and an additional 2.6% and 0.3%, respectively, had done so with patients within 3 months of terminating treatment. Pope et al. (1979) found that 0.7% of the psychologists surveyed had been sexually involved with patients. Bouhoustos et al. (1983) found 4.8% of male and 0.8% of female respondents had been sexually involved with patients. Gartrell et al. (1986) found 6.4% of their psychiatrist respondents, 7.1% of the males and 3.1% of the females, had had sexual contact with patients. Of the psychiatrists they surveyed, Derosis et al. (1987) found that 6.6% of American psychiatrists overall, 7.9% of the males and 2.2% of the females had had sexual contact with patients.

Relatively few reports have studied the circumstances of those incest victims who later experience sexual contact with therapists. Although I have been told of many such cases by therapists who presented this type of situation to me in consultation, the literature on the subject remains quite limited. Voth (1972) described such a case, noting

> the effects of the affair were disastrous at the time of its occurrence and proved to be a serious complication for subsequent treatment. As a consequence of the affair, her illness was aggravated to the extent that a year's hospitalization became necessary, much time and money was spent, her marriage was strained, and a deep distrust formed toward psychiatrists and psychoanalysts. (p. 394)

DeYoung's (1981) cases fared poorly as a result. Herman and Schatzow (1984) mentioned that they had evaluated such a patient and found her too unstable to be suitable for time-limited group psychotherapy. They speculated that the incest victim might prove differentially vulnerable to seduction by a therapist.

The current study expands the observations above by exploring findings in 12 patients who suffered both incest and sexual exploitation by at least one therapist. To my best knowledge, it constitutes the first description of a fairly large group of thusly exploited individuals and is fairly unique in that there is some degree of confirmation for the allegations made by the majority of the patients involved.

METHODS

The records of all patients in my practice who had reported sexual contact with one or more therapists were selected for review. For the purposes of this study, an event or events between therapist and patient had to fulfill the requirements of two definitions. The first was that used by Gartrell et al. (1986) in their study of psychiatrist-patient sexual contact: "contact which was intended to arouse or satisfy sexual desire in the patient, therapist, or both" (p. 1127). The second was Herman's (1981) definition of a sexual relationship: "Any physical contact that had to be kept a secret" (p. 70).

The latter was added specifically to guard against inadvertent inclusion of instances in which a patient knowingly had entered a treatment in which highly eroticized or stimulating events might occur. While such "treatments" are ethically repugnant, many have been and continue to be practiced. If a patient-consumer knowingly elects such a situation, his or her circumstances differ from those of the individual who enters what he or she believes will be a conventional therapy and encounters transgressions of the boundaries that a reasonable person would assume should exist.

Several patients failed to meet these criteria and were eliminated from further consideration. For example, a patient who tried to mutilate herself in the course of a session was restrained by her male psychiatrist. As she writhed in his grasp, she was aware that his hand touched her breast as she struggled to free herself and slash herself with a razor blade she had brought. She protested the touching of her breast with great vehemence, but acknowledged that it had occurred in a context that was far from erotic. Another patient maintained that her female psychiatrist had tried to seduce her, but acknowledged that all the psychiatrist actually had done was to look at her in a manner that she interpreted as homosexual.

A male patient protested that his female social worker was deliberately arousing him by disrobing, inviting him to disrobe, and rubbing him in a way that led him to have an erection. However, the social worker openly practiced what she called "nude Reichian massage therapy," and the patient understood that nudity and massage would be part of the treatment. Still others spoke about being seduced or sexually approached by a therapist, but further inquiry revealed that no professional relationship had existed or had been contemplated between them. They were describing real or potential liaisons with someone whom they knew or came to know was a therapist. Often it appeared that they had met the therapist in a social context, brought up some of their personal concerns in the course of conversation, and assumed/hoped that they could get some help in the course of an interaction with the therapist.

I also excluded the records of consultation notes on cases involving therapist-patient sex in which I had consulted to a sexually exploitive therapist who was seeking help. Further, I omitted instances in which I consulted to the current nonexploiting therapist of a patient who had had such an experience, but had not seen the patient. In addition, I omitted situations in which I had seen a patient without being told of this type of history, and learned of it later from another source, or through telephone or letter contact with the patient after she had left my care. For example, a woman whom I had seen briefly decided that she did not want to work with a male therapist. I inquired as to whether she had had an unfortunate experience with another male therapist and received a negative answer. I referred her to a female colleague. Some months later the patient sent me a letter confessing that she had not told me the truth— that she had been seduced by a male therapist, had feared a repetition of this experience with me, and felt obliged to request a transfer to a woman colleague.

I also excluded instances in which the reliability of the patient was suspect, not merely on impressionistic grounds, but on the basis of rather compelling evidence. Furthermore, I elected to exclude those patients who had sought me out because they had heard or heard about my presentation on the first cohort of such patients at the American Psychiatric Association in 1986. They were almost all colleagues or the spouses of colleagues, mental health professionals who could easily compare the initial presentation of these materials to a revised form and might identify themselves or information about them. The safeguarding of their treatments took priority over the expansion of the data base. Suffice it to say that the patients' material that will be presented constitutes less than one-third of the relevant material in my possession. The expansion of the data base would not alter the findings that will be shared, but might strengthen their credibility.

Twelve patients gave reports that satisfied the above definitions and exclusions. Their charts were reviewed once again for evidence of childhood mistreatment. Definitions of physical and psychological child abuse were taken from the work of Goldstein et al. (1979) and Wilbur (1984), respectively. The definition of incest used was that of Herman (1981): "any sexual relationship between a child and an adult in a position of parental authority" (p. 70). Following Herman further, the crucial issue is the power differential between the parent and the dependent child and its use to bring about a physical contact that had to remain clandestine. It was realized that the use of such a definition might prove problematic in some sorts of incest scenarios.

The charts of those patients whose histories included both incest and therapist-patient sexual contact were further reviewed for evidence of documentation of the stigmata of a number of mental disorders and syndromes, particular phenomena of interest, and the presence of certain experiences and historical features. Whenever possible, standard definitions, such as those of DSM-III and DSM-III-R (American Psychiatric Association 1980, 1987), were employed, but this often proved frustrating, especially since a considerable amount of the data was collected prior to 1980. Many definitions and criteria now perceived as useful simply were not available at the time of data collection and had to be applied retrospectively. For this reason, a consultant advised against performing statistical analyses, lest I risk giving the appearance that the findings of the study were overly robust with respect to the quality of the available data.

FINDINGS

Twelve patients, 11 female and 1 male, constitute the final study group of incest victims who later suffered sexual exploitation at the hands of at least one therapist. A brief description of these patients is given in Table 13-1. The patients averaged 32.5 years of age when they entered treatment with me. Although (not surprisingly) I never received the complete records in any case, the available data indicate that they had received at least 54 aggregate diagnoses, an average of 4.5 per patient. They had seen an average of 6.9 therapists (range, 1 to 28); omitting the one remarkably traveled patient, this still leaves an average of 5 prior therapists for this group. This is consistent with Gelinas' (1983) observations on the disguised presentation of incest victims and how their superficial symptoms often decree that they receive a treatment that may never explore for or help

Table 13-1.   Patient characteristics

Patient no.	Gender	Age	Occupation	Prior diagnoses
1	F	32	Counselor	Depression, alcoholism
2	M	32	Businessman	Depression, anxiety, sexual dysfunction
3	F	36	Counselor	Eating disorder, alcoholism, mixed substance abuse, depression, anxiety, borderline personality
4	F	27	Secretary	Depression, multiple personality disorder
5	F	37	Physical therapist	Schizophrenia, depression, borderline personality, hysteria
6	F	36	Homemaker	Alcoholism, drug abuse, hysteria, depression, schizophrenia
7	F	42	Counselor	Depression, schizophrenia, eating disorder, borderline personality
8	F	33	Teacher	Depression, hysteria
9	F	36	Executive	Alcoholism, drug abuse, eating disorder, borderline personality, depression
10	F	27	Disabled	Schizophrenia, manic-depressive, temporal lobe epilepsy, alcoholism, drug abuse, borderline personality
11	F	26	Celebrity	Schizophrenia, manic-depressive, temporal lobe epilepsy, drug abuse, borderline personality
12	F	26	Prostitute	Temporal lobe epilepsy, eating disorder, borderline personality, depression, hysteria, multiple personality disorder

the patients cope with their incest trauma. This in turn may beget a series of unsatisfactory treatment experiences.

Despite the wide range of occupations found in this group, it is noteworthy that 25% of this cohort had become therapists after being violated by a therapist. Could this be a sampling artifact, or could it indicate that one mechanism by which these individuals had coped was identification with the aggressor?

The most striking finding was that each victim of therapist-patient sexual exploitation had not only been an incest victim, but that each had had intercourse with the incestuous abuser. No individual simply had been fondled or stimulated in a less extreme manner; all had had vaginal and/or anal intercourse, and all but one had been forced to perform fellatio. In each case, the incestuous use had been prolonged over a period of months; in many cases, it had continued for years. Of the 12, 11 had been violated by their fathers and one by an older brother in whose care she was left. In one case, there had been additional sexual abuse by the mother and an older brother; in one by the mother, two uncles, and a sister; in one by a parent surrogate; and in one by a stepfather.

These patients reported sexual contacts with an aggregate of 23 prior therapists, whose professional identifications are indicated in Table 13-2. One perpetrator was a general physician who may or may not have had some psychiatric training, but whose practice was largely devoted to counseling and psychotherapy. Two patients were unsure of the professional affiliation of their abusers; their therapists had been assigned to them on admission to an inpatient substance abuse program and had been addressed on a first-name basis.

The 12 patients encountered 23 therapist perpetrators, an average of 1.9 perpetrators/patient. Six patients had encountered 1 such therapist, 4 had encountered 2, 1 had encountered 3, and the last had been exploited by 6.

It is unsettling to reflect that of the 83 therapists that these patients had seen, 23 (27.7%) had proven to be sexual misadventurers. The patient who was used by 6 therapists herself became a therapist of exceptional ability.

The therapist perpetrators' alleged behaviors could not be construed as overinterpreted minor indiscretions or overenthusiastic expressions of good will, caring, or agape. While 21 fondled their patients' clothed breasts or genital areas, only 3 restricted themselves to such expressions. Seventeen had intercourse with their patient subject. One perpetrator suffered a myocardial infarction as he dropped his pants and died within 72 hours. His indiscretion is classified as "attempted intercourse."

One psychiatrist repeatedly asked his then-adolescent female patient to disrobe and suggested things that she might like to do both heterosexually and homosexually, encouraging the latter form of experimentation. She became a polysubstance addict, extremely confused over her

Table 13-2.   Therapist perpetrators

Total number	23
Male	22
Female	1
Profession	
Psychiatrist	11
General physician	1
Psychologist (Ph.D.)	2
Psychologist (M.A.)	4
Addiction counselor	2
Pastoral counselor	1
Unknown	2

sexual identity, who sexually exploited a series of male patients in her practice as a therapist. One female psychologist observed her handsome, tall, and well-muscled male patient pull out his penis and urinate, under the mutually accepted rationalization that this would give him a greater sense of acceptance and approval with regard to this part of his anatomy. Other motives are suspected.

Of the 23 perpetrators, 22 began sexual behaviors while the therapy was in progress. In most cases, the sexual behaviors occurred repeatedly throughout the therapy, during sessions, and, occasionally, during hospital visits. In the last case, the therapist and patient agreed to defer sex until after termination; they consummated their relationship within a week of ending therapy. In only one instance did the sexualization of the therapy lead to the rather rapid transfer of the patient to a colleague, who was fully informed of what had occurred.

It is often thought that such accounts by patients are fantasies or confabulations. However, two studies have begun to offer new credibility to their accounts. Coons and Milstein (1986) were able to document abuse allegations in 85% of a series of 20 patients with multiple personality disorder. Herman and Schatzow (1987) found 74% of a group of incest survivors were able to get excellent corroboration of their recollections, and an additional 9% obtained suggestive but less telling data.

In this study, there was some degree of documentation in 9 (75%) of the 12 cases for the behaviors of at least one perpetrator (Table 13-3). Six therapists directly admitted that the sexual contact had occurred. Four did so explicitly to me. One straight-forwardly said that he had fallen in love with his patient and hailed her professionally. Once jolted (by his own realization) into a clear awareness of what he had done, he transferred her to a colleague. He and the patient subsequently underwent therapy to deal with how their relationship began, and married.

Three others made open admissions, but perhaps were less than on the road to rehabilitation. One said that he had seduced the patient, but had become a "born-again Christian" and was forgiven. He later persuaded the patient to leave treatment with me and resumed both the sexual liaison and her "treatment." Another admitted his acts in the course of a telephone contact in which he asked me to treat him, and then commented that since he now was my patient, he was protected by confidentiality from my revealing his admissions. My response was not

Table 13-3.   Nature of documentation of perpetrators' behaviors

Direct admission	6
Indirect admission	2
Confirmed by party to whom therapist confessed	3

what he had hoped. Yet another became my patient and admitted (and rationalized) his indiscretions with one of these patients, who had herself refused to identify her abuser. Another wrote a love letter to the patient who was then in treatment with me. He explicitly referred to their hours of love in his office.

I have classified as indirect admissions two cases in which colleagues, on learning that I had begun to treat a former patient of theirs, called me and begged me to bear in mind that I was "holding their careers in my hands." In three cases, therapists in treatment with me mentioned that they were treating individuals who had sexually exploited patients, and mentioned by name the perpetrators and their exploitation of one of the patients in this series. One such revelation occurred a dozen years after the patient first told me of her experience.

The legal aspects of these revelations will not be discussed in this chapter.

The frequency with which these patients fulfilled DSM-III diagnostic criteria for certain mental disorders is noted in Tables 13-4 and 13-5. Virtually all could be said to have atypical anxiety and depression, and dissociative features. Fully developed multiple personality disorder was

Table 13-4. Patients meeting DSM-III criteria for selected Axis I disorders

Disorder	Patients meeting criteria	
	n	Percentage
Atypical depression	12	100
Atypical anxiety disorder	12	100
Atypical dissociative disorder or multiple personality disorder	12	100
Posttraumatic stress disorder	11	92
Psychosexual dysfunctions	10	83
Somatoform disorders	10	83
Eating disorders	9	75
Substance use disorders—total[a]	8	67

[a]All were mixed and included alcoholism.

Table 13-5. Patients meeting DSM-III criteria for selected Axis II disorders

Disorder	Patients meeting criteria	
	n	Percentage
Borderline personality disorder	10	83
Histrionic personality disorder	5	42
Narcissistic personality disorder	1	8

encountered, and less well-defined dissociative syndromes were universal. There was a high incidence of the features of posttraumatic stress disorder, but it is of note that it almost invariably became evident in the course of treatment with me once the denial and minimization of the incest and therapist sexual exploitation was punctured. Prior to this point, these patients had many chronic posttraumatic features, and several showed features of posttraumatic decline, but only a few had a florid posttraumatic stress disorder picture of diagnosable intensity. The process of therapy often triggered the abrupt emergence of acute and sometimes disabling symptomatology. One woman virtually decompensated when she began to experience flashbacks of her mother's genitalia coming closer to her face, and recalled being held down until she completed performing cunnilingus. Another, after amnesia for a (later confirmed) sexual encounter with a therapist was removed, misperceived me as that therapist whenever the subject came under discussion, and several times ran from my office in a state of abject terror.

It is of no small interest that the chaotic manifest behavior of most of these patients led to behaviors that, on a phenomenological level, fulfilled criteria for borderline personality disorder. This is clearly related to the symptom complexes detailed in Table 13-6. As a group, these patients intermittently displayed a range of symptoms that strongly suggested that they were borderline or frankly psychotic. Virtually all had experienced some variety of hallucinations or related phenomena and/or could periodically misperceive their environment to the extent that they appeared delusional. The overlap of posttraumatic, borderline, and dissociative symptoms and the confusion that this engenders in the evaluation of trauma and abuse victims (Gelinas 1983; Herman and van der Kolk 1987; Kluft 1987a, 1987b) is a frequent contribution to the misdiagnosis and

Table 13-6. Prevalence of selected symptoms/experiences

Symptom/experience	Patients with symptom	
	n	Percentage
"Psychotic" symptoms	12	100
Passive influence symptoms	12	100
Distorted self-image	12	100
Dissociative symptoms	12	100
"Hypnotic" symptoms	11	92
Identity fragmentation/dysphoria	11	92
Suicide attempt	11	92
Self-mutilation		
Total	10	83
Severe	7	58
Rape as adult	8	67

mistreatment of the incest survivor population. In fact, none suffered psychoses.

Taken as a whole, the findings communicated above are a striking validation of Gelinas' (1983) contention that "the usual disguised presentation of the undisclosed victim [of incest] is a characterological depression with complications and with atypical impulsive and dissociative elements" (p. 325).

As a group, these patients frequently had begun treatment with me amnestic for, withholding information about, or minimizing the existence and implications of the incest and the sexual exploitation by therapists (Table 13-7). Almost invariably, the patients' first estimation of the damage they had suffered (taken from their first report or recollection of their history of incest) increased as they processed the experience. Initially, there appeared to be two exceptions, patients 2 and 4. Patient 2 was considered explicable because it was believed that his traumatization had been restricted to a few episodes of genital fondling when his father was intoxicated. However, as this text was being revised, he returned for further treatment, having begun to get flashbacks of having been sodomized. Patient 4, who minimized the impact of her prior therapist's misuse of her, left treatment with me to resume their liaison.

Despite my raising the issue of reporting the perpetrators and/or pressing charges, it is of interest that these patients were most reluctant to press charges or file complaints against the therapist perpetrators, for reasons detailed in Table 13-8. The protective stance the patients have taken toward their abusers and their convictions that they would suffer if they pursued any redress of grievances contributes to their passive tolerance of what had occurred. Two patients continued to have a relationship with the therapist who had exploited them. In one case, the

Table 13-7.   Patients' estimate of damage at hands of perpetrators

Patient no.	Incest		Sex with therapist	
	Initial	Final	Initial	Final
1	Minimal	Severe	Minimal	Severe
2	Moderate	Severe	Minimal	Severe
3	Severe	Severe	Minimal	Severe
4	Unknown	Unknown	Minimal	Minimal
5	Minimal	Severe	Moderate	Severe
6	Minimal	Severe	Minimal	Severe
7	Severe	Severe	Severe	Severe
8	Unknown	Unknown	Minimal	Severe
9	Moderate	Severe	Severe	Severe
10	Severe	Severe	Minimal	Severe
11	Severe	Severe	Unknown	Unknown
12	Minimal	Severe	Minimal	Severe

Table 13-8.   Reasons given for not filing grievances or charges

Reason	Patients endorsing reason	
	n	Percentage
Wish to defend therapist	9	75
Incident long ago	6	50
Patient felt unable to bear stress of filing and pursuing complaints	6	50
Patient has continued personal and sexual relationship with therapist	2	17
Patient has become colleague of therapist	2	17
Family member in therapy with therapist	1	8
Therapist deceased	1	8
Lawyer felt case unwinnable	1	8

patient was transferred and help was sought for both, individually and as a couple. This became a committed relationship. In the other, a totally chaotic mixture of sex and therapy was elected by both participants in the face of most vigorous protest from myself and concerned others. Tragically, in one instance in which the wish to press charges was strong and the perpetrator had confessed, several law firms refused to take the case, maintaining that the patient's instability rendered the case unwinnable. Confronted by these circumstances, the patient decompensated. The actual legal steps that ensued will not be discussed here.

In my review of these patients' situations, it seemed appropriate, in the interest of objectivity, to explore to what extent they may have contributed to their own revictimization; that is, what behaviors occurred in connection with erotic and other transferences, and with traumatic re-enactments. This in no way is meant to exculpate the therapists involved or to cast guilt on the patients. No matter how flagrant the temptation, it is the therapist's task to maintain a therapeutic atmosphere rather than to enter into a gross breach of ethics, however well rationalized.

It is difficult to reconstruct the context in which the exploitations occurred. Clearly, many of the therapists' statements were self-serving, and, to the contrary, many of the patients' statements were self-blaming, and rather similar to the statements that they had offered in defense of those who had misused them incestuously. Therefore, I elected to enumerate and discuss those aspects of the patients' behavior in their work with me that seemed relevant to this issue (Table 13-9). These observations are offered in the spirit of Yates' (1982) classic description of the erotization of sexual abuse victims. It must be realized that one cannot be sure whether such behaviors may have initially occurred prior to any actual sexual events in the therapies in which they were exploited, or occurred for the first time in their work with me, in reenactment of what they had

Table 13-9.   Overt seductive behavior

Patient no.	Gender	Age	Behavior
2	Male	32	Repeatedly waited in men's room with genitals exposed, hoping to encounter and arouse therapist
5	Female	37	Disrobed partially on several occasions, made repeated efforts to touch therapist erotically
6	Female	36	Repeatedly offered to pay for therapy with sexual favors
7	Female	27	Repeatedly offered to trade sexual favors for drugs
9	Female	26	Repeatedly offered to fellate therapist, told sexual fantasies while staring at his crotch, repeatedly undid and removed articles of clothing
12	Female	26	Repeatedly offered to pay for therapy with sexual favors

experienced in those previous therapies. Very often, the patients felt that they could not be sure about their own actions. Many had come to distrust their own memories. Several had been accused of active collusion by the therapists and had felt compelled to accept these charges.

The behaviors described in Table 13-9 were generally repetitive and insistent. They were highly disruptive to the therapy. Patients' explanations for their behaviors included 1) the belief that only by having sex with me would they be sure I liked them or was interested in them, 2) the wish to demean me and prove I was "no better than the rest," 3) a compelling need to test my "safety," 4) a misguided belief that they needed such a guilty secret to guarantee my involvement with them (fear of abandonment), and 5) a pressure to distract themselves from their painful past by sidetracking their therapy. Virtually all the dynamics described by Dujovne (1983) were encountered on occasion. I regarded them all as attempted reenactments within the transference.

DISCUSSION

This report should not be understood to suggest that all victims of therapist-patient sex have been incest victims, although, as noted above, incest is a frequent historical antecedent. Nor should the association of these two situations be totally discounted as a sampling artifact, however, since I was not known to specialize either in the treatment of incest victims or in the survivors of therapist sexual exploitation at the time I collected the materials for this study. The patients described above are not presented as typical of all incest victims, although their clinical presentations and problem areas are consistent with those Gelinas (1983) described as char-

acteristic in this population. They do, however, offer a discouraging illustration of the vulnerability of the incest victim to further victimization.

It is worth noting that many have questioned whether incest is always
associated with significant psychiatric impairment, a literature reviewed
by Herman (1981) and Russell (1986). The available data indicate that
some individuals appear to survive incest reasonably intact. Many incest
victims report minimal impairment in community surveys, but such findings generally exclude those who are impaired enough to be inpatients;
rely on self-reports, which characteristically are prone to minimization
and cannot control for denial; and group the infrequently and minimally
abused with those exposed to profound and prolonged exploitation. The
most impaired members of community samples begin to approximate the
distress levels of patient populations (Herman et al. 1986).

My own experience in evaluating individuals who staunchly maintain
that incest has left them unscarred is that they are reporting their wish
rather than the clinical reality that I perceive. All too often their disavowal
and/or dissociation remains intact, and they are vulnerable to future mis-
hap. Not infrequently they suffer from more of the restrictive than the
intrusive signs of trauma (Horowitz 1976); such signs often are not defined
as indicators of discomfort. It is of note that many of the study patients,
despite their profound difficulties, minimized the impact of incest and
therapist exploitation on them. They also seemed unable to conceptualize
what the trajectory of their life might have been but for their misuse and
did not understand deficits with respect to their potential as consequences
of their exploitation.

The individuals described in this study experienced definitive retrau-
matization in the form of an incest scenario within their treatments. Although
most had functioned at a high level for long periods of their life, 10 had
been hospitalized for psychiatric disorders on at least one occasion, 5 had
had long hospital stays, and they all clearly were distressed and vulnerable
individuals. Indeed, 67% had been raped as adults. It is useful to begin to
explore some of the factors that contribute to this excess vulnerability.

Although the categories used below are neither comprehensive nor mutually exclusive, they serve to organize a number of observations that, together, may be described as "the sitting duck syndrome." The sitting duck
syndrome is a condition of heightened vulnerability to revictimization due
to the conjunction of: 1) severe symptoms and traits, 2) dysfunctional individual dynamics, 3) pathologic object relations and family dynamics, and
4) deformation of the observing ego/debased cognition.

Severe Symptoms and Traits

These patients were polysymptomatic and extremely distressed (Tables
13-4 to 13-6). The individual who is highly symptomatic and appears to

have compromised ego strengths is at risk for further misadventure. This has been recognized as a high predictor of sexual exploitation, second only to prior sexual victimization (Feldman-Summers and Jones 1984).

The impact of their distress is severalfold. Their therapists may fear to destablize them by exploring beyond the surface in the face of their severe symptoms. Unfortunately, few clinicians look beyond the apparent signs of psychosis and preoedipal pathology to consider the dissociative and posttraumatic psychopathologies with which they overlap (Gelinas 1983; Herman and van der Kolk 1987; Kluft 1987a, 1987b; Spiegel and Fink 1979). Therefore, it is likely that such patients will be misdiagnosed and misunderstood, and their treatments will fail to address the core of their psychopathology (Gelinas 1983). Consequently, these patients are treated for what Gelinas described as "the disguised presentation of incest," (p. 312) come to despair of achieving mastery of their situations and acquire a certain degree of learned helplessness (Seligman 1975; Seligman and Peterson 1986). They find themselves and their situations largely overwhelming and incomprehensible. In consequence, they come to value their attachment to the therapist more highly than any hopes of recovery, begetting a regressive dependency that increases their vulnerability.

Their dissociative defenses may cloud their consciousness, leading to a characteristic proclivity to confusion and autohypnotic withdrawal, which, in the process of blocking out or attenuating painful events and sensations, leaves these patients with a discontinuous experience of themselves. They may have numerous passive-influence experiences, which further decrease their sense of being in control of themselves and their mental functioning. They may doubt their perceptions and distrust their own ego strengths. Kramer (1983) described the development of compulsive doubting, and especially object-coercive doubting (in which the patient tries to make another confirm or disconfirm the perceptions they themselves find disruptive), which further diminishes their trust of themselves. Also, both Gelinas' (1983) observations and the findings of this study suggest that one likely consequence of beginning to work with incestuous material is the development of a delayed posttraumatic stress disorder.

The fragmentation of self and identity that such patients experience (Carmen and Rieker 1989; Gelinas 1983; Putnam, Chapter 6, this volume; Ulman and Brothers 1987, 1988) both results from and compels them to use defenses that have in common with what Bowlby (1979, 1980) described as "defensive exclusion." As a result, these patients are likely to compartmentalize rather than integrate their experience, via splitting, dissociation, repression, and the defensive entry into altered states of consciousness. This further enhances their perplexity in the world.

In consequence of the above, the patient's initial efforts to master what has befallen her leads to a sense of decompensation, despair, and helplessness. She is left with the impression that she is not the master of her

own psychological house, that help is unlikely, and that her own perceptions are not reliable guides to future actions. Under these circumstances,
the patient is vulnerable to anyone who can take control, offer the promise
of resolution or structure, gratify dependency needs, and, in effect, serve
as a self-object to stabilize her shaky sense of self. Relief and rapid and
uncritical reliance can progress quite easily under the influence of an
unscrupulous individual to the virtual submission seen in many of these
patients and noted by Pope and Bouhoutsos (1986).

This is compounded by another phenomenon that accompanies the
dissociation-proneness and/or high hypnotizability that is quite common
in incest victims. It is not clear whether abused patients develop such an
aptitude in the context of severe discipline (Hilgard 1970) or child abuse
itself (Nash et al. 1984), fail to replace dissociative defenses with others
because they have been excessively mobilized due to trauma (Hicks 1985),
or whether only those patients with an innately high capacity for hypnosis
develop such responses. In any case, intrinsic to the hypnotic response
is an element of perceived involuntariness, most familiar in terms of the
compelling and involuntary quality of the posthypnotic suggestion (Mott
1979). The incest victim often experiences a sense of perceived involuntary
helplessness (in addition to the learned helplessness noted above), evoked
transferentially, situationally, and/or symbolically, that leads to a regressive reconfiguration of their pattern of response to events. This reconfiguration involves the experience that the locus of control of her responses
is external to herself.

Dysfunctional Individual Dynamics

Certainly a major factor in the recurrent vulnerability of the abused patient is the repetition compulsion. It may be that this venerable psychodynamic construct is founded on biologic underpinnings (van der Kolk
and Greenberg 1987). Although it may appear too obvious to require
mention, many of the identifications that the incest victim may make are
identifications with those who have hurt her or facilitated her abuse (i.e.,
identifications with the aggressor or with those who have failed to protect
her). The sense of self that emerges is most unlikely to serve the patient's
own best interests. Furthermore, virtually every victim of therapist-patient sexual exploitation has a masochistic character structure (Dujovne
1983), and the patients in this study were no exceptions. Succumbing to
a therapist's advances or initiating advances to a therapist may be reenactment, an effort to actualize a fantasy, a form of resistance to more
threatening issues, a defense against and/or an expression of hostility or
envy (in the latter case, often with the wish to bring the therapist down
to the patient's level), a need to reassure oneself that the therapist is not
a separate and autonomous individual (and thereby cannot be lost), an

effort to control, a means of getting dependency needs fulfilled, an anxiety release, an expression that relating in nonsexual ways is intolerable (and destabilizing to one's highly sexualized identity), a power maneuver, a way of trying to feel special, a way of asking for acceptance, and a way of rejecting the potency of the therapy (derived from Dujovne 1983). In addition, it may be a way of merging with a self-object to stabilize a shaky sense of self, a regression to or fixation at levels of oedipal triumph and narcissistic fulfillment, and so on. This list is far from comprehensive. It serves most usefully to underline the myriad determinants of a patient's vulnerability and cautions against simplistic single-factor formulations.

Pathologic Object Relations and Family Dynamics

Incest victims' relationships are characterized by what Zelen (1985) described as *anxious attachments*. They often are preoccupied with the state of their relatedness to those perceived as important, often to the point of becoming oblivious to their own needs and interests. Carmen and Rieker (1989) stated that incest victims have been raised in families in which they have been taught to sacrifice themselves to gratify the perceived needs of others, and

> sustain severe narcissistic disturbances because their own emotional lives are directed soley toward adapting to or conforming to parental wishes or expectations. They become adept and empathic in reading parental clues for appropriate as well as inappropriate affects, behavior, and thoughts, including redefinition of reality if necessary. (p. 434)

A similar configuration has been described by Summit (1983) as "the child sexual abuse accommodation syndrome." As children they were systematically taught to disregard their own needs and, hence, are devoid of the usual self-protective mechanisms and are more vulnerable to abuse in all settings.

Carmen and Rieker (1989) also noted that the incest victim learns to disconfirm and transform the abuse in the interest of family loyalty and secrecy. Self-sacrifice, often reinforced with dire threats regarding the consequences of disclosure, is characteristic. The abuse is denied with the use of extreme defensive adaptations. Reality is disavowed. In addition, the affective responses to abuse are altered because a normal response is unacceptable. The child remains dependent on the abusers for soothing, comfort, and protection. As Shengold (1979) observed:

> If the parent who abuses and is experienced as bad must be turned to for relief of the distress that parent has caused, then the child must break with what he has experienced, and must, out of desperate need, register the parent—delusionally—as good. (p. 539)

The alternative means the annihilation of the child's self, so reality is discounted in the service of survival.

Carmen and Rieker (1989) further showed that the victim tries to change the meaning of the abuse to make the abuse appear an appropriate response, such as discipline or merited punishment. The young child tends to define whatever is punished as bad.

In addition, the child in the incest family is perforce parentified; that is, she is given roles and duties to minister to the needs of the adults, who decline to acknowledge and minister to her own needs. This role reversal, the task of sacrificing herself to preserve the stability of the family, this learned protectiveness of the abuser(s) at her own expense, induces a character stance of altruistic surrender. Paradoxically, with no real sense of self or of mastery, and with an awareness that the locus of control of her actions is external to herself, the incest victim nonetheless feels responsible for circumstances that she cannot truly control and feels obliged to bend herself to the task regardless. This is a major determinant to later victimization and to the likelihood that whatever befalls her will be experienced as of her own making (i.e., as "her fault").

Deformation of the Observing Ego/Debased Cognition

Unable to tolerate her helplessness in the face of mistreatment or the horror of the realities that have befallen her, the incest victim tries to make sense of her world within the allowable rules of understanding; that is, those that permit her some sense of mastery consistent with the maintenance of the family's "pseudo-normal veneer" (Kluft et al. 1984). These adaptations deform the objectivity of the observing ego and debase the cognitive functions. Much of this process is implicit in remarks made above, but other mechanisms come into play.

There is evidence that trauma disrupts the sequences of cognitive maturation described by Piaget (Fine, Chapter 8, this volume; Fish-Murray et al. 1987). The very building blocks of thought can be disarranged, with deleterious consequences for the child's mentation, perception, and abilities to make a correct assessment of reality. Furthermore, the victim of trauma often resequences events and becomes convinced that events that occurred later in a sequence of events had, in fact, occurred earlier (Terr 1979, 1983). From this distorted memory structure emerges a preoccupation with omens; that is, the victim believes she saw hints of what would occur in advance of the event and comes to believe that if she had done so and so a thing instead of another, no harm would have befallen her. As a result, the child, ex post facto, takes responsibility and blame for events in which she could not have played a causative role.

The incest victim, who is frequently reminded of the dysfunctional nature of accurate recall and perception, lives in a decontextualized world.

As Carmen and Rieker (1989) indicated, the child, by obliterating or disconnecting knowledge of her abuse, remains able to maintain powerful attachments to those who have abused her. Furthermore, by systematically blocking out evidences that could correct the initial faulty cognitions and assessments, the incest victim is condemned to repeat rather than learn from painful experiences. With a combination of decontextualization (Carmen and Rieker 1989); accommodation to a more palatable pseudoreality (Kluft et al. 1984; Summit 1983); tenacious adherence to the delusion or promise of a good parent (Shengold 1979); and derealization, doubting, and obfuscation of the actual events that are not repressed or dissociated (Kramer 1983), the child faces the world unprepared to see danger as danger. Instead, she is likely to interpret the warning signs that most would appreciate as ominous as reasonable and compelling instructions to comply with "reality" as it is defined by the sort of person(s) or situation(s) that most would take vigorous steps to avoid.

CONCLUSION

The study of 12 patients who suffered both incestuous abuse and sexual exploitation by at least one therapist offers some insights into the mechanisms by which the incest victim becomes differentially susceptible to revictimization. It is arguable that in many individuals incest induces 1) severe symptoms and problematic traits, 2) a wide range of idiosyncratic dynamic determinants, 3) socialization to atypical object relations and family dynamics that discourage the individual's caring for herself, and 4) the traumatic deformation of the observing ego and debasement of the mind's cognitive structures and schemata. These factors combine to make the incest victim accept as normative, familiar, and even necessary and/or desirable, situations and relationships that most would perceive as dangerous and exploitive, and attribute to herself responsibility for the actions of those who have taken steps to exploit her. Repetitive revictimization follows naturally. In sum, these four clusters of characteristics constitute what might be called "the sitting duck syndrome," which is highly predisposing for repetitive revictimization.

Although it cannot be said that this syndrome is specific for incest victims, the observation of this syndrome in a patient without a known incest history should alert the clinician that the patient may well be an incest victim or have suffered some other form of "soul murder" (Shengold 1979). The presence of this syndrome in an incest victim should alert the clinician to consider that the welter of symptoms that the patient presents should not preclude an attempt to work through the incest trauma in the course of the therapy. The patient's overwhelmed appearance may be more reflective of an untreated posttraumatic state than of profound and fixed psychopathology. The excellent prognosis of many cases of the most severe dissociative disorders (Kluft 1987b) strongly suggests that the severely distressed and highly symptomatic incest victim may have a more optimistic treatment outcome than might at first appear to be the case.

REFERENCES

American Psychiatric Association: Diagnostic and Statistical Manual of Mental Disorders, 3rd Edition. Washington, DC, American Psychiatric Association, 1980

American Psychiatric Association: Diagnostic and Statistical Manual and Mental Disorders, 3rd Edition, Revised. Washington, DC, American Psychiatric Association, 1987

Beck JC, van der Kolk BA: Reports of childhood incest and current behavior of chronically hospitalized psychotic women. Am J Psychiatry 144:1426–1430, 1987

Benward J, Densen-Gerber J: Incest as a causative factor in anti-social behavior: an exploratory study. Contemporary Drug Problems 33:323–340, 1975

Bouhoutsos J, Holroyd J, Lerman H, et al: Sexual intimacy between psychotherapists and patients. Professional Psychology 14:185–196, 1983

Bowlby J: On knowing what you are not supposed to know and feeling what you are not supposed to feel. Can J Psychiatry 24:403–408, 1979

Bowlby J: Attachment and Loss, Vol 3: Sadness and Depression. New York, Basic Books, 1980

Briere J: The long-term effects of childhood sexual abuse: defining a post-sexual abuse syndrome. Paper presented at the Third National Conference on the Sexual Victimization of Children, Washington, DC, April 1984

Bryer JB, Nelson BA, Miller JB, et al: Childhood sexual and physical abuse as factors in adult psychiatric illness. Am J Psychiatry 144:1426–1430, 1987

Carmen E(H), Rieker PP: A psychosocial model of the victim-to-patient process: implications for treatment. Psychiatr Clin North Am 12:431–444, 1989

Carmen E(H), Rieker PP, Mills T: Victims of violence and psychiatric illness. Am J Psychiatry 14:378–383, 1984

Coons PM, Milstein V: Psychosexual disturbances in multiple personality: characteristics, etiology, treatment. J Clin Psychiatry 47:106–110, 1986

Craine LS, Henson CE, Colliver JA, et al: Prevalence of a history of sexual abuse among female psychiatric patients in a state hospital system. Hosp Community Psychiatry 39:300–304, 1988

Davidson V: Psychiatry's problem with no name: therapist-patient sex. Am J Psychoanal 37:43–50, 1977

Derosis H, Hamilton J, Morrison E, et al: More on psychiatrist-patient sexual contact. Am J Psychiatry 144:688–689, 1987

DeYoung M: Case reports: the sexual exploitation of incest victims by health professionals. Victimology 6:92–101, 1981

Dujovne B: Sexual feelings, fantasies, and acting out in psychotherapy. Psychotherapy: Theory, Research, Practice 20:243–250, 1983

Enslie GJ, Rosenfeld A: Incest reported by children and adolescents hospitalized for severe psychiatric problems. Am J Psychiatry 140:708–710, 1983

Feldman-Summers S, Jones G: Psychological impacts of sexual contact between therapists or other health care practitioners and their clients. J Consult Clin Psychol 52:1054–1061, 1984

Fish-Murray CC, Koby E, van der Kolk BA: Evolving ideas: the effect of abuse on children's thought, in Psychological Trauma. Edited by van der Kolk BA. Washington, DC, American Psychiatric Press, 1987, pp 89–110

Fritz G, Stoll K, Wagner NA: A comparison of males and females who were sexually molested as children. J Sex Marital Ther 7:54–59, 1981

Gartrell N, Herman JL, Olarte S, et al: Psychiatrist-patient sexual contact: results of a national survey, 1: prevalence. Am J Psychiatry 143:1126–1131, 1986

Gelinas DJ: The persisting negative effects of incest. Psychiatry 46:312–332, 1983

Goldstein J, Freud A, Solnit A: Before the Best Interests of the Child. New York, Free Press, 1979

Greenacre P: The role of transference. J Am Psychoanal Assoc 2:671–684, 1954

Harlan S, Rodgers L, Slattery B: Male and female adolescent prostitutes: Huckleberry House Sexual Minority Youth Services Project. Washington, DC, Youth Development Bureau, U.S. Department of Human Services, 1981

Herman JL: Father-Daughter Incest. Cambridge, MA, Harvard University Press, 1981

Herman JL, Schatzow E: Time-limited group therapy for women with a history of incest. Int J Group Psychother 34:605–616, 1984

Herman JL, Schatzow E: Recovery and verification of memories of childhood sexual trauma. Psychoanalytic Psychology 4:1–14, 1987

Herman JL, van der Kolk BA: Traumatic antecedents of borderline personality disorder, in Psychological Trauma. Edited by van der Kolk BA. Washington, DC, American Psychiatric Press, 1987, pp 111–126

Herman JL, Russell D, Trocki K: Long-term effects of incestuous abuse in childhood. Am J Psychiatry 143:1293–1296, 1986

Herman JL, Gartrell N, Olarte S, et al: Psychiatrist-patient sexual contact: results of a national survey, II: psychiatrists' attitudes. Am J Psychiatry 144:164–169, 1987

Hicks R: Discussion: a clinician's perspective, in Childhood Antecedents of Multiple Personality. Edited by Kluft RP. Washington, DC, American Psychiatric Press, 1985, pp 239–258

Hilgard J: Personality and Hypnosis. Chicago, IL, University of Chicago Press, 1970

Holroyd J, Brodsky A: Psychologists' attitudes and practices regarding erotic and non-erotic contact with patients. Am Psychol 32:843–849, 1977

Horowitz MJ: Stress Response Syndromes. Northvale, NJ, Jason Aronson, 1976

Husain A, Chapel JL: History of incest in girls admitted to a psychiatric hospital. Am J Psychiatry 140:591–593, 1983

James J, Myerding J: Early sexual experiences and prostitution. Am J Psychiatry 134:1381–1385, 1977

Kardener S, Fuller M, Mensh I: A survey of physicians' attitudes and practices regarding erotic and non-erotic contact with patients. Am J Psychiatry 130:1077–1081, 1973

Katlan A: Children who were raped. Psychoanal Study Child 28:208–224, 1973

Kaufman L, Peck A, Tagiuri C: The family constellation and overt incestuous relations between father and daughter. Am J Orthopsychiatry 24:266–279, 1954

Kluft RP: First-rank symptoms as a diagnostic clue to multiple personality disorder. Am J Psychiatry 144:292–298, 1987a

Kluft RP: An update on multiple personality disorder. Hosp Community Psychiatry 38:363–373, 1987b

Kluft RP, Braun BG, Sachs RG: Multiple personality, intrafamilial abuse, and family psychiatry. International Journal of Family Psychiatry 5:283–301, 1984

Kramer S: Object-coercive doubting: a pathological defensive response to maternal incest. J Am Psychoanal Assoc 31(Suppl):325–352, 1983

Marmor J: Sexual acting-out in psychotherapy. Am J Psychoanal 32:3–8, 1972

McCartney J: Overt transference. Journal of Sex Research 2:227–237, 1966

Mills T, Rieker PP, Carmen E(H): Hospitalization experiences of victims of abuse. Victimology 9:436–449, 1984

Moore R: Ethics in the practice of psychiatry: update on the results of enforcement of the code. Am J Psychiatry 142:1043–1046, 1985

Mott T: The clinical importance of hypnotizability. Am J Clin Hypn 21:263–269, 1979

Nash M, Lynn S, Givens D: Adult hypnotic susceptibility, childhood punishment, and child abuse: a brief communication. Int J Clin Exp Hypn 32:6–11, 1984

Peters JJ: Children who are victims of sexual assault and the psychology of offenders. Am J Psychother 30:398–421, 1976

Pope KS, Bouhoutsos JC: Sexual Intimacy Between Therapists and Patients. New York, Praeger, 1986

Pope KS, Levenson H, Schover LR: Sexual intimacy in psychology training: results and implications of a national survey. Am Psychol 34:682–689, 1979

Pope KS, Schover LR, Levenson H: Sexual behavior between clinical supervisors and trainees: implications for professional standards. Professional Psychology 11:157–162, 1980

Russell DEH: The Secret Trauma: Incest in the Lives of Girls and Women. New York, Basic Books, 1986

Sansonnet-Hayden H, Haley G, Marriage K, et al: Sexual abuse and psychopathology in hospitalized adolescents. Journal of the American Academy of Child Psychiatry 26:753–757, 1987

Seligman M: Helplessness: On Depression, Development, and Death. San Francisco, CA, WH Freeman, 1975

Seligman M, Peterson C: A learned helplessness perspective on childhood depression: theory and research, in Depression in Young People: Developmental and Clinical Perspectives. Edited by Rutter M, Izard C, Read P. New York, Guilford, 1986

Shengold LL: Child abuse and deprivation: soul murder. J Am Psychoanal Assoc 27:533–559, 1979

Silbert M, Pines A: Sexual abuse as an antecedent to prostitution. Child Abuse Negl 5:407–411, 1981

Sloan P, Karpinski E: Effects of incest on the participants. Am J Orthopsychiatry 12:666–673, 1942

Spiegel D, Fink R: Hysterical psychosis and hypnotizability. Am J Psychiatry 136:777–781, 1979

Stone AA: Sexual misconduct by psychiatrists: the ethical and clinical dilemma of confidentiality. Am J Psychother 140:195–197, 1983

Stone M: Boundary violations between therapist and patient. Psychiatric Annals 6:670–677, 1976

Summit RC: The child sexual abuse accommodation syndrome. Child Abuse Negl 7:177–193, 1983

Summit RC, Kryso JA: Sexual abuse of children: a clinical spectrum. Am J Orthopsychiatry 48:237–251, 1978

Terr LC: Children of Chowchilla: a study of psychic terror. Psychoanal Study Child 34:547–623, 1979

Terr LC: Chowchilla revisited: the effects of psychic trauma four years after a school-bus kidnapping. Am J Psychiatry 140:1543–1550, 1983

Tsai M, Wagner N: Therapy groups for women sexually molested as children. Archives of Sexual Behavior 7:417–427, 1978

Tsai M, Feldman-Summers S, Edgar M: Childhood molestation: variables related to differential impacts on psychosexual functioning in adult women. J Abnorm Psychol 88:407–417, 1979

Ulman RB, Brothers D: A self-psychological reevaluation of posttraumatic stress disorder (PTSD) and its treatment: shattered fantasies. J Am Acad Psychoanal 15:175–203, 1987

Ulman RB, Brothers D: The Shattered Self: A Psychoanalytic Study of Trauma. Hillsdale, NJ, Analytic Press, 1988

van der Kolk BA, Greenberg MS: The psychobiology of the trauma response: hyperarousal, constriction, and addiction to traumatic reexposure, in Psychological Trauma. Edited by van der Kolk BA. Washington, DC, American Psychiatric Press, 1987, pp 63–87

Voth HM: Love affair between doctor and patient. Am J Psychother 26:394–400, 1972

Wilbur CG: Multiple personality and child abuse. Psychiatr Clin North Am 7:3–7, 1984

Yates A: Children eroticized by incest. Am J Psychiatry 139:482–485, 1982

Zelen SL: Sexualization of therapeutic relationships: the dual vulnerability of patient and therapist. Psychotherapy 22:178–185, 1985

CHAPTER 14

Discussion

Judith Lewis Herman, M.D.

The ordinary human response to atrocities is to banish them from consciousness. Complex psychological mechanisms are mustered to keep the reality of horrible events far from ordinary awareness. Certain violations of the human social compact, notably incest, are judged to be too terrible to utter aloud: this is the meaning of the word *unspeakable*.

Atrocities, however, refuse to be buried. Equally as powerful as the desire to deny atrocities is the human conviction that denial does not work. Our folk wisdom is filled with ghosts who refuse to rest in their graves until their stories are told. Incest will out. It appears that remembering and telling the truth about terrible events are prerequisites for the restoration of social order and for the healing of individual victims.

The conflict between these opposite imperatives, to deny horrible events and to proclaim them aloud, is the central preoccupation of traumatized people. Victims often tell their stories in a highly emotional, contradictory, and fragmented manner that undermines their credibility, thus serving the twin imperatives of truth telling and secrecy. When the truth is recognized, victims can begin their recovery in a relatively uncomplicated fashion. But far too often, secrecy prevails, and the story of the traumatic event surfaces not as verbal narrative but as a reenactment or symptom.

Like the stories of atrocities, the symptoms of traumatized people simultaneously call attention to the existence of an unspeakable secret and deflect attention from it. This dialectic of trauma is most apparent in the alternations of numbing and intrusive symptoms in patients with post-traumatic stress disorder. It results in complicated, sometimes uncanny feats of altered consciousness, which Orwell (1949), one of the committed truth-tellers of our century, called *doublethink*, and which professionals, searching for a calm, precise language, call *dissociation*. It results in the protean, dramatic, and often bizarre symptoms of hysteria, which Freud recognized a century ago as disguised communications about sexual abuse.

Witnesses as well as victims are subject to the dialectic of trauma. It is very difficult for the observer to remain clearheaded and calm, to see more than a few fragments of the picture at one time, to retain all the pieces, and to fit them together. It is even more difficult to find a language that conveys persuasively what one has seen. Denial, repression, and dissociation operate on a social as well as an individual level. The knowledge of horrible events periodically intrudes into public consciousness, but is rarely retained for long. To speak publicly about one's knowledge of atrocities is to invite the stigma that attaches to victims. Those who attempt to describe atrocities that they have witnessed also risk their credibility.

This volume represents the best efforts of a group of sophisticated clinicians and researchers to venture into knowledge of the unspeakable and to communicate their findings in the dispassionate language of the professional. It appears at a time when public discussion of the common atrocities of sexual and domestic life has been made possible by the women's liberation movement. In the past 10 years, basic facts about the epidemiology of child sexual abuse have been established beyond reasonable doubt (Finkelhor 1979; Russell 1984). Increased public awareness has resulted in an exponential increase in reported and substantiated cases of incest (see Goodwin, Chapter 4). Clinical descriptions of sexually abused children and their families have proliferated, and prospective studies following these children from the time of disclosure are in their early stages (see Schetky, Chapter 3). If these studies persevere, we may have a much clearer picture 10 or 20 years from now of the full range of human adaptations to early incestuous abuse.

But even then, prospective studies will tell us only about the long-range effects of incest that has been discovered, and therefore interrupted. For obvious reasons, it is not possible to conduct a longitudinal study of abused children without intervening to put a stop to the abuse. Even with today's improved case finding, the majority of incest victims reach adulthood with their secrets undisclosed. We have no way of knowing what proportion of incest victims eventually come to psychiatric attention. But we do know now that our psychiatric clinics and hospitals are filled with incest victims (Beck and van der Kolk 1987; Bryer et al. 1987; Carmen et al. 1984; Herman 1986; Jacobson and Richardson 1987). In addition, we are beginning to understand the connections between early incestuous abuse and the complex psychopathology we find in our adult patients. We are beginning to understand what I have called the *dialectic of trauma*.

Our patients challenge us to reconnect fragments, to reconstruct history, and to develop theories that make meaning of their present symptoms in the light of past events. These are risky ventures, given everything we know about the deceptions of memory and the frailty of retrospective reasoning. Yet if the connection between present symptoms and the underlying early trauma is lost, these patients may be condemned to an endless round of incomplete or ineffective treatments. We are all too familiar with patients who have developed lifelong careers as treatment failures, who have accumulated multiple psychiatric diagnoses, who have been tried on every class of psychopharmacologic agent (often in large doses and in combination), who have been hospitalized on numerous occasions, who have been treated by numerous psychotherapists of varying schools (including the orthodox and the highly unorthodox), and whose medical charts may weigh almost as much as they do. Eventually helping professionals may be drawn into a reenactment of the original abusive relationship, venting our frustrations in verbal abuse and pejorative labeling of the patient, getting into heated disputes with other professionals (the well-known phenomenon of "staff splitting"), or even, as Kluft demonstrated in Chapter 13, violating sexual boundaries.

I have often wondered why these patients keep seeking help despite repeated failures and disappointments. One might view this behavior as simply another repetition compulsion. Or, taking a more affirmative view, one might consider their persistence as a testimony to their virtues of determination and hope. Many of us who work with these patients have been inspired by their courage. Their endurance in the pursuit of treatment reflects a conviction, often unarticulated but nonetheless very powerful, that recovery can begin if only the right connection—between patient and caregiver, and between symptom and trauma—can be found. Our role in the healing process is to bear witness and thus to make it possible for the patient to bear a reality that cannot be borne in isolation. By our presence, we enable our patients to tell what has happened to them and to make sense out of the unspeakable events of the past.

The chapters in this volume, then, are unified by their attempt to reconstruct connections that have been lost. At the simplest level, they attempt to alert the clinician to particular diagnostic categories where an incest history is often found: multiple personality disorder and other dissociative disorders (Braun, Chapter 11), borderline personality disorder (Stone, Chapter 9), and somatoform disorders (Loewenstein, Chapter 5). As Loewenstein correctly pointed out, these diagnostic categories taken together reconstruct the picture of what was once called *hysteria* and remind us that both Freud and Briquet originally described the connection between hysterical symptoms and traumatic events in sexual and domestic life. This connection was subsequently lost in a wave of social repression and has only relatively recently been rediscovered (Herman 1981; Masson 1984; Rush 1980).

Many of the authors in this volume also attempt to describe a hypothetical mechanism by which incestuous abuse produces the complex symptomatology seen in adult survivors. In each case, repeated trauma in childhood is found to affect the course of normal development by disconnecting its ordinarily indivisible component parts. One might view the abusive home as something like a linear accelerator of the psyche that, in fracturing the processes of normal development, allows us a privileged insight into their organization. Just as subatomic particles are not ordinarily seen in nature and defy ordinary rules of common sense, the fragments of human memory, cognition, and personality produced in abusive environments are not ordinarily seen in nature and may seem fantastic when we discover them in our patients. It is probable, as Braun (Chapter 11) proposed, that the more severe and unremitting the childhood trauma, the greater the splintering of developmental processes, and the more bizarre and extraordinary fragments will be observed. Perhaps we should call them "neutrinos" or "quarks."

Braun (Chapter 11) described the effects of repeated trauma as a disconnection of the ordinary components of memory (behavior, affect, sensation, and knowledge), resulting in varied forms of memory disturbance in dissociative disorders. Spiegel (Chapter 12) also explored the relationship between trauma, induction of hypnotic states, and dissociation. Putnam (Chapter 6) described the effect of treated trauma on the development of the self, and Schultz (Chapter 7) focused particularly on the distortions produced by the incest secret on the process of identity formation in adolescence. Fine (Chapter 8) described the effects of repeated trauma on the Piagetian stages of cognitive development, with resultant cognitive distortions seen in adult life. Spiegel (Chapter 12) reminded us that the process of adaptation to trauma is continuous and that even patients with a very severe dissociative disorder (i.e., multiple personality disorder) may respond to new traumas in adult life without resorting to established dissociative defenses.

Several authors also attempted to delineate a spectrum of complicated posttraumatic conditions and to correlate the severity of the abuse history with the resultant psychopathology. Braun (Chapter 11) postulated three preconditions for the formation of the most severe form of dissociative disorder (i.e., multiple personality disorder) and presented a series of case histories that relate the degree of ego fragmentation to the severity of the abuse. Goodwin (Chapter 4) contributed the useful FEARS mnemonic to describe moderate and severe forms of posttraumatic disorder. Goodwin also described a relationship between a history of severe incestuous abuse and the fragmentation of memory, cognition, and personality.

Finally, these chapters represent an attempt to overcome the processes of denial, repression, and dissociation that the authors have observed in themselves. Using the techniques of self-analysis and consciousness raising, Kluft (Chapter 2) uncovered many instances from his own quite ordinary, even sheltered, adolescence, in which he encountered girls and women who had been incestuously abused. This courageous venture into truth telling without the protection of professional objectivity provides invaluable insight into the adolescent socialization of male sexuality and makes explicit the unspoken rules by which certain women are exploited and sacrificed, *with the knowledge and complicity of other men.*

Kluft (Chapter 2) described his painful moral dilemma when challenged to participate in a male bonding ritual of intercourse with a prostitute, and his resourceful compromise that allowed him to treat the prostitute respectfully while still preserving some status with his friends. Those of us who attempt to treat incest survivors often find ourselves in a similar dilemma, torn between alliance with the victim and alliance with our peers. In bearing witness to the atrocities that our patients have suffered, we discover more than anyone wants to know about human evil. We seek continually to find a mode of communication that can withstand the imperatives of *doublethink*; a language that preserves connections—with our patients and with our colleagues—and allows all of us to come a little closer to facing the unspeakable.

REFERENCES

Beck JC, van der Kolk BA: Reports of childhood incest and current behavior of chronically hospitalized psychotic women. Am J Psychiatry 144:1474–1476, 1987

Bryer JB, Nelson BA, Miller JB, et al: Childhood sexual and physical abuse as factors in adult psychiatric illness. Am J Psychiatry 144:1426–1430, 1987

Carmen E, Rieker PP, Mills T: Victims of violence and psychiatric illness. Am J Psychiatry 141:378–383, 1984

Finkelhor D: Sexually Victimized Children. New York, Free Press, 1979

Herman JL: Father-Daughter Incest. Cambridge, MA, Harvard University Press, 1981

Herman JL: Histories of violence in an outpatient population: an exploratory study. Am J Orthopsychiatry 56:137–141, 1986

Jacobson A, Richardson B: Assault experiences of 100 psychiatric inpatients: evidence of the need for routine inquiry. Am J Psychiatry 144:908–913, 1987

Masson J: The Assault on Truth. New York, Farrar, Straus, & Giroux, 1984

Orwell G: Nineteen Eighty Four. San Diego, CA, Harcourt Brace Jovanovich, 1949

Rush F: The Best Kept Secret. Englewood Cliffs, NJ, Prentice-Hall, 1980

Russell DEH: Sexual Exploitation: Rape, Child Sexual Abuse, and Workplace Harassment. Beverly Hills, CA, Sage, 1984

Index